Benign Tumors of the Liver

Luca Aldrighetti • Francesco Cetta
Gianfranco Ferla
Editors

Benign Tumors of the Liver

Forewords by Gennaro Nuzzo and Antonio Daniele Pinna

In collaboration with Francesca Ratti

Springer

Editors
Luca Aldrighetti
Hepatobiliary Surgery
San Raffaele Hospital
Milano
Italy

Gianfranco Ferla
Hepatobiliary Surgery
San Raffaele Hospital
Milano
Italy

Francesco Cetta
IRCCS MultiMedica Hospital
Sesto San Giovanni
Milano
Italy

ISBN 978-3-319-12984-6 ISBN 978-3-319-12985-3 (eBook)
DOI 10.1007/978-3-319-12985-3

Library of Congress Control Number: 2015934364

Springer Cham Heidelberg New York Dordrecht London

Printed on acid-free paper

Springer is part of Springer Science+Business Media (www.springer.com)

Foreword I

It is a great pleasure for me to introduce the book *Benign Tumors of the Liver.*

Luca Aldrighetti, Francesco Cetta, and Gianfranco Ferla are surgeons with a dedicated commitment to hepatobiliary surgery and also valued friends, so I wish to thank them for the invitation to write this foreword. They deserve praise both for stimulating interest in the role of liver surgery, and especially minimally invasive techniques, in patients with benign liver tumors and for having decided to address this topic despite being well aware of all the associated difficulties.

The topic was a good choice because the extensive use of abdominal ultrasound has led to incidental detection of an increasing number of focal liver lesions that, in the absence of chronic liver disease and previous cancer, are almost always benign. Nevertheless, for patients such findings mark the beginning of an "odyssey", on which they undergo an infinite number of tests, often unnecessary and expensive, before a definitive diagnosis is obtained. The optimal management of benign tumors of the liver thus remains an open issue, and Drs. Aldrighetti, Cetta, and Ferla have called upon the best Italian and foreign specialists to consider each aspect.

This book provides a wealth of up-to-date information that will enable every physician to provide patients with safe and appropriate care whenever a focal lesion is discovered. It will enable readers:

1. To understand the nature of benign tumors of the liver. Some of these tumors (such as liver adenoma and biliary cystadenoma) have indeed been extensively investigated in recent years thanks to progress in molecular biology, genetics, and histochemistry, and this has proved valuable in deepening understanding of disease characteristics and assisting in choice of therapy.
2. To obtain a correct diagnosis based on the clinical, biologic, radiologic, and pathologic features of each tumor. In particular, current imaging techniques allow very accurate diagnostic definition of benign tumors in most cases, thus reducing the need for a biopsy and avoiding unnecessary interventions. The collaboration between radiologists and surgeons is therefore important, and of course this synergy is even more fruitful if both are especially dedicated to these pathologies.

3. To correctly identify the need for surgical treatment of these tumors, which is rarely required. Indeed, many studies have demonstrated the low risk of development of malignancies and the low incidence of complications such as hemorrhage in the majority of benign tumors. The need for surgical treatment should be reevaluated when changes in terms of lesion volume and number are registered, taking into account their topography within the liver and potential technical difficulties related to their removal.
4. To define the steadily increasing role of new techniques in interventional radiology and minimally invasive surgery (laparoscopic and robotic). Today the initial fear that the lower invasiveness of these techniques could lead to a broadening of surgical indications has disappeared, especially thanks to the guidance and control provided by scientific societies and national registries, in which Luca Aldrighetti has himself played a fundamental role.

Before closing I wish to congratulate the three editors: Francesco and Gianfranco, who are of similar age to me, lived through the era of discussions on gallstones and odditis and I now find them involved, with unflagging enthusiasm, in a topic that would have seemed very distant from us in that period. Luca, far younger than myself, has devoted much attention to the laparoscopic technique, "accurate" in all gestures and resembling the art of open surgery; furthermore, he has displayed an all-round interest in scientific topics relating to liver surgery and drawn attention to lesser-known aspects of various diseases.

My hope is that doctors who are faced with an incidental focal liver lesion will be able to turn to this book as a reliable guide that will aid them in reassuring patients and in advising them appropriately while acknowledging the duty to refer complex cases to those centers where all the skills required to correctly deal with them are available.

Rome, Italy Gennaro Nuzzo, MD, MH AFC

Foreword II

Benign tumors of the liver are quite frequent lesions affecting approximately 20 % of the population, and their diagnosis has been increasing in frequency lately, owing to the routine use of contrast-enhanced abdominal ultrasound.

To differentiate diagnosis between the several benign and malignant hepatic lesions is a real challenge for radiologists. This difficulty has recently become easier to overcome, by virtue of the improvement in diagnostic tools, in particular to the worldwide availability of magnetic resonance, now considered the gold standard technique for a correct identification of any hepatic lesion.

The need for a precise diagnosis is the key point for the subsequent treatment. Though surgical resection remains the treatment of choice for malignant nodules and some of the benign lesions, most of the latter, such as small haemangiomas, focal nodular hyperplasia, and asymptomatic simple cysts, do not require any treatment. However, data from ELTR and UNOS show that in the last 20 years about 1 % of all liver transplantations in the world have been performed for benign liver tumors. Therefore, these patients should be managed in specialized centres, and a few selected cases may require aggressive surgical strategy.

The development of laparoscopic and robotic surgery has found an interesting application in this field. Although these technologies should not extend surgical indication in any way, benign liver tumors requiring surgery are optimal indications for a mini-invasive approach.

In my opinion, Aldrighetti, Cetta and Ferla have done an excellent job in this book in focusing on all types of benign liver tumors; they have endeavored to summarize the epidemiology and the molecular biology aspects, explained how to reach a precise diagnosis among these different entities, illustrated the available surgical techniques and even the alternative treatments by percutaneous approaches.

This handy and complete volume, covering all the aspects of benign liver tumors, is a state-of-the-art review not to be missed by all professionals and physicians involved in this specific field.

Bologna, Italy — Antonio Daniele Pinna, MD

Preface

When I was first asked to choose a topic for a book regarding liver surgery, I realized that one of the less systematically investigated areas of liver pathology is benign tumors. This is despite the fact that up to two-thirds of patients seen at the outpatient clinic have benign lesions and well-defined multidisciplinary management is still lacking.

In editing this book, I wanted to provide an instrument that would be of practical value not only for hepatobiliary specialists but also for surgeons without a specific commitment to liver surgery who are frequently asked for an opinion regarding surgical indications and follow-up of focal hepatic lesions and for general practitioners, who need to correctly refer the patient.

Diagnosis of benign tumors of the liver is now experiencing exponential growth, mainly owing to the diffusion of more accurate imaging techniques, the role of which is precisely described, providing guidance on differential diagnosis. The full range of benign liver tumors and conditions is then systematically reviewed and surgical indications are accurately analyzed with a view to assisting in the avoidance of useless interventions. Transplantation, laparoscopic resection, and robotic surgical techniques are described and illustrated, emphasizing the optimization of intra- and postoperative management in order to avoid potential complications and degeneration.

I asked many well-known and esteemed experts to contribute as authors of this book on the basis of their outstanding knowledge in the field, and I think that the quality of the end product bears testimony to all their efforts. I therefore firstly wish to express my gratitude to the authors, and then to compliment them on the excellent work that they have done.

I would also like to thank the other editors, Prof. Ferla and Prof. Cetta, for their helpfulness and remarkable dedication in the whole field of liver surgery and for their huge enthusiasm in book supervision.

Finally, it is impossible to forget to acknowledge the contribution of Prof. Capussotti, who is surely the pioneer of scientific and technical education of hepatobiliary surgeons in Italy and who represents a model of integrity and accuracy for present and future generations.

Milan, Italy Luca Aldrighetti

Contents

Contributors

Luca Aldrighetti Hepatobiliary Surgery Unit, IRCCS San Raffaele Hospital, Milan, Italy

Hepatobiliary Surgery Unit, San Raffaele Hospital, Vita-Salute San Raffaele University, Milan, Italy

Sergio Aloia Department of Transplantation, Unit of Hepatobiliary Surgery and Liver Transplant, Cardarelli Hospital, Naples, Italy

Nicolò Bassi IV Divisone Chirurgica, II Dipartimento Chirurgico, Centro Regionale di Riferimento per la Chirurgia epatobiliopancreatica Ospedale Regionale, Treviso, Italy

Luigi Beretta Anesthesia and Neurointensive Care, S. Raffaele University Hospital, Milan, Italy

Fulvio Calise Department of Transplantation, Unit of Hepatobiliary Surgery and Liver Transplant, Cardarelli Hospital, Naples, Italy

Lorenzo Capussotti Department of General and Oncologic Surgery, Ospedale Mauriziano, Torino, Italy

Luciano Casciola Division of Minimally Invasive Surgery, Casa di Cura Città di Roma, Rome, Italy

Marco Catena Hepatobiliary Surgery, San Raffaele Hospital, Milan, Italy

Matteo Cescon Department of Emergency, Surgery and Transplantation, Sant'Orsola Hospital, University of Bologna, Bologna, Italy

Francesco Cetta IRCCS MultiMedica, Milan, Italy

Federica Cipriani Hepatobiliary Surgery Unit, IRCCS San Raffaele Hospital, Milan, Italy

HPB Surgery, Southampton General Hospital, Southampton, UK

Enrico Crolla Department of Transplantation, Unit of Hepatobiliary Surgery and Liver Transplant, Cardarelli Hospital, Naples, Italy

Francesco De Cobelli Department of Radiology, San Raffaele Hospital, Milan, Italy

Agostino Maria De Rose Hepatobiliary Surgery Unit, Catholic University of the Sacred Heart – A. Gemelli Hospital, Rome, Italy

Alessandro Del Maschio Department of Radiology, San Raffaele Hospital, Milan, Italy

Ambra Licia di Prima Anesthesia and Intensive Care, S. Raffaele University Hospital, Milan, Italy

Giorgio Ercolani Department of Emergency, Surgery and Transplantation, Sant'Orsola Hospital, University of Bologna, Bologna, Italy

Antonio Esposito Department of Radiology, San Raffaele Hospital, Milan, Italy

Alessandro Ferrero Department of General and Oncologic Surgery, Ospedale Mauriziano, Torino, Italy

Renato Finazzi Hepatobiliary Surgery Unit, IRCCS San Raffaele Hospital, Milan, Italy

CAA Epatologia Medica e Infettivologia, Chirurgia Generale Epatobiliare, Liver Unit, Dipartimento di Scienze Chirurgiche, IRCCS Ospedale San Raffaele, Milan, MI, Italy

Antonio Giuliani Department of Transplantation, Unit of Hepatobiliary Surgery and Liver Transplant, Cardarelli Hospital, Naples, Italy

Felice Giuliante Hepatobiliary Surgery Unit, Catholic University of the Sacred Heart – A. Gemelli Hospital, Rome, Italy

Mohammad Abu Hilal Southampton General Hospital, University Hospital, Southampton, UK

Gabriele Ironi Department of Radiology, San Raffaele Hospital, Milan, Italy

Ihab Kamel Department of Radiology, The Johns Hopkins School of Medicine, Baltimore, MD, USA

Serena Langella Department of General and Oncologic Surgery, Ospedale Mauriziano, Torino, Italy

Paolo Marra Department of Radiology, San Raffaele Hospital, Milan, Italy

Marco Massani IV Divisone Chirurgica, II Dipartimento Chirurgico, Centro Regionale di Riferimento per la Chirurgia epatobiliopancreatica Ospedale Regionale, Treviso, Italy

Massimo Memoli General Medicine and Clinical Immunology, San Raffaele Hospital, Milan, Italy

C. Nistri IV Divisone Chirurgica, II Dipartimento Chirurgico, Centro Regionale di Riferimento per la Chirurgia epatobiliopancreatica Ospedale Regionale, Treviso, Italy

Gennaro Nuzzo Hepatobiliary Surgery Unit, Catholic University of the Sacred Heart – A. Gemelli Hospital, Rome, Italy

Michele Paganelli Hepatobiliary Surgery, San Raffaele Hospital, Milan, Italy

Andrew J. Page Division of Surgical Oncology, Department of Surgery, The Johns Hopkins School of Medicine, Baltimore, MD, USA

Alberto Patriti Division of General Minimally Invasive and Robotic Surgery, Department of Surgery, ASL2 Umbria – San Matteo degli Infermi Hospital, Spoleto, Perugia, Italy

B. Pauletti IV Divisone Chirurgica, II Dipartimento Chirurgico, Centro Regionale di Riferimento per la Chirurgia epatobiliopancreatica Ospedale Regionale, Treviso, Italy

Timothy M. Pawlik Division of Surgical Oncology, Department of Surgery, The Johns Hopkins School of Medicine, Baltimore, MD, USA

Enrico Pinotti Hepatobiliary Surgery Unit, IRCCS San Raffaele Hospital, Milan, Italy

Antonio Daniele Pinna Department of Emergency, Surgery and Transplantation, Sant'Orsola Hospital, University of Bologna, Bologna, Italy

Fabio Procopio Department of Hepatobiliary Surgery, Humanitas Research Hospital, University of Milan-School of Medicine, Rozzano, Milan

Carlo Pulitanò Department of HPB and Transplantation Surgery, Royal Prince Alfred Hospital, Sydney, NSW, Australia

Francesca Ratti Hepatobiliary Surgery, San Raffaele Hospital, Milan, Italy

Raffaella Reineke Anesthesia and Intensive Care, S. Raffaele University Hospital, Milan, Italy

Aldo Rocca Department of Transplantation, Unit of Hepatobiliary Surgery and Liver Transplant, Cardarelli Hospital, Naples, Italy

Nadia Russolillo Department of General and Oncologic Surgery, Ospedale Mauriziano, Torino, Italy

Claudio Sallemi Department of Radiology, San Raffaele Hospital, Vita-Salute University, Milan, Italy

Vincenzo Scuderi Department of General and Hepato-Biliary Surgery, Liver Transplantation Service, Ghent University Hospital Medical School, Ghent, Belgium

Vishal G. Shelat HPB Surgery, Southampton General Hospital, Southampton, UK

Kevin C. Soares Division of Surgical Oncology, Department of Surgery, The Johns Hopkins School of Medicine, Baltimore, MD, USA

Loredana Sodano Department of Transplantation, Unit of Hepatobiliary Surgery and Liver Transplant, Cardarelli Hospital, Naples, Italy

Federico Tomassini Department of General and Hepato-Biliary Surgery, Liver Transplantation Service, Ghent University Hospital Medical School, Ghent, Belgium

Guido Torzilli Department of Hepatobiliary Surgery, Humanitas Research Hospital, University of Milan-School of Medicine, Rozzano, Milan

Roberto Ivan Troisi Department of General and Hepato-Biliary Surgery, Liver Transplantation Service, Ghent University Hospital Medical School, Ghent, Belgium

Massimo Venturini Department of Radiology, San Raffaele Hospital, Vita-Salute University, Milan, Italy

Chiara Zanfi Department of Emergency, Surgery and Transplantation, Sant'Orsola Hospital, University of Bologna, Bologna, Italy

Part I

General Perspective

Epidemiology and Histopathology 1

Francesco Cetta

Benign liver tumors of the liver comprise a wide range of "mass-forming lesions," including tumors deriving from the hepatocyte, the cholangiocyte, and the various cells of the vascular system, as well as various tumors of mesenchymal origin and a group of cystic or polycystic diseases of various origin [1–3].

The present chapter deals with epidemiology and histopathology of the most frequent benign liver tumors, focusing specifically on those deriving from hepatocytes and vascular structures, including, on the basis of their prevalence in the general population, hemangiomas, focal nodular hyperplasia (FNH), and hepatic adenoma (HA) [1–3].

1.1 Hemangiomas

Hepatic hemangiomas (also referred to as cavernous hemangiomas) are the most common benign neoplasms of the liver [2–8].

Estimates of the prevalence range from 0.4 to 10 % of the population, although one autopsy series specifically searching for hepatic lesions suggested a prevalence as high as 20 %. A 1.4–7 % prevalence has been reported in necropsy or surgical series [2–4].

The extensive use of noninvasive abdominal imaging modalities has led to an increased detection of asymptomatic lesions. In a series of 549 patients who underwent MRI for evaluation of focal hepatic lesions, 585 of 805, i.e., 72 %, resulted to be hemangiomas [3, 4].

F. Cetta
IRCCS MultiMedica, Milan, Italy
e-mail: cetta_francesco@libero.it

L. Aldrighetti et al. (eds.), *Benign Tumors of the Liver*,
DOI 10.1007/978-3-319-12985-3_1

Hepatic hemangiomas are usually small (<5 cm) and incidentally discovered during abdominal studies for unrelated causes. Lesions larger than 5 cm have been arbitrarily termed "giant hemangiomas."

Hepatic hemangiomas may occur at all ages. However, 60–80 % of cases are diagnosed in patients who are in their fourth and fifth decade of life, and the average age of patients presenting with symptomatic lesions is approximately 45 years. Patients presenting for evaluation of hepatic hemangioma are predominantly female F:M ratio 2: 1 to 6: 1. In particular, female patients often have a younger age and present with larger tumors. History of multiparity seems to have a facilitating role. Hepatic hemangiomas can also occur in the infancy and have also been detected in a growing fetus.

The prevalence of hemangiomas in patients with focal nodular hyperplasia (FNH) resulted higher than in the general population. It has been suggested that both lesions may have common causative factors, including focal alteration of the hepatic blood supply that somehow facilitates the hyperplastic lesions f FNH [6].

The cause of hepatic hemangiomas is unknown, but they are considered to be vascular malformations or hamartomas of congenital origin. Enlargement occurs by ectasia rather than hypertrophy or hyperplasia.

No definite familial or genetic mode of inheritance has been described. However, a large family of Italian origin has been reported, in which three female patients in three generations had large hepatic hemangiomas. The exclusive presence of hemangiomas in females could be explained by sex-dependent differences in penetrance, by a different expression of a putative liver-hemangioma gene, or by an increase of gender-related growth factors or hormones [7, 8].

In particular, enlargement of existing hemangiomas has been reported during pregnancy. This again suggests a relationship with female hormonal factors such as an endogenous or exogenous exposure to estrogens or progesterone [7, 8].

Glinkova et al. reported that enlargement occurred over time in 23 % of patients receiving estrogen therapy as compared to only 10 % in of the control group. On the other hand, estrogen receptors have not been detected in all tumors, and tumor growth has also been demonstrated in the absence of estrogen therapy and in postmenopausal women [8].

As such, the risk associated with the use of contraceptives or pregnancy is poorly understood. In particular there is still insufficient evidence to conclusively link estrogens to the development or progression of hepatic hemangiomas.

Kasabach–Merritt syndrome was originally described as purpura associated with thrombocytopenia and "capillary hemangioma." Recent studies have identified these lesions as tufted angioma or kaposiform hemangioendothelioma rather than typical hemangioma. It is a rare disease in which a vascular tumor leads to decreased platelet levels (consumption coagulopathy) and possible bleeding.

Hereditary hemorrhagic telangiectasia (HHT), also known as Rendu–Osler–Weber disease, is an autosomal dominant genetic disorder that leads to abnormal blood vessel formation in the skin, in the mucous membranes, and often in the liver, lung, and brain. Five genetic types of HHT have been recognized. Three of them have been linked to particular genes. More than 80 % of all cases are due to germ line mutations in either the ENG gene, mapped at 9q34.1, or ACVRL1. A total of over 600 different mutations have been detected. In about 2 % of cases, mutations in the gene MADH4, have been found cause colonic polyposis in addition to HHT.

Histopathology: Macroscopically, hemangiomas may vary in size from a few millimeters to many centimeters. They are dark purple, soft, compressible lesions that are well demarcated and frequently surrounded by a thin capsule (blood-filled "cysts").

Histologically, they consist of cavernous vascular spaces lined by endothelium and separated by connective tissue, totally lacking biliary or portal structures. By immunohistochemistry, the endothelium displays vascular as opposed to sinusoidal differentiation. Large tumors can have central thromboses, necrotic areas, or dystrophic calcifications.

1.2 Hepatic Adenoma

Hepatic adenoma (HA) is a benign tumor usually occurring in an otherwise normal liver [9–15]. Solitary adenoma, usually associated with the use of contraceptives or anabolic steroids, should be distinguished from hepatic adenomatosis (multiple adenomas, usually 10 or more).

HAs consist of hepatocytes which are arranged in liver cell plates that are only mildly thickened or irregular. The tumor parenchyma is supplied by numerous arteries, which are not accompanied by bile ducts. Hepatocytes are of normal size.

The association between HA and contraceptives has long been established. The incidence of HA is approximately 0.1 per 100,000 in non-OCP users versus 4 per 100,000 in OCP users. Two-thirds of HA express estrogen and progesterone receptors, and enlargement or even rupture has been reported during pregnancy. Distribution in HA incidence is different across the world. Whereas a marked female predominance has been reported in Europe, North America, and South Asia, accounting for 91, 78, and 73 %, respectively, in China only 37 % of HA patients are female, and only 11 % of them have a personal history of OCP or anabolic steroid use.

A precise mechanism underlying the role of estrogen in the pathogenesis of HA has not yet been clarified. However, the exogenous estrogen exposure has been considered by most studies as a stimulating growth factor for HA. Furthermore, HAs are more common in females than in males, with a F:M ratio of 11:1. This gender discrepancy is likely due to a combination of unregulated estrogen stimulation on hepatocytes, with variable effects of estrogens on liver metabolism, immunity, and response to cell injury.

An increased risk of hepatic adenoma has also been noted with the use of androgen preparations, such as in aplastic anemia, hypogonadism, hypopituitarism, and other endocrine disorders. Furthermore, the widespread use of androgens by bodybuilders has also been reported to promote HA formation.

In addition to steroid use, other risk factors associated with HA include hereditary diseases such as glycogenosis (namely, type I and type III glycogen storage disease, where HAs predominantly affect male patients), galactosemia, hepatic iron overload related to beta thalassemia, and maturity-onset diabetes of the young type (MODY 3).

HAs are benign monoclonal tumors occurring essentially in young women taking oral contraceptives (OCs). They frequently bleed but rarely transform into hepatocellular carcinoma (HCC).

Several molecular features associated with HA have been described (See Chap. 2). Recurrent mutations were identified in the TCF1 (transcription factor 1) gene, encoding the hepatocyte nuclear factor 1 alpha (HNF1 alpha), in the CTNNB1 (catenin beta 1) gene coding for beta-catenin, and in the IL6ST (interleukin 6 signal transducer) gene, which encodes for the signaling coreceptor gp 130 and is important for the activation of the JAK/STAT pathway.

In particular, HNF1A is a key transcription factor involved in liver development. It controls hepatocyte differentiation as well as glucose and lipid metabolism. Transcriptomic analysis of H-HAs revealed the dysregulation of genes involved in glucose and lipid metabolism. The main features observed included repression of gluconeogenesis, activation of glycolysis, and stimulation of aberrant fatty acid synthesis. Moreover, in human H-HA, several oncogenic factors lead to mTOR activation, angiogenesis, cell cycle activation, and cell proliferation.

Pathological analysis showed that inactivating biallelic mutations of HNF1A define a very homogeneous subgroup of HA characterized by a marked steatosis. However, steatosis alone is insufficient to diagnose H-HA. In fact, it is also detected in more than 35 % of inflammatory and unclassified HAs. In particular, expression of liver fatty acid-binding protein (LFABP) is specifically downregulated in H-HAs and has been included in the panel of immunohistological markers used to classify H-HAs (100 % specificity and 100 % specificity).

Concerning beta-catenin-mutated HAs, genotype–phenotype correlation revealed striking hallmarks of these adenomas. First, few male subjects develop HAs. However, when it occurs, it is usually a beta-catenin-mutated adenoma. At the pathological level, these adenomas exhibit cholestasis and cell dysplasia. Interestingly, beta-catenin mutations are associated with a high risk of malignant transformation. Beta-catenin-mutated adenomas show strong overexpression of GLUL (coding for glutamine synthase) and LGR5 (coding for leucine-rich repeat-containing G-protein-coupled receptor 5), which are 2 beta-catenin target genes.

By immunohistochemistry, diagnosis of a beta-catenin-mutated adenoma is performed using beta-catenin and glutamine synthase immunostaining. Beta-catenin-mutated HA are characterized by a nuclear localization of beta-catenin and a strong homogeneous expression of glutamine synthase in the cytoplasm. This pattern is homogeneous and diffuse in beta-catenin-mutated Has and differs from the "map-like pattern" that is usually observed in FNH. Due to difficult interpretation, because beta-catenin is detectable only in a few nuclei, analysis of beta-catenin expression has to be combined with glutamine synthase staining, in order to increase detection sensitivity for beta-catenin activation.

Concerning "inflammatory adenomas," IL6ST/gp130, STAT3, or GNAS were discovered as oncogenes activated by mutations in IHA. In tumors, each mutation is exclusive of the 2 others, and the 3 genes can explain more than 75 % of the overall IHAs. This suggests that other driver genes leading to JAK/STAT3 activation remain to be identified. Mutations in IL6ST/gp130, STAT3, or GNAS act by a similar mechanism called "oncogene-induced inflammation" that leads to constitutive STAT3 activation. Uncontrolled activation of the JAK/STAT pathway in tumor hepatocytes explains the inflammatory phenotype observed at both the histologic and clinical levels. Cytokines and chemokines induced by STAT3 and secreted by hepatocytes act as chemoattractants that promote tumor infiltration by lymphocytes. The origin of dystrophic artery and sinusoidal dilatation that is usually observed in the tumor is unknown, but a direct or indirect role of the release of inflammatory proteins by the mutated hepatocytes could be hypothesized. All of these data highlight that hepatocytes are major inflammatory cells and that inflammation is a key mechanism in liver tumorigenesis.

In summary, concerning HAs, genotyping allowed the identification of three subtypes: HNF1 alpha inactivated (accounting for 35–50 % of cases), beta-catenin activated (15–18 % of cases), and inflammatory (40–55 % of cases) HA, which can be identified by immunohistochemistry on paraffin-embedded material. Furthermore, HNF1 alpha and inflammatory adenomas (IHA) often display associated pathologic characteristics. In particular, IHA patients are frequently overweight, with high alcohol intake, as compared to patients with HNF1 alpha HA.

Finally, less than 10 % of HA do not express any of these markers (See Chap. 2).

Additional remarks include the following: adenomatosis has been considered since 1985 as a different entity from HA; the so-called telangiectatic FNH [16] is not anymore considered as atypical FNH but as a group of HAs, today classified as IHA with specific clinical biological features as a high BMI and raised gamma glutamyl transpeptidase and CRP. In particular, genetic mutations are able to identify the various HA subgroups.

Recently, Sasaki et al. surveyed HA in a consecutive series of 13 patients (7 females) in Japan, where HA is comparatively less frequent than in Western countries. There were 2 HNF 1A inactivated HA (15 %), 2 beta-catenin activated (15 %), 5 inflammatory HA (39 %), and 4 unclassified (29 %) [15].

1.3 FNH

Focal nodular hyperplasia (FNH), first described by Edmondson in 1958 [1], is the second most common benign liver tumor, outnumbered only by hemangioma. FNH is more prevalent in women (F:M ratio = 8:1) and usually occurs in the third to fifth decades of life [16–25]. A link between FNH and oral contraceptive use has been reported but is disputed [20, 21].

Lesions are usually less than 5 cm in diameter and solitary in 80 % of cases. Only 3 % are larger than 10 cm, although FNH of up to 19 cm have been reported. Macroscopically, FNH appears as a light brown, well-circumscribed lobulated tumor. In contrast to hemangiomas, FNH lacks a capsule.

Classical FNH is characterized by a central starlike fibrous region containing malformed vascular structures. The solitary central artery with high flow and the absent portal vein give the lesion a characteristic radiologic appearance, in more than 70–80 % of cases. However, some classical FNHs, mainly those smaller than 3 cm, have no central scar at pathological examination.

FNH typically occurs in normal or almost normal liver. The lesion is multinodular, composed of nearly normal hepatocytes arranged in 1–2-cell-thick plates. Bile ductules are usually found in the interface between hepatocytes and fibrous regions. It is thought that increased arterial flow hyperperfuses the local parenchyma, leading to secondary hepatocellular hyperplasia. FNH is therefore considered a hyperplastic response to increased blood flow, rather than a true neoplastic process. Various vascular abnormalities such as telangiectasia, hereditary hemorrhagic telangiectasia (Kasabach–Merritt syndrome), and arteriovenous malformation and anomalous venous drainage, as well as portal vein aplasia (Abernethy syndrome), may be present, especially in patients with multiple FNHs.

The generally accepted hypothesis concerning the genesis of FNH lesions has been initially proposed by Wanless et al. in 1995 [17]. According to this theory, arterial malformation disturbs the local blood flow, thus causing a hyperplastic response of normal liver cells to either hyperperfusion or hypoxia [18]. The notion that FNH lesions develop secondary to vascular abnormalities is supported by several observations [22]. In some adults, the liver contains both hemangiomas and FNH. A study among 247 patients with hepatic masses identified 148 patients with FNH, of which 20 % had concomitant hemangiomas of the liver [6]. Another indication is the differential prevalence of FNH in families with hereditary hemorrhagic telangiectasia (HHT), an autosomal dominant genetic disorder characterized by vascular malformations. In a study of 275 family members, FNH was found in 5 individuals. Recently, anecdotal evidence was published on the proposed sequence from hemangioma to FNH, probably starting with thrombosis of the hemangioma followed by involution of the lesion and subsequent occurrence of a hyperplastic regenerative reaction. A child that was analyzed at the age of 6 months for a palpable hemangioma of the liver presented 5 years later with a lesion of unknown origin in the same topographic area of the organ. Surgical excision and pathological examination revealed an FNH [24].

Clonal analysis demonstrated the reactive polyclonal nature of liver cells in FNH in 60–100 % of cases. Unlike HA, which is characterized by monoclonal expansion, FNH arises by polyclonal cell proliferation. This polyclonal origin, that is detectable in most of cases, further proves the benign nature of FNH. In FNH, gene expression data reveal activation of the beta-catenin pathway. In particular, beta-catenin shows a heterogeneous distribution along the hepatocellular nodules in the absence of an activating mutation of the gene.

In normal hepatocytes, beta-catenin and its known targeted genes are expressed exclusively in the immediate perivenous areas. This zonated defined pattern of expression differs from that observed in beta-catenin-activated HA or HCC, which usually shows more diffuse cytoplasmic GS staining and nuclear beta-catenin staining.

Gene expression studies have revealed molecular features supporting the theory of vascular abnormalities as a driving event in the formation of FNH. FNH presents abnormal expression of genes involved in angiogenesis with an increased expression of the ANGPT1/ANGPT2 ratio, promoting angiogenesis. In fact, AGPT is classically responsible for vessel formation, and ANGPT2 acts as an antagonist of ANGPT1.

1.4 Other Benign Tumors

In contrast to hepatocellular tumors, the benign variant of a biliary tumor is exceedingly rare, accounting for a small proportion (less than 2 %) of all benign tumors of the liver. Bile duct adenoma is usually asymptomatic, but obstructive jaundice can be the presenting symptom depending on the location and size. Actually, in one study, the clinical, gross, and histological features of 152 cases have been reviewed [26]. All of them were asymptomatic nodules, incidentally discovered during surgery ($n=103$) or at autopsy ($n=49$). They were usually subcapsular, ranged in size from 1 to 20 mm (mean 5.8 mm), and well circumscribed, but nonencapsulated. Authors believe that bile duct adenoma is a reactive process to a focal injury rather than a true neoplasm or a developmental anomaly [26].

Biliary hamartomas (von Meyenburg complexes) are more common benign malformations of the biliary tract. They are small lesions (usually <1 cm) consisting of cystic spaces and fibrous stroma. The main relevance is to distinguish them from metastases [27].

Angiomyolipomas are tumors derived from perivascular epithelioid cells, which are associated with tuberous sclerosis and mostly occur in the kidney. Hepatic angiomyolipomas are difficult to diagnose correctly by imaging procedures. They are premalignant lesions and should then undergo surgical treatment [28].

Peliosis hepatis refers to a vascular disorder that can appear as a tumor. It is associated with the use of steroid hormones, malignancy, transplantation, and chronic inflammation. Histology reveals multiple blood-filled cysts of different sizes. The natural history is not known, but rupture has been reported.

Conclusion

Recent development in molecular biology, together with genotype–phenotype correlation, has given a clue for a deeper insight into benign liver tumors, facilitating new nosographic grouping and classification. In particular, (1) FHN can be considered a mainly vascular lesion, more similar to hemangioma than to adenoma; (2) adenomas have been classified on the basis of peculiar genetic mutations, differing from one type to another and having crucial implications not only for biological behavior and prognosis (evolution into HCC) but also for classification refinement, using new immunohistochemical methods, based on most recent technical advancement.

All three lesions can coexist together in the same subject. In fact, in about 20 % of cases, hemangiomas have been found in association with adenomas and/or FNH, suggesting a "common background," at least for some types of these pathological entities. In particular, metabolic alterations (namely, in glucose metabolism or glycogen synthesis), estrogen exposure, or endogenous secretion and also disruption of the Wnt–beta-catenin pathway, which is responsible for hepatocyte zonation but is also playing a crucial role in liver regeneration, emerge as pathogenetic factors from a combined epidemiologic and histopathologic analysis.

A final comment concerns "diffuse inflammation" of the environment surrounding benign liver tumors, involving not only canonical inflammatory cells (macrophages, Kupffer cells, stellate cells) but also the hepatocyte, which has recently been considered as an additional "inflammatory cell" that could be responsible for both local and systemic inflammation.

References

1. Edmondson HA (1958) Tumors of the liver and intrahepatic bile ducts. In: Atlas of tumor pathology. Armed Forces Institute of Pathology, Washington, DC
2. Ishak KG, Robin L (1975) Benign tumors of the liver. Med Clin North Am 59:995–1013
3. John TG, Greig JD, Crosbie JL et al (1994) Superior staging of liver tumors with laparoscopy and laparoscopic ultrasound. Ann Surg 220:711–719
4. Gandolfi L, Leo P, Solmi L et al (1991) Natural history of hepatic hemangiomas: clinical and ultrasound study. Gut 32:677–680
5. Mathieu D, Zafrani ES, Anglade MC et al (1989) Association of focal nodular hyperplasia and hepatic hemangioma. Gastroenterology 97:154–157
6. Vilgrain V, Uzan F, Brancatelli G et al (2003) Prevalence of hepatic hemangioma in patients with focal nodular hyperplasia: MR imaging analysis. Radiology 229:75–79
7. Van Malenstei H, Maleux G, Monhalis D et al (2011) Giant liver hemangioma : the role of female sex hormones and treatment. Eur J Gastroenterol Hepatol 23:438–443
8. Glinkova V, Shevah O, Boaz M et al (2004) Hepatic hemangiomas. Possible association with female sex hormones. Gut 53:1352–1355
9. Rooks JB, Ory HW, Ishak KG et al (1979) Epidemiology of hepatocellular adenoma. The role of oral contraceptive use. JAMA 242:644–648
10. Laurent C, Trillaud H, Lepreux S et al (2003) Association of adenoma and focal nodular hyperplasia: experience of a single French academic center. Comp Hepatol 2:6
11. Labrune P, Trioche P, Duvaltier I et al (1997) Hepatocellular adenomas in glycogen storage disease type I and III: a series of 43 patients and review of the literature. J Pediatr Gastroenterol Nutr 24:276–279
12. Nault J-C, Bioulac-Sage P, Zucman-Rossi J (2013) Hepatocellular benign tumors-from molecular classification to personalized clinical care. Gastroenterology 144:888–902
13. Flejou JF, Barge J, Menu Y et al (1985) Liver adenomatosis. An entity distinct from liver adenoma? Gastroenterology 89:1132–1138
14. Cherqui D, Rahmouni A, Charlotte F et al (1995) Management of focal nodular hyperplasia and hepatocellular adenoma in young women: a series of 41 patients with clinical, radiological, and pathological correlations. Hepatology 22:1674–1681
15. Sasaki M, Nakanuma Y (2012) Overview of hepatocellular adenoma in Japan. Int J Hepatol. doi:10.1155/2012/648131
16. Paradis V, Champault A, Ronot M et al (2007) Telangiectatic adenoma: an entity associated with increased body mass index and inflammation. Hepatology 46:140–146
17. Wanless IR, Mawdsley C, Adams R (1985) On the pathogenesis of focal nodular hyperplasia of the liver. Hepatology 5:1194–1200

18. Wanless IR (1990) Micronodular transformation (nodular regenerative hyperplasia) of the liver: a report of 64 cases among 2,500 autopsies and a new classification of benign hepatocellular nodules. Hepatology 11:787–797
19. Mortelé KJ, Praet M, Van Vlierberghe H et al (2000) CT and MR imaging findings in focal nodular hyperplasia of the liver: radiologic-pathologic correlation. Am J Roentgenol 175:687–692
20. Mathieu D, Kobeiter H, Cherqui D et al (1998) Oral contraceptive intake in women with focal nodular hyperplasia of the liver. Lancet 352:1679–1680
21. Mathieu D, Kobeiter H, Maison P et al (2000) Oral contraceptive use and focal nodular hyperplasia of the liver. Gastroenterology 118:560–564
22. Fukukura Y, Nakashima O, Kusaba A et al (1998) Angioarchitecture and blood circulation in focal nodular hyperplasia of the liver. J Hepatol 29:470–475
23. Chandler TM, Heran MK, Chang SD et al (2011) Multiple focal nodular hyperplasia lesions of the liver associated with congenital absence of the portal vein. Magn Reson Imaging 29:881–886
24. Turowski C, Feist H, Alzen G et al (2009) Conversion of a neonatal hepatic hemangioma to focal nodular hyperplasia. Pathol Int 59:251–254
25. Nguyen BN, Fléjou JF, Terris B et al (1999) Focal nodular hyperplasia of the liver: a comprehensive pathologic study of 305 lesions and recognition of new histologic forms. Am J Surg Pathol 23:1441–1454
26. Allaire GS, Rabin L, Ishak KG et al (1998) Bile duct adenomas. A study of 152 cases. Am J Surg Pathol 12:708–715
27. Troltzsch M, Borte G, Kahn T et al (2003) Non invasive diagnosis of von Meyenburg complexes. J Hepatol 39:129
28. Flemming P, Lehmann U, Becker T et al (2000) Common and epithelioid variants of hepatic angiomyolipoma exhibit clonal growth and share a distinctive immunophenotype. Hepatology 32:213–217

Molecular Biology and Genetics

2

Francesco Cetta

Hepatocellular benign tumors are characterized by benign proliferation of hepatocytes with a mass-forming presentation and mainly consist of hepatocellular adenoma (HA) and focal nodular hyperplasia (FNH) [1, 2]. HA and FNH share common features. First, a large female preponderance has been found in both diseases, with a female/male ratio = 8:1 for FNH and 9:1 for HA. In addition, FNH and HA derive from the proliferation of mature hepatocytes and arise on an otherwise normal liver. Therefore, they represent a model to study liver tumorigenesis outside the classic background of cirrhosis [2].

Has have been classified into four major molecular subgroups according to their genetic and phenotype characteristics [2–8].

2.1 HNF1A-Mutated Adenomas

This group includes 30–40 % of HAs and is defined by HNF1A (coding for hepatocyte nuclear factor 1 alpha) mutations. In most of cases, both inactivating HNF1A mutations are somatic and are thus found only in tumoral cells. However, some patients carry a germline inherited HNF1A mutation in one allele. In these cases, there is an association with maturity-onset diabetes type 3 (MODY3), a monogenic non-insulin-dependent diabetes. Adenomas that develop in patients with MODY3 have another somatic mutation inactivating the second allele of HNF1A in the tumor hepatocytes according to the 2-hit model described by Knudson for inactivation of tumor suppressor genes. In particular, patients with germline mutations of HNF1A are predisposed to develop liver adenomatosis. Genetic studies performed in mouse models suggest a necessary cooperation between HNF1A inactivation and

F. Cetta
IRCCS MultiMedica, Milan, Italy
e-mail: cetta_francesco@libero.it

L. Aldrighetti et al. (eds.), *Benign Tumors of the Liver*,
DOI 10.1007/978-3-319-12985-3_2

additional genetic alterations to promote liver tumorigenesis. However, until now in humans, no additional genetic alterations have thus far been identified in HNF1A-mutated adenomas (H-HAs), and biallelic inactivating mutations of HNF1A are exclusive of CTNNB1, IL6ST, GNAS, and STAT3 mutations classically found in other HCA subtypes [2–8].

HNF1A belongs to the hepatocyte nuclear factor family and is a key transcription factor involved in liver development. In addition, HNF1A controls hepatocyte differentiation as well as glucose and lipid metabolism. Transcriptomic analysis of H-HAs revealed the dysregulation of genes involved in glucose and lipid metabolism. The main features observed included repression of gluconeogenesis, activation of glycolysis, and stimulation of aberrant fatty acid synthesis. Moreover, in human H-HA, several oncogenic factors lead to mTOR activation, angiogenesis, cell cycle activation (CCND1), and cell proliferation (PDGFRA and B, ERRB2). Interestingly, these observations were also observed on HNF1A silencing in different hepatocellular cell lines, thereby showing the specific role of HNF1A inactivation in inducing the metabolic and pro-proliferative disorders observed in H-HA [2–8].

Genotype/phenotype correlations further support these observations. Indeed, pathological analysis showed that inactivating biallelic mutations of HNF1A define a very homogeneous subgroup of adenomas characterized by a marked steatosis. However, steatosis alone is insufficient to diagnose H-HA. In fact, it can be detected in more than 35 % of inflammatory and unclassified HAs. Expression of liver fatty acid-binding protein (LFABP) is specifically downregulated in H-HAs. LFABP staining has been included in the panel of immunohistological markers used to classify H-HAs (with 100 % specificity and 100 % sensitivity). Finally, HNF1A can be considered at the crossroads between metabolism and tumorigenesis in the liver [2].

2.2 Beta-Catenin-Activated Adenomas

Mutations of beta-catenin are localized at hot spots in exon 3 of the CTNNB gene. Beta-catenin-mutated HAs constitute approximately 10–15 % of all HAs. Interestingly, beta-catenin-activated mutations are exclusive of HNF1A mutations but can be combined with gp130 or GNAS mutations, and half of the beta-catenin-activated adenomas (bHAs) are also inflammatory (bIHA) [2].

Under physiological conditions, in the absence of activating ligand, the Wnt/beta-catenin pathway is inactivated, and beta-catenin is phosphorylated by the GSKB/APC/AXIN complex. Phosphorylation of beta-catenin leads to its ubiquitination and subsequent degradation by the proteasome. In tumors, mutations of beta-catenin impair phosphorylation by the GSK3B/APC/AXIN complex and decrease its degradation; as a consequence, beta-catenin accumulates and translocates to the nucleus to act as a co-transcription factor via the association with the T-cell factor/lymphoid-enhancing complex. The Wnt/beta-catenin pathway plays a key role in amino acid metabolism, cell–cell interactions, liver regeneration, and zonation [2, 9].

Wnt is also a well-known oncogenic pathway involved in several types of cancer, namely, HCC. However, a genetically engineered mouse model harboring liver-specific expression of beta-catenin-activating mutations developed neither HA nor HCC. On the contrary, liver-specific deletion of the APC gene or co-expression of HRAS with CTNNB1 mutant leads to formation of HCC. These results show that activation of beta-catenin is not sufficient alone to induce liver carcinogenesis but can cooperate with other pathways to promote tumor development.

Genotype/phenotype correlation revealed striking hallmarks of beta-catenin-mutated HAs. First, few male subjects develop Has. However, when it occurs, it is usually a bHA. At the pathological level, these adenomas exhibit cholestasis and cell dysplasia. Importantly, beta-catenin mutations are associated with a high risk of malignant transformation. Beta-catenin-mutated adenomas show strong overexpression of GLUL (coding for glutamine synthase) and LGR5 (coding for leucine-rich repeat-containing G-protein-coupled receptor 5), which are 2 beta-catenin target genes [2].

By immunohistochemistry, diagnosis of a beta-catenin-mutated adenoma is performed using beta-catenin and glutamine synthase immunostaining. bHAs are characterized by a nuclear localization of beta-catenin and a strong homogeneous expression of glutamine synthase in the cytoplasm. This pattern is homogeneous and diffuses in bHAs and differs from the "maplike pattern" observed in FNH. Due to difficult interpretation, because beta-catenin is detectable only in a few nuclei, analysis of beta-catenin expression has to be combined with glutamine synthase staining to increase detection sensitivity for beta-catenin activation. However, although these two markers have very good specificity (approximately 100 %), they show insufficient sensitivity (75–85 %) for the diagnosis of beta-catenin mutations. Because of the high risk of malignant transformation, HAs without overexpression of beta-catenin target genes and not mutated for HNF1A (mutually exclusive with beta-catenin mutations) should be screened for beta-catenin mutations [2, 8].

2.3 Inflammatory Adenomas

The third group of HAs is composed of inflammatory adenomas and accounts for 40–50 % of all adenomas. The peculiar feature of IHAs is the activation of the JAK/STAT pathway.

At the histologic level, IHAs are characterized by polymorphic inflammatory infiltrates, dystrophic vessels, and sinusoidal dilatations. They also exhibit overexpression of serum amyloid A (SAA) and C-reactive protein, 2 proteins of the acute phase of inflammation.

Identification of IHAs reveals obesity and high alcohol intake as two new risk factors for occurrence of inflammatory adenomas but not for the other subtypes. Importantly, a subset of IHAs also harbors an activating mutation of beta-catenin and, consequently, shows an increased risk of malignant transformation [2, 11–13]. Recently, three different molecular drivers, namely, IL6ST (coding for gp130), STAT3, and GNAS, were discovered as oncogenes activated by mutations in

IHCA. In tumors, each mutation is exclusive of the two others, and the three genes (IL6ST, STAT3, and GNAS) can explain more than 75 % of the overall IHAs.

In the canonical IL-6/JAK/STAT pathway, interleukin (IL)-6 binds to gp80, the IL-6 receptor (IL6R) that dimerizes with gp130, the co-receptor signal transducer (IL6ST); then, 2 IL-6/gp130/gp80 complexes associate and form an hexameric complex at the cell membrane88. This leads to the recruitment of JAK1 and JAK2, which phosphorylate in turn STAT3 and STAT1. Activated phospho-STAT3 and phospho-STAT1 homodimerize and/or heterodimerize and translocate to the nucleus to act as transcription factors. Somatic heterozygous mutations activating gp130 are found in 65 % of inflammatory adenomas. Mutations of gp130 are mainly small in-frame deletions targeting the IL-6 binding site. Gp130 mutant leads to gp130 dimerization and constitutive STAT3 activation in the absence of IL-6. Rare cases of HCC also harbor gp130-activating mutations. Interestingly, these HCCs develop on normal livers and also show beta-catenin-activating mutations, suggesting malignant transformation of HCAs [2].

The second oncogene mutated in IHCA, STAT3, is mutated in 5 % of IHAs. These mutations lead to amino acid substitutions mainly localized in the SH2 domain involved in STAT3 dimerization. STAT3 mutants are phosphorylated and activated in the absence of IL-6 and lead to an uncontrolled constitutive activation of the inflammatory pathway. The third gene, GNAS, is also found to be mutated in 5 % of IHAs. GNAS encodes the alpha subunit of the Gs protein. The Gs protein complex is composed of the alpha and beta/gamma subunits. In their inactive forms, alpha and beta/gamma subunits are associated. When a stimulus leads to G-protein-coupled receptor activation, guanosine triphosphate replaces guanosine diphosphate on the subunit. Then, the latter dissociates and activates the adenylate cyclase, thereby increasing levels of intracellular cyclic adenosine monophosphate, which acts as an intracellular second messenger. Thus, the alpha subunit is inactivated due to an intrinsic guanosine triphosphatase activity that converts guanosine triphosphate into guanosine diphosphate [2].

Activating mutations of GNAS localize at hot spots in the guanosine triphosphatase domain. Guanosine triphosphatase activity of the subunit is consequently impaired and leads to aberrant activation of adenylate cyclase and accumulation of cyclic adenosine monophosphate. GNAS is considered an oncogene recurrently mutated in benign lesions such as pituitary and thyroid adenomas, myelodysplastic syndrome, and intraductal papillary mucinous neoplasm but also in cancers such as cholangiocarcinoma. Typical GNAS-activating mutations have been identified in sporadic HCAs and in adenomas arising in patients with McCune–Albright syndrome. McCune–Albright syndrome is a rare disease defined by "café au lait" skin macula, fibrous dysplasia of bone, and high risk of pituitary and thyroid adenomas. McCune–Albright syndrome is caused by somatic mosaic-activating mutations of GNAS genes and is a condition that promotes occurrence of HCAs. GNAS-activating mutations lead to mild STAT3 activation in hepatocellular cell lines, which underlines a cross talk between the cyclic adenosine monophosphate and JAK/STAT pathways. Finally, in approximately 25 % of IHAs, it was not possible to identify any gene defect that could explain the phenotype [2].

This suggests that other driver genes leading to JAK/STAT3 activation remain to be identified. Mutations in IL6ST/gp130, STAT3, or GNAS act by a similar mechanism called "oncogene-induced inflammation" that leads to constitutive STAT3 activation. Uncontrolled activation of the JAK/STAT pathway in tumor hepatocytes explains the inflammatory phenotype observed at both the histologic and clinical levels. Cytokine and chemokine induced by STAT3 and secreted by hepatocytes act as chemoattractants that promote tumor infiltration by lymphocytes. The origin of dystrophic artery and sinusoidal dilatation observed in the tumor is unknown, but a direct or indirect role of the release of inflammatory proteins by the mutated hepatocytes could be hypothesized.

All of these data highlight that hepatocytes are major inflammatory cells and that inflammation is a central mechanism of liver tumorigenesis. Animal models would be very useful to dissect the roles of the inflammatory pathway in benign tumorigenesis, to understand the cooperation between the IL-6/JAK/STAT and beta-catenin pathways in malignant transformation, and to test for new biotherapies. However, liver-specific animal models are lacking [2].

Unclassified adenomas include approximately 10 % of all HCAs. Different genetic and environmental factors can predispose to development of HCAs. First, several rare genetic syndromes are strongly associated with the occurrence of adenomas. Some patients with MODY3 (monoallelic germline mutations of HNF1A) develop liver adenomatosis with biallelic H-HCA. Following this mechanism, HNF1A meets the criteria of a classic tumor suppressor gene with a transmitted predisposition to develop tumors as defined by Knudson. To our knowledge, currently all familial transmission of liver adenomatosis identified worldwide is associated with germline HNF1A mutations. In these patients, familial genetic counseling is required to propose screening for diabetes and HCA [2].

However, liver adenomatosis could also be related to other molecular subtypes. Other genetic disorders associated with the occurrence of adenomas are glycogen storage diseases and particularly type 1a glycogenosis. Glycogenosis 1a is a rare recessive metabolic disease characterized by germline mutations inactivating glucose-6-phosphatase [14–16]. More than 50 % of these patients develop HAs during follow-up [14–16]. As a mirror of the human disease, mice with a liver-specific deletion of glucose-6-phosphatase harbored the same metabolic disorder and developed HCA. A recent study showed that gene therapy using adenovirus could correct the metabolic disorder and prevent development of HCA in this mouse model. Two studies have recently shown that all HAs observed in patients with glycogenosis were bHCAs, IHCAs, or unclassified, whereas no HNF1A mutations were identified. Furthermore, metabolic disorders induced by HNF1A and G6PC inactivation appear to be very similar, at least partly explaining the exclusive occurrence of these genetic defects in patients. Finally, McCune–Albright syndrome, an orphan disease characterized by mosaic somatic GNAS-activating mutations, predisposes patients to the development of IHA. Strikingly, these genetic diseases predispose to the development of specific molecular subtypes: H-HA in patients with MODY3 [10], IHA in patients with McCune–Albright syndrome, and absence of H-HA in glycogenosis [14–17]. However, whereas genetic diseases constitute strong risk factors, penetrance of the HCA phenotype is incomplete and particularly rare in patients with MODY3. Thus, additional modifier genes or environmental factors remain to be identified to fully understand which patients will develop HA.

Most cases of HA are not associated with rare genetic diseases, but a clinical study conducted at a hospital in Bordeaux showed that 39 % of HCAs are multifocal macroscopically. In addition to the macroscopic tumors, pathological studies have revealed the presence of multiple microscopic foci of IHCA easily identified using SAA immunostaining. Microscopic adenomas inactivated for HNF1A and negative for LFABP are also observed in patients with adenomatosis developed on a germline mutation of HNF1A background or in multiple H-HAs without MODY3. We can hypothesize that a modifier genetic background associated with environmental factors could favor multiple occurrences of HA. Oral contraception is also strongly associated with occurrence of HCAs. Indeed, a dose-dependent association has been described, and estrogen exposure could act as promoting HNF1A gene mutations. Spontaneous regression of HCAs after withdrawal of estrogen has also been described, thereby suggesting that development of HCAs could be in particular cases dependent on the hormonal context.

Androgen consumption is a well-known risk factor for HCAs, particularly bHCAs. HCAs have been reported in patients with Fanconi anemia treated with an androgen, in cases of anabolic androgen steroid abuse in athletes, or due to an endogenous high level of androgen such as in Klinefelter's syndrome or polycystic ovary syndrome. Dramatic regression of HCAs after withdrawal of androgen has been recurrently described. Several associations between HCA and antiepileptic drugs have been reported, but a causative effect remains to be shown. However, only a small number of patients using oral contraceptives develop HCA (about 3 per 100,000 in exposed patients). A role for an additional unknown minor allele associated with environmental factors is of concern. Supporting this hypothesis, it was observed that some patients with HHCAs also harbor germline heterozygous mutations of CYP1B1 [17]. These mutations lead to decrease enzymatic activity and could play a role in estrogen metabolism.

Moreover, patients with adenomatosis in a large French family harbored two monoallelic germline mutations inactivating HNF1A and CYP1B1. These results support possible cooperation between genetic and environmental factors to modulate the risk of HA occurrence. The last risk factors significantly associated with occurrence of IHA are alcohol consumption and obesity. The mechanisms linking these two metabolic disorders with the occurrence of HCA showing an autonomous IL-6/JAK/STAT3 activation remain to be investigated, taking into account both environmental factors and genetic backgrounds. The direct toxic role of alcohol or a role of cytokine production observed during long-term alcohol consumption and in obese patients cannot be excluded.

In summary, these data sustain a model in which the liver could be predisposed to the development of multiple HCAs in association or not with a major genetic syndrome. This model challenges the current dogma according to which the nontumor liver surrounding adenomas is really normal. Because a "carcinogenic field effect" is proposed in cirrhosis to explain development of HCC, we propose that appearance of multiple adenomas could be caused by a "benign tumorigenic field effect." This predisposition could be the result of a conjunction between genetic and genotoxic factors leading to proliferation of benign hepatocytes. Benign hepatocellular tumors can be classified using immunohistochemical analyses. Studies of genotypes and phenotypes of FNH and HCAs have led to the identification of risk factors and improved invasive and noninvasive diagnostic techniques, evaluation of prognosis, and treatment.

Focal nodular hyperplasia (FNH) is a polyclonal lesion that is characterized by local vascular abnormalities and heterogeneous activation of Wnt/beta-catenin and transforming growth factor signaling.

FNH is the second most common benign liver tumor, outnumbered only by hemangioma [18]. Clonal analysis demonstrated the reactive polyclonal nature of liver cells in FNH in 60–100 % of cases, depending on the series. In particular, Paradis et al. concluded from their analyses that FNH lesions arise by polyclonal cell proliferation, unlike HA which is characterized by monoclonal expansion [19, 20]. In addition, other studies [2, 21–26], analyzing chromosome gains and losses by comparative genomic hybridization, allelotyping, or karyotyping, identified chromosome alterations indicating a clonal origin of the FNH nodules in 14–50 % of cases. However, genetic analysis of FNH did not demonstrate somatic gene mutations in CTNNB1, TP53, TCF1, or APC, which is the gene responsible for FAP. This polyclonal origin, that is detectable in most of cases, further proves the benign nature of FNH and supports the strategy not to treat FNH in asymptomatic cases [2, 19, 20].

Gene expression data reveal an activation of the beta-catenin pathway in FNH. Beta-catenin is regarded as a pivotal stimulus for proliferation of hepatocytes and a master actor of liver development and liver regeneration after injury, as well as a master regulator of liver zonation. In FNH, beta-catenin shows a heterogeneous distribution along the hepatocellular nodules in the absence of an activating mutation of the gene and in the absence of alterations in the Wnt signaling pathway.

In normal hepatocytes, beta-catenin and its known target genes, such as GS, are expressed exclusively in the immediate perivenous areas. This zonated defined pattern of expression differs from that observed in beta-catenin-activated HCA or HCC, which usually shows more diffuse cytoplasmic GS staining and nuclear beta-catenin staining, in accordance with the monoclonal origin of the beta-catenin-activating mutations in these tumors [2, 9].

In FNH, beta-catenin activation showed a heterogeneous distribution along the hepatocellular nodules, with a characteristic architectural distribution over relatively large areas, sometimes centered on visible veins and usually remaining at a distance from fibrous bands. This specific beta-catenin expression pattern may be interpreted as the result of an altered hepatocyte zonation in FNH leading to increased beta-catenin gradient, starting from the veins,

Activation of the beta-catenin pathway in FNH could consequently contribute to tumor formation as beta-catenin may promote hepatocyte proliferation and regeneration. However, in contrast to an activating mutation, hepatocytes in FNH remain sensitive to repression of the beta-catenin pathway in regions surrounding fibrosis.

There is agreement on the view that (1) FNH could originate from a hyperplastic lesion composed of reactive polyclonal proliferating hepatocytes and (2) this proliferation of abnormal hepatocytes could be caused by an increased blood flow due to local vascular malformation [27, 28].

Gene expression studies have revealed molecular features supporting the theory of vascular abnormalities as a driving event in the formation of FNH. In fact, FNH presents abnormal expression of genes involved in angiogenesis with an increase in expression of the ANGPT1/ANGPT2 ratio. ANGPT1 is classically responsible for vessel formation, and ANGPT2 acts as an antagonist of ANGPT1. Therefore, increased expression of ANGPT1/ANGPT2 is expected to promote angiogenesis. In addition, genome expression using microarray in FNH identified an overexpression of several genes of the extracellular matrix, particularly at the central fibrous scar, related to activation of the transforming growth factor pathway. Another major finding was the overexpression of Wnt/beta-catenin target genes, including *GLUL* coding for glutamine synthase. In the normal liver lobule, beta-catenin is activated in 2–3 cells thick layers of hepatocytes around the central vein and repressed in hepatocytes in the portal area. On the contrary, in FNH, overexpression of glutamine synthase is enlarged and shows a specific location with a maplike pattern predominantly in the periphery of the nodules. The heterogeneous distribution of glutamine synthase is caused by beta-catenin activation without beta-catenin-activating mutations in accordance with FNH polyclonal origin. Again, this could result from an abnormal arterial blood flow. Because this maplike pattern of glutamine synthase expression is characteristic, easy to recognize, and specifically observed in FNH, it is presently used for diagnosis.

In conclusion, FNH is usually an asymptomatic benign tumor with normal liver enzyme levels and tumor markers (AFP, CA19-9, ACE) that are mostly found incidentally using imaging. FNH is frequently associated with liver hemangioma (20 % of cases 35), with other FNH (multiple FNH in 20–30 % of cases), and more rarely with HCA. Some rare diseases such as Rendu–Osler disease, Budd–Chiari syndrome, Kasabach–Merritt syndrome, and portal vein agenesis are also associated with FNH. Interestingly, these diseases are characterized by vascular abnormalities in the liver and constitute a strong link with the vascular hypothesis, explaining the origin of FNH. However, the vast majority of patients with FNH do not have any of those known risk factor

Conclusion

The overall amount of data suggests a model in which the liver could be predisposed to the development of adenomas (or to other benign – and malignant – liver tumors), in association or not with a major genetic syndrome.

Inherited genetic syndromes are rare diseases but very useful from a molecular point of view, because they can often give the clue for a better knowledge of more frequent sporadic tumors.

There are three new concepts that deserve to be outlined, because they are apparently contrary to "the current opinion":

1. Even in patients with inherited multitumoral syndromes (See also Chap. 3), such as FAP and Beckwith–Wiedemann, but also with congenital metabolic diseases, such as glycogenosis, galactosemia, and MODY3, the inherited germline mutation is not sufficient by itself to determine the occurrence of the tumoral phenotype (as occurs in patients with germline mutations of the APC gene, which determine colonic cancer in 100 % of affected patients), but the cooperation of other genetic mutations or epigenetic and/or environmental factors is always required.
2. (a) In all types of hepatic adenomas associated with inherited disease or germline mutations, the lesion is almost never unique, but – even if typical adenomatosis is not detectable – multiple lesions are going to develop, so challenging the "current dogma," according to which the non-tumoral liver surrounding adenomas is really normal; (b) as "inflammation-related adenomas too suggest, analogously to malignant HCC-which usually develop from chronically inflamed cirrhotic livers-also benign adenomas frequently have a local or systemic "inflammatory" environment.
3. Tumors occur because of the cooperation between inherited and environmental factors. In rare genetic diseases (which account for less than 10–15 % of all liver tumors), the germline predisposing mutation is usually unique and well defined. In the vast majority of sporadic tumors (i.e., those without any known risk factor or even those related with exposure to estrogen or drugs) without associated predisposing conditions, there is an oligogenic group of germline mutations which is responsible for "inherited predisposition" or "tumor susceptibility" [29]."

This model of "private genetic epidemiology" has been recently demonstrated as "proof of concept" in nonsmokers developing lung adenocarcinoma [29] and is likely to work in the great majority of the most frequent sporadic tumors, including liver tumors.

According to this model, in common sporadic cancers, each individual finds his/her own way to cancer that also depends on congenital predisposing factors, which vary from an individual to another. This concept could have important implications for the "personalized medicine" and could be used to reduce the burden of expectations from genome-wide association studies (GWAS) aimed at detecting single predisposing locus. As there is no major common susceptibility locus, but many and different loci among individuals, it is not possible to identify them by population-based GWAS.

References

1. Shaked O, Siegelman ES, Olthoff K, Reddy KR (2011) Biologic and clinical features of benign solid and cystic lesions of the liver. Clin Gastroenterol Hepatol 9:547–562
2. Nault J-C, Bioulac-Sage P, Zucmann-Rossi J (2013) Hepatocellular benign tumors- from molecular classification to personalized clinical care. Gastroenterology 144:888–902
3. Bioulac-Sage P, Cubel G, Balabaud C et al (2011) Revisiting the pathology of resected benign hepatocellular nodules using new immunohistochemical markers. Semin Liver Dis 31:91–103
4. Bioulac-Sage P, Rebouissou S, Sa Cunha A et al (2005) Clinical, morphologic, and molecular features defining so-called telangiectatic focal nodular hyperplasias of the liver. Gastroenterology 128:1211–1218
5. Bioulac-Sage P, Blanc JF, Rebouissou S et al (2007) Genotype phenotype classification of hepatocellular adenoma. World J Gastroenterol 13:2649–2654
6. Zucman-Rossi J, Jeannot E, Nhieu JTV et al (2006) Genotype-phenotype correlation in hepatocellular adenoma: new classification and relationship with HCC. Hepatology 43:515–524
7. Bioulac-Sage P, Laumonier H, Couchy G et al (2009) Hepatocellular adenoma management and phenotypic classification: the Bordeaux experience. Hepatology 50:481–489
8. Bioulac-Sage P, Rebouissou S, Thomas C et al (2007) Hepatocellular adenoma subtype classification using molecular markers and immunohistochemistry. Hepatology 46:740–748
9. Benhamouche S, Decaens T, Godard C et al (2006) Apc tumor suppressor gene is the "zonation-keeper" of mouse liver. Dev Cell 10:759–770
10. Reznik Y, Dao T, Coutant R et al (2004) Hepatocyte nuclear factor- 1 alpha gene inactivation: co-segregation between liver adenomatosis and diabetes phenotypes in two maturity-onset diabetes of the young (MODY) 3 families. J Clin Endocrinol Metab 89:1476–1480
11. Bunchorntavakul C, Bahirwani R, Drazek D et al (2011) Clinical features and natural history of hepatocellular adenomas: the impact of obesity. Aliment Pharmacol Ther 34:664–674
12. Bioulac-Sage P, Taouji S, Possenti L et al (2012) Hepatocellular adenomas subtypes. The impact of overweight and obesity. Liver Int 32:1217–1221
13. Watkins J, Balabaud C, Bioulac-Sage P et al (2009) Hepatocellular adenoma in advanced-stage fatty liver disease. Eur J Gastroenterol Hepatol 21:932–936
14. Lerut JP, Ciccarelli O, Sempoux C et al (2003) Glycogenosis storage type I diseases and evolutive adenomatosis: an indication for liver transplantation. Transpl Int 16:879–884
15. Calderaro J, Labrune P, Morcrette G et al (2013) Molecular characterization of hepatocellular adenomas developed in patients with glycogen storage disease type I. J Hepatol 58:350–357
16. Mutel E, Abdul-Wahed A, Ramamonjisoa N et al (2011) Targeted deletion of liver glucose-6 phosphatase mimics glycogen storage disease type 1a including development of multiple adenomas. J Hepatol 54:529–537
17. Jeannot E, Poussin K, Chiche L et al (2007) Association of CYP1B1 germ line mutations with hepatocyte nuclear factor 1 alpha mutated hepatocellular adenoma. Cancer Res 67:2611–2616
18. Vilgrain V, Fléjou JF, Arrivé L et al (1992) Focal nodular hyperplasia of the liver: MR imaging and pathologic correlation in 37 patients. Radiology 184:699–703
19. Paradis V, Laurent A, Flejou JF et al (1997) Evidence for the polyclonal nature of focal nodular hyperplasia of the liver by the study of X-chromosome inactivation. Hepatology 26:891–895
20. Paradis V, Bièche I, Dargère D et al (2003) A quantitative gene expression study suggests a role for angiopoietins in focal nodular hyperplasia. Gastroenterology 124:651–659
21. Rebouissou S, Bioulac-Sage P, Zucman-Rossi J (2008) Molecular pathogenesis of focal nodular hyperplasia and hepatocellular adenoma. J Hepatol 48:163–170
22. Bioulac-Sage P, Laumonier H, Rullier A et al (2009) Over-expression of glutamine synthetase in focal nodular hyperplasia: a novel easy diagnostic tool in surgical pathology. Liver Int 29:459–465

23. Chen Y-W, Jeng Y-M, Yeh S-H, Chen P-J (2002) P53 gene and Wnt signaling in benign neoplasms: beta-catenin mutations in hepatic adenoma but not in focal nodular hyperplasia. Hepatology 36:927–935
24. Rebouissou S, Couchy G, Libbrecht L et al (2008) The beta-catenin pathway is activated in focal nodular hyperplasia but not in cirrhotic FNH-like nodules. J Hepatol 49:61–71
25. Gaffey MJ, Iezzoni JC, Weiss LM (1996) Clonal analysis of focal nodular hyperplasia of the liver. Am J Pathol 148:1089–1096
26. Cai Y-R, Gong L, Teng X-Y et al (2009) Clonality and allelotype analyses of focal nodular hyperplasia compared with hepatocellular adenoma and carcinoma. World J Gastroenterol 15:4695–4708
27. Turowski C, Feist H, Alzen G et al (2009) Conversion of a neonatal hepatic hemangioma to focal nodular hyperplasia. Pathol Int 59:251–254
28. Scoazec JY, Flejou JF, D'Errico A et al (1995) Focal nodular hyperplasia of the liver: composition of the extracellular matrix and expression of cell-cell and cell-matrix adhesion molecules. Hum Pathol 26:1114–1125
29. Renieri A, Mencarelli MA, Cetta F et al (2014) Oligogenic germline mutations identified in early non-smokers lung adenocarcinoma patients. Lung Cancer 85:168–174

Genetic Syndromes and Benign Liver Tumors

3

Francesco Cetta, Giuseppe Fusai, and Massimo Malagò

A wide range of inherited syndromes or diseases related with congenital genetic alterations include liver tumors as a part of the syndrome [1–10].

Deficit of alpha 1 antitrypsin has been typically related to the occurrence of hepatocellular carcinoma (HCC), during early life, requiring liver transplantation. However, since A1AT is so closely associated with HCC, it will not be included in the present chapter, dealing specifically with benign liver tumors, even if genetic diseases due to a single gene alteration, determining a single enzymatic protein malfunction, which is subsequently responsible for hepatocellular carcinoma, could be one of the few examples of tumors that could be cured or prevented by genetic engineering. In fact, the possibility of substituting the mutated gene with its wild-type variant could represent a veritable example of HCC cured or prevented by genetic engineering.

One of the most important genetic syndromes associated with benign liver tumors is glycogen storage disease (GSD) [1–3]. Genetic GSD is caused by any inborn error of metabolism (genetically defective enzymes) involved in these processes. In the USA is it is estimated to occur in 1 per 20–25,000 births. GSD is an inherited autosomal recessive disorder characterized by intracellular accumulation of glycogen. There are 11 distinct diseases that are commonly considered to be GSD [1–3].

F. Cetta (✉)
IRCCS MultiMedica, Milan, Italy
e-mail: cetta_francesco@libero.it

G. Fusai • M. Malagò
HPB Surgery and Liver Transplant Unit, Royal Free Hospital, University College of London, London, UK

L. Aldrighetti et al. (eds.), *Benign Tumors of the Liver*,
DOI 10.1007/978-3-319-12985-3_3

Type I GSD is the most common form and results from genetic mutations determining deficits in the glucose-6-phosphatase system. On the other hand, type III GSD is due to a defective glycogen debranching enzyme. Both diseases determine glycogenolysis alterations with increased glycogen accumulations in various districts, namely, in the liver and in the kidney [1, 2].

Epidemiologic studies showed that 22–75 % of patients with type I GSD develop hepatic adenomas, which are usually diagnosed by the second decade of life. On the contrary, the prevalence of hepatic adenomas is lower in type III GSD, where only 4.4–25 % of affected siblings develop HA. The estimated risk of malignant transformation of hepatic adenomas related with type I GSD is as high as 10 %, whereas the risk for malignant transformation is much lower in patients with type II GSD. In fact, only six patients have been reported up to now in the literature.

All these findings suggest that increased glycogen storage in the liver seems to induce hepatic tumorigenesis, likely altering glucose metabolism and glycogen synthesis. However, there is no detailed pathophysiological hypothesis concerning liver tumorigenesis from "metabolic alterations."

Other hereditary diseases, acting as risk factors associated, namely, with hepatic adenomas [5–8] include: (1) galactosemia, (2) hepatic iron overload related to beta thalassemia, and (3) maturity-onset diabetes of the young type 3 (MODY3) [4].

Galactosemia is a rare autosomal recessive metabolic disorder, occurring in about 1 per 60.00 births. In individual with galactosemia, the enzymes needed for further metabolism of galactose are severely diminished or missed entirely, leading to toxic levels of galactose 1-phosphate in the various tissues, resulting in hepatomegaly and subsequent cirrhosis but also in an increased occurrence of benign liver tumors. Gene responsible for galactosemia include GALT, GALK1, and GALE, which are responsible for galactosemia type 1, 2, and 3, respectively.

Thalassemia is caused by variant or missing genes that affect hemoglobin synthesis. They include different variants considered as autosomal recessive blood disorders. People with thalassemia have microcytic anemia and develop significant complications, including iron overload, bone deformities, and cardiovascular diseases. Since it confers a degree of protection against malaria (selective survival advantage of heterozygous carriers), it is more frequent in the Mediterranean region where malaria was endemic. Iron overload determines the occurrence of liver alterations, also including hepatic adenomas.

MODY3 is determined by heterozygous germline mutations of the HNF1 alpha gene that is mapped at chromosome 12q24.2. This gene encodes for the hepatocyte nuclear factor 1 (HNF1) alpha, a 681 AA homeodomain transcription factor that is involved in hepatocyte differentiation. HNF1 alpha controls the expression of some liver-specific genes, such as beta fibrinogen, alpha 1 antitrypsin, and albumin. It has currently been considered as a tumor suppressor gene involved in liver tumorigenesis. In particular, biallelic inactivating mutations of HNF1 alpha have been reported in 35–40 % of HA. HNF1alpha mutations occurring in sporadic HAs are somatic in 90 % of cases. However, when occurring in patients with MODY3, they are related to the germline gene variant determining the disease [4].

Another type of genetic alteration that is strictly related with liver tumorigenesis, frequently determining the occurrence of benign hepatic tumors, is the complex termed "vascular alterations." In addition to be responsible for the two most frequent benign liver tumors, i.e., hemangiomas and focal nodular hyperplasia (FNH), vascular alterations are integral to some genetic syndromes, determining congenital vascular malformations, also showing peculiar liver tumors or alterations.

Congenital vascular malformations associated with benign liver tumors include:

1. Portal vein agenesis and/or extrahepatic congenital portosystemic shunts (Abernethy syndrome) [9]. It is a very rare congenital condition. The term "syndrome" means that there is a wide range of possible malformations, including partial or complete agenesis of the portal vein, associated with a different flow from the splanchnic district to the vena cava. In particular, the flow from splanchnic viscera usually bypasses the liver and drains directly into the inferior vena cava, left renal vein, iliac veins, or right atrium. This alteration is frequently associated with live tumors (up to 40 % of patients), including focal nodular hyperplasia, liver adenoma, and hepatocellular carcinoma. These lesions may coexist together in the same subject.

   It has been hypothesized that alterations of the liver vascular perfusion can be responsible for the occurrence of all types of lesions, making the Abernethy syndrome an intriguing model for "alternative" liver tumorigenesis. In these patients, who may require surgery during childhood or the second decade of life, liver transplantation has been suggested.
2. Hereditary hemorrhagic telangiectasia (HHT) (Rendu–Osler–Weber disease). Kasabach–Merritt syndrome, ataxia telangiectasia, and peliosis hepatis are other genetically determined vascular abnormalities, also involving the liver. HTT is an autosomal dominant genetic disorder characterized by widespread vascular malformations, including cutaneous, mucosal, and visceral telangiectasias that can involve the lung, brain, and liver. In patients with HHT, the liver shows increased hepatocellular regenerative activity. This could act as a potent stimulus for the development of FNH. In fact, in subjects affected by HHT, the prevalence of FNH is 100-fold greater than in the general population [10].

The putative role of vascular disturbances in the genesis of FNH is also supported by the observation of FNH-like lesions in patients with cirrhosis. In explanted livers of 130 cirrhotic patients, the presence of esophageal varices was significantly associated with the presence of FNH-like nodules, suggesting a contribution of portal hypertension to the formation of nodular hyperplastic lesions.

Recently, anecdotal evidence was published on the proposed sequence from hemangioma to FNH, probably starting with thrombosis of the hemangioma, followed by involution of the lesion and subsequent occurrence of a hyperplastic regenerative reaction. A child that was analyzed at the age of 6 months for a palpable hemangioma of the liver presented 5 years later with a lesion of unknown origin in the same topographic area of the organ. Surgical excision and pathologic examination revealed an FNH [11].

On the basis of these findings, therefore, the association between HHT and FNH further supports the vascular etiology not only of hemangiomas but also of FNH. The notion that FNH lesions develop secondary to vascular abnormalities is suggested by several observations. In some adults, the liver contains both hemangiomas and FNH. A study among 247 patients with hepatic masses identified 148 patients with FNH, of which 20 % had concomitant hemangiomas of the liver [12].

Benign liver tumors in patients with activating mutations of the beta-catenin gene or of the gp 130 gene. Beta-catenin-activating mutations have been identified in a number of HAs [5–8]. Beta-catenin mutations lead to an activation of the Wnt pathways, which plays a key role in liver development and physiology, involving functions such as lineage specification, differentiation, stem cell renewal, epithelial–mesenchymal transition, zonation, proliferation, cell adhesion, and liver regeneration. With mutation of the beta-catenin gene, there is an inappropriate upregulation of many of its targets, including glutamine synthetase (GS) and the G-protein-coupled receptor 49. This subsequent aberrant upregulation contributes to the development of cellular atypia and an increased risk of malignant transformation to HCC that is more frequent in this type of HA than other HA subtypes [5].

Beta-catenin mutations may determine similar effects as germline mutation of the APC gene, causing familial adenomatous polyposis (FAP) – an inherited multitumoral syndrome, responsible for the occurrence of hundreds to thousands of colonic polyps, evolving invariably toward colonic cancers, and of a wide range of other extracolonic manifestations, also including benign and malignant liver tumors. Beta-catenin and APC cooperate together in the Wnt pathway. Interestingly, patients with APC germline mutations do not have beta-catenin mutations, i.e., APC, and beta-catenin are mutually excluding of each other in disrupting the Wnt pathway. In addition, no HA cases with both beta-catenin-activating and HNF1 alpha biallelic inactivating mutations have been observed, suggesting that these two tumorigenic pathways are also mutually exclusive. Finally, it is of interest that beta-catenin mutations are also found in 20–34 % of patients with HCC [5–8].

Gene expression data reveal an activation of the beta-catenin pathway in FNH. Beta-catenin is regarded as a pivotal stimulus for the proliferation of hepatocytes and a master actor of liver development and liver regeneration after injury, as well as a master regulator of liver zonation. In FNH, beta-catenin shows a heterogeneous distribution along the hepatocellular nodules in the absence of inactivating mutations of the gene and in the absence of alterations in the Wnt signaling pathway [5].

In normal hepatocytes, beta-catenin and its known target genes, such as GS, are expressed exclusively in the immediate perivenous areas. This zonated defined pattern of expression differs from that observed in beta-catenin-activated HA or HCC, which usually shows more diffuse cytoplasmic GS staining and nuclear beta-catenin staining, in accordance with the monoclonal origin of the beta-catenin-activating mutations in these tumors. In FNH, beta-catenin activation shows a characteristic architectural distribution on relatively large areas, centered on visible veins. In contrast to activating mutations, hepatocytes in FNH remain sensitive to repression of the beta-catenin pathway in regions surrounding fibrosis [5–8].

In addition, it has been shown that some hepatocellular adenomas (HA) are associated with gain-of-function mutations caused by in-frame somatic deletions in the IL6 signal transduction gene that encodes for the signaling co-receptor gp 130 [5]. The recurrent gain of function gp 130 mutations fully explains activation of the acute inflammatory phase that has been observed in tumor hepatocytes. Interestingly, gp 130 and beta-catenin mutations may coexist in the same HA [5–8].

In addition to activating mutations in the interleukin-6 receptor gene, activating mutations have also been identified in the Janus kinase –signal transducer and activator of transcription (JAK-STAT) pathway. In particular, in "inflammatory" adenomas, which are related to activating mutations of these genes – also as an effect of a congenital alteration – and which make up to 50 % of all HA, there is also a characteristic high expression of C-reactive protein and the inflammatory serum amyloid-associated (SAA) protein. Androgen consumption is a well-known risk factor for HA, particularly the beta-catenin mutation-associated HA. HA have been reported in patients with Fanconi anemia, treated with androgen, but also, likely due to a similar mechanism – because of endogenous high levels of androgen – in inherited diseases or syndromes such as Klinefelter's syndrome (XXY) or congenital polycystic ovary syndrome [5].

Inherited multitumoral syndromes include benign liver tumors as a part of the syndrome. Liver is not the main target of any of the most frequent inherited multitumoral syndromes, due to germline mutations of tumor suppressor genes (RB, p53, Lynch syndrome, Cowden syndrome).

Anyway, liver involvement, as a peculiar target of the syndrome, even if not the main involved organ, has been observed in ataxia telangiectasia (AT) [13, 14], Beckwith and Wiedemann syndrome (BWS), and familial adenomatous polyposis (FAP) [15–24].

AT is characterized by ataxia (due to cerebellum impairment), telangiectasia (namely, in the sclera), chronic lung diseases, and immune system alterations, including an increased incidence of leukemia and lymphomas, but also of primary cancers in various sites, also including malignant and benign tumors of the liver [13, 14]. Interestingly, AT patients frequently show increased levels of alpha fetoprotein. AT is a rare autosomal recessive disease, caused by mutations of the ATM gene, located at 11q22.3. Its incidence ranges between 1 per 40,000 and 1 per 100,000. Carriers of AT, i.e., the parents of an AT-affected individual, have an increased risk of breast cancer [13]. AT is considered as a "genome instability syndrome." The gene ATM encodes for a protein which coordinates the cellular response to DNA double-strand breaks, cooperating with other genes responsible for mismatch repair genes (such as those responsible for Lynch syndrome or Werner syndrome.)

BWS is an overgrowth disorder usually present at birth and characterized by abdominal wall defect and exomphalos, macrosomia, macroglossia, gigantism, and neonatal hypoglycemia and hemihypertrophy, as well as genitourinary or cardiac anomalies [25, 26]. BWS has an estimated incidence of 1 in 13,700 and is increased among children conceived through in vitro fertilization. BWS has been related with the locus 11p15 that leads to overactivity of the IGF2 gene (growth factor) and no active copy of CDKN1C (inhibitor of cell proliferation). Over five distinct errors have been identified, including IGF-2, CDKN1C, H19, and KCNQ1OT1. Children with BWS have a 600-fold greater risk to develop childhood cancers, such as Wilms' tumor, pancreatoblastoma, and hepatoblastoma, and less frequently adrenal cortical carcinoma, neuroblastoma, and rhabdomyosarcoma. In addition to hepatomegaly and hepatoblastoma, children with BWS may also develop adenomas and other benign liver tumors [25, 26].

FAP actually includes two different subtypes determined by two genes: APC, responsible for 85 % of cases, and MUTYH, responsible for the remaining 15 %.

APC is a tumor suppressor gene, mapped at chromosome 5q21, which is responsible for the production of the APC protein that plays a key role in the Wnt pathway. APC is a large multifunction tumor suppressing protein which acts as a "gatekeeper" to prevent development of tumors. APC regulates beta-catenin, a protein that plays a crucial role in cell communication, signaling, growth, and apoptosis. The APC protein is present both in the cell nucleus and in the membrane. The canonical tumor suppressor function of APC is suppression of beta-catenin (a protein that also plays a crucial role in liver regeneration), but other tumor suppressor functions of APC may be related to cell adherence and cytoskeleton organization [15–22].

Germline mutations of APC determine the occurrence of FAP, which is an autosomal dominant disease, occurring in 1 per 10,000 births. It is characterized by hundreds to thousands of colonic polyps, evolving invariably into colonic cancer before age 50. Germline mutations of the APC gene determine two different types of FAP, the diffuse and the sparse phenotype, on the basis of the number of colonic polyps. Genotype–phenotype correlation studies have shown that some clinical manifestations are strictly related to the site of the APC germline mutation. In particular, the "diffuse polyposis variant" is associated with mutations 5′ to codon 1,440, whereas the "sparse variant" more frequently occurs in patients with APC mutations 3′ to 1,440 [15–22].

A third type of FAP is determined by another gene MUTYH, which encodes the DNA repair enzyme MYH glycosylase. Mutations in the MUTYH gene are inherited in an autosomal recessive pattern.

In addition to colonic polyps and cancers, patients with FAP may develop a wide range of tumoral and non-tumoral extracolonic manifestations, including retinal pigment epithelium hypertrophy, sebaceous cysts or dental abnormalities, osteomas, as well as benign and malignant brain tumors, gastric and duodenal polyps and cancers, pancreatic and periampullary tumors, and thyroid tumors. Interestingly, patients with FAP and APC germline mutations also develop a wide range of liver tumors [15–17].

In particular, original research from our group showed that genotype–phenotype correlations are not restricted to the number of colonic polyps but also involve the variable risk of occurrence of extracolonic tumors [17–24].

In fact, it has been suggested that desmoids are more frequent in patients with APC mutations beyond codon 144, even if somatic mutations often occur at a codon different from that involved by the germline mutation. On the contrary, papillary thyroid carcinoma (PTC) is restricted to patients with mutations in exon 15 and 5′ to codon 1,220 (in 14 of 16 cases, with the remaining 2 having mutations at codon 1,309) and the female gender (F:M ratio =80:1 vs. F:M ratio 2.5–3:1 in sporadic tumors) [19, 20], suggesting the required involvement of gender-related factors for PTC occurrence.

Interestingly, PTC co-segregates with congenital hypertrophy of the retinal pigment epithelium (CHRPE) and with hepatoblastoma (HB) and a wide range of other benign and malignant liver tumors [21–24]. In particular, HB (as well as other liver tumors) mainly occurs in patients with mutations in exon 15 (mainly at codon 1,061) but has also been observed in patients with mutations in the 5′ portion of the APC gene, such as mutations at codons 141, 215, 302, and 541, respectively [21–24].

In addition, FAP-associated PTC and HB usually, but not always, show nuclear and cytoplasmic expression of beta-catenin (maybe because of the Wnt pathway disruption due to APC germline mutation), and this feature is mutually exclusive with the BRAF mutation in thyroid tumors and CTNNB1 (gene coding for beta-catenin) mutation in liver tumors, respectively [20–24].

It is likely that FAP-associated thyroid tumors and liver tumors represent a veritable example of cooperation between purely inherited factors (APC germline mutations) and epigenetic or environmental factors, namely, factors strictly related to the female sex, analogously to what occurs in hepatic adenomas, in which inherited mutations also have been found [20–24].

In FAP patients, hepatoblastoma usually occurs before age 4 (with an 800-fold increased risk) [15, 16]. However, also hepatic adenomas (HA) and FNH have been reported. In anecdotal cases the concomitant presence of hepatocellular and cholangiocellular tumors has been reported in the same patient [21–24]. We have recently reported a girl, with a germline mutation of the APC gene at codon 1,061, who was diagnosed with hepatoblastoma before age 3, had right hepatectomy at age 5, and subsequently developed typical HCC in the liver remnant at age 14 [23, 24].

Conclusion

Genetic alterations and inherited syndromes are rare disease, affecting a small proportion of the population. However, since they have a well-defined causative mechanism, they could be useful for a deeper insight into the pathophysiologic mechanisms and pathways which are responsible for benign and malignant liver tumors and also give a clue for a better knowledge of the pathogenesis of some types of the most frequent sporadic tumors.

The most frequent risk factors determining liver alterations and cancers are viral infections (HBV, HCV), alcohol abuse, or exposure to xenobiotics (aflatoxin, drugs, hormones). Only a minority of liver tumors have genetic mutations and inherited alterations as the main causative factors. In the present overview, we have shown that there are 3–6 main types of genetic alterations facilitating the occurrence of benign (and also malignant) liver tumors. They include: (1) metabolic disorders, in particular those affecting glucose metabolism (HNF1 alpha mutations, MODY3 diabetes) and glycogen storage (glycogenosis); (2) genes involving vascular alterations, telangiectasia, etc.; (3) genes involving chronic inflammation; (4) a wide range of genes, including growth factors such as IGF-2 (BWS) and oncogenes (beta-catenin, which also plays a pivotal role specifically in liver regeneration); (5) tumor suppressor genes, such as APC, which is responsible for FAP and controls beta-catenin function in the Wnt pathway, and ATM, which act as a tumor suppressor but is frequently associated with increased levels of alpha fetoprotein; and (6) mismatch "repair genes" (Lynch syndrome) or other genes involved in the DNA repair (MUTYH, ATM). Germline mutations of these DNA repair genes facilitate the occurrence of "early aging" syndromes also including benign and malignant tumors in a wide range of tissues.

The liver is a complex organ with complex and integrated functions, requiring various types of specialized cells. This complexity mirrors the wide variety of benign liver tumors and also the variety and complexity of genetic alterations that can be involved in their development.

References

1. Lee PJ (2002) Glycogen storage disease type I. Eur J Pediatr 161(Suppl 1):S46–S49
2. Labrune P, Trioche P (1997) Hepatocellular adenomas in glycogen storage disease type I and III. J Pediatr Gastroenterol Nutr 24:276–279
3. Demo E et al (2007) Glycogen storage disease III HCC. J Hepatol 46:492–498
4. Reznik Y, Dao T, Coutant R et al (2004) Hepatocyte nuclear factor- 1 alpha gene inactivation: co-segregation between liver adenomatosis and diabetes phenotypes in two maturity-onset diabetes of the young (MODY) 3 families. J Clin Endocrinol Metab 89:1476–1480
5. Nault J-C, Bioulac-Sage P, Zucman-Rossi J (2013) Hepatocellular benign tumors – from molecular classification to personalized clinical care. Gastroenterology 144:888–892
6. Bioulac-Sage P et al (2007) Hepatocellular adenoma subtype classification using molecular markers and immunohistochemistry. Hepatology 46:740–748
7. Rebouissou S, Bioulac-Sage P, Zucman-Rossi J (2008) Molecular pathogenesis of focal nodular hyperplasia and hepatocellular adenoma. J Hepatol 48:163–170
8. Rebouissou S et al (2007) Frequent in –frame somatic deletions activate gp 130 in inflammatory hepatocellular tumours. Nature 457:140–146
9. Murray CP, Yoo SJ, Babyn PS (2003) Congenital extrahepatic portosystemic shunts. Pediatr Radiol 33:614–620
10. Buscarini E, Danesino C, Plauchu H, de Fazio C, Olivieri C, Brambilla G et al (2004) High prevalence of hepatic focal nodular hyperplasia in subjects with hereditary hemorrhagic telangiectasia. Ultrasound Med Biol 30:1089–1097
11. Turowski C, Feist H, Alzen G et al (2009) Conversion of neonatal hepatic hemangioma to focal nodular hyperplasia. Pathol Int 59:251–254
12. Vilgrain V, Flejou JF, Arriv L et al (1992) Focal nodular hyperplasia of the liver: MR imaging and pathologic correlations in 37 patients. Radiology 184:699–703
13. Reiman A, Srinivasan V, Barone G et al (2011) Lymphoid tumours and breast cancer in ataxia telangiectasia; substantial protective effect of residual ATM kinase activity against childhood tumours. Br J Cancer 105:586–591
14. Thompson D, Duedal S, Kirner J et al (2000) Cancer risks and mortality in heterozygous ATM mutation carriers. J Natl Cancer Inst 97:813–822

15. Giardiello F, Petersen G, Bresinger J et al (1996) Hepatoblastoma and APC gene mutation in familial adenomatous polyposis. Gut 39:867–869
16. Hirschman BA, Pollock BH, Tomlison GE (2005) The spectrum of APC mutations in children with hepatoblastoma from familial adenomatous polyposis kindreds. J Pediatr 147:263–266
17. Cetta F, Dhamo A, Civitelli S et al (2008) Extraintestinal manifestations of familial adenomatous polyposis. Ann Surg Oncol 15:1446–1448
18. Cetta F, Gori M, Baldi C et al (1999) The relationships between phenotypic expression in patients with familial adenomatous polyposis (FAP) and the site of mutations in the adenomatous polyposis coli(APC) gene. Ann Surg 229:445–446
19. Cetta F, Montalto G, Gori M et al (2000) Germline mutations of the APC gene in patients with familial adenomatous polyposis –associated thyroid carcinoma: results from a European operative study. J Clin Endocrinol Metab 85:286–292
20. Cetta F, Ugolini G, Martellucci J, Gotti G (2015) Screening for thyroid cancer in patients with familial adenomatous polyposis. Ann Surg 261(1):e13–e14
21. Cetta F, Cetta D, Petracci M et al (1997) Childhood hepatocellular tumors in FAP. Gastroenterology 113:1051–1052
22. Cetta F, Montalto G, Petracci M (1997) Hepatoblastoma and APC gene mutation in familial adenomatous polyposis. Gut 41:417
23. Montalto G, Cetta F, Baldi C et al (2000) A wide range of primary liver tumors can be found in patients with familial adenomatous polyposis. J Pediatr Hematol Oncol 22:90–91
24. Cetta F, Mazzarella L, Bon G et al (2003) Genetic alterations in hepatoblastoma and hepatocellular carcinoma associated with familial adenomatous polyposis. Med Pediatr Oncol 41:496–497
25. De Baun MR, Tucker MA (1998) Risk of cancer during the first four years of life in children from the Beckwith –Wiedemann Syndrome Registry. J Pediatr 132:398–400
26. Elliott M, Bayly R, Cole T, Temple IK, Maher ER (1994) Clinical features and natural history of Beckwith-Wiedemann syndrome: presentation of 74 new cases. Clin Genet 46:168–184

Liver Pathophysiology: Liver Regeneration, Vascular Alterations, and Ischemia/Reperfusion

4

Francesco Cetta, Giuseppe Fusai, and Massimo Malagò

The liver is the only solid organ that has a tremendous capacity for restoration of tissue loss by regeneration. Liver regeneration is a highly controlled process and stops once the volume of the lost tissue is restored [1–11].

Also, the liver is unique in a sense that it is the only organ that receives dual blood supply from two different sources, one of which is portal circulation. It has been assumed that liver functions, including the regenerative capacity, are remotely controlled by the splanchnic organs, including intestine and intestinal microbiota, pancreas, and also the spleen [1–6].

Surgical resection of hepatic lobes or hepatocyte loss caused by viral or chemical injury triggers hepatocyte replication, while enlarged liver mass is corrected by apoptosis. Hepatocytes have a great replicative capacity and are capable of repopulating the liver. However, "stem-like" cells proliferate when hepatocyte replication is blocked or delayed [1–3].

Detailed studies of the mechanisms that regulate liver growth have been done in animals subjected to partial hepatectomy or chemical injury. Substantial progress have been achieved by (1) using appropriate transgenic and knockout mouse models and (2) studying liver vascularization and experimental changes such as those induced by portal vein embolization, portal vein ligation [6–8], or, more recently, by the use of the ALPPS procedure [12, 13].

The liver receives its dual blood supply from the portal vein and the hepatic artery. The normal liver receives approximately 80 % of its blood from the portal vein and 20 % from the hepatic artery. Blood flow from the two vessels follows a

F. Cetta (✉)
IRCCS MultiMedica, Milan, Italy
e-mail: cetta_francesco@libero.it

G. Fusai • M. Malagò
HPB Surgery and Liver Transplant Unit, Royal Free Hospital, University College of London, London, UK

L. Aldrighetti et al. (eds.), *Benign Tumors of the Liver*,
DOI 10.1007/978-3-319-12985-3_4

different pattern intrahepatically but drains into a terminal hepatic venule as the common drainage vessel [6].

A decrease in portal venous flow is compensated for by an increase in hepatic arterial flow. Although the underlying physiopathology is still unclear, adenosine, a vasodilator agent, has been suggested as a contributing factor. In normal portal venous flow, adenosine accumulates in the space of Mall but is constantly being washed away by the portal venous flow [9, 10].

When the portal blood flow is severely reduced, such as following portal vein embolization (PVE), less adenosine is washed into the portal blood and adenosine accumulates. Induced adenosine concentrations cause dilatation of the hepatic artery and increase hepatic arterial flow [6, 9, 10].

A dramatic change in hepatic blood flow, in particular from the portal vein, induces a rapid change in liver volume. This feature is observed either after PVE or partial hepatectomy (PH). Because hepatic arterial flow is preserved in the non-embolized lobe, hepatic hemodynamics following PVE slightly differ from those following PH. Hepatic arterial flow in the non-embolized lobe increases immediately secondary to intrinsic blood flow regulation by the liver, the so-called hepatic arterial buffer response (HABR) [6, 9, 10]. This may preserve hepatic viability, and marked atrophy of the embolized lobe occurs due to a reduction in total blood flow. On the contrary, portal venous flow to the non-embolized lobe increases because venous return from the splanchnic system is unchanged. The overall effect is to induce marked hypertrophy of the non-embolized lobe [6, 9, 10].

Experimental studies using rats have shown that after complete ligation of the left portal vein, left hepatic arterial flow increases by 210 %, whereas right hepatic arterial flow decreases by 67 %. Overall, total left hepatic flow decreases by 45 %, whereas total right hepatic flow increases by 230 % [11]. This finding suggests that attenuation of the increased hepatic arterial flow to the embolized lobe further decreases blood flow and enhances the effect of PVE. Nagino et al. reported the effect of dual embolization (PVE followed by arterial embolization) to enhance hepatic regeneration when insufficient hypertrophy was achieved by PVE alone. This procedure is a veritable "in situ partial hepatectomy" and carries the risk of massive necrosis in the embolized lobe [8].

Recently developed ALPPS (associating liver partition and portal vein ligature for staged hepatectomy) induces faster hypertrophy of the future liver remnant (FLR) compared to both the conventional two-stage hepatectomy and portal vein ligature or embolization [12, 13].

In addition to hemodynamic changes, upregulation of various humoral mediators and subsequent activation of intrahepatocyte signal transduction occur in the process of liver regeneration.

In brief, stimulation by PH or PVE increases circulating interleukin-6 (IL6) and tumor necrosis factor alpha (TNF-alpha). These pro-inflammatory cytokines prepare hepatocyte for growth [2, 14–18].

Further stimulation by various growth factors, such as hepatocyte growth factor (HGF), transforming growth factor alpha (TGF-alpha), and epidermal growth factor (EGF), stimulates DNA synthesis through the activation of transcriptional factors (nuclear factor kappa B (NFkB), activator protein-1 (AP-1), CCAAT enhancer-binding protein beta (C/EBP-beta)) and signal transducers and activators of transcription 3 (STAT3) [2, 6, 14–18].

Gene expression in the regenerating liver can be divided into several phases, starting with the expression of a large number of immediate early genes [2, 14–18].

The first phase of gene expression after PH, referred as "the immediate early phase," occurs very rapidly after the operation and lasts for approximately 4 h. The proto-oncogenes c-fos, c-jun, and c-myc were the first genes to be identified in this group. Subsequently, it was shown that as many as 70 genes participate in the immediate early response to PH. These genes do not share a common function and include, among others, transcription factors, tyrosine phosphatases, as well as secreted and intracellular metabolic proteins. Surprisingly, although the mitogen-activated protein (MAP) kinases ERK1 and 2 increase in activity after PH, their elevation is relatively modest compared to that of JNK. JNK is likely to play an important role in liver regeneration through the phosphorylation of c-jun, a gene that is required for hepatic development. JNK and p38 activation after partial hepatectomy may be components of a "stress" response, but it is not known to what extent such response is required for hepatocyte replication.

After PH there is activation of transcription factors. They are proteins which bind specific recognition sites in genes to initiate or enhance their transactivation. A transcription factor can bind and activate multiple target genes. Conversely, single genes bind multiple transcription factors. Thus, transcription factors can propagate signals by activating many different genes.

After PH the following transcription factors, NFkB, AP-1 C/EBP-beta, and STAT 3, have been found activated. In particular, NFkB is a transcription factor that transactivates genes involved in (1) inflammation, (2) cell adhesion, (3) proliferation, and (4) apoptosis.

TNF through the production of reactive oxygen species (ROS) at the mitochondrial level is a potent activator of NFkB in the liver. The critical step of NFkB activation is the removal of the inhibitor IkB from the NFkB heterodimer formed by the p65 and p 50 subunits. The IKK complex phosphorylates IkB and initiates its degradation. NFkB heterodimer, free of the inhibitor, migrates to the nucleus and binds to genes containing the NFkB recognition sequences.

The second phase of gene expression after PH is referred to as "delayed early gene response."

Bcl-Xl is an interesting example of these genes. It is the main antiapoptotic gene expressed in the liver (bcl2 is expressed only in biliary cells), and its mRNA increases after PA, reaching a maximum at 8 h after PH. One possibility is that Bcl-X1 functions as an antioxidant to prevent damage from reactive oxygen species (ROS) generated by mitochondria [1, 2]. Cell cycle genes are activated between 8 and 20 h after PH. They include p53, mdm2, p21, cyclins, and cyclin-dependent kinases. The induction of cyclin D1 is the most reliable marker for cell cycle (G1 phase) progression in hepatocytes. Overexpression of cyclin D1 in primary hepatocytes causes DNA replication even in the absence of growth factors. Therefore, hepatocytes that express CD1/cdk4 have passed the G1 restriction point and enter the G1/S transition [1, 2].

However, in liver regeneration after PH, not only stimulators but also repressors are activated. Examples of cell cycle repressor activation after PH include TGF-beta, activin, p21, and p53 [6, 18–20]. TGF-beta 1 is a multifunctional cytokine that works as both proponent and inhibitor of cell proliferation depending on the cell type, differentiation status, and milieu in which the cell works [20]. It is considered as one of the most potent growth inhibitors for hepatocytes in vitro but exerts a pivotal role during liver regeneration [2, 20]. The liver is housed by different categories of cells of hepatic, biliary, and mesenchymal origin. During liver regeneration, all of these cells restore the liver volume through a concerted action in which TGF-beta 1 seems to produce the platform for the newly divided hepatocytes by cementing them to the reconstructed extracellular matrix, thus inhibiting further growth of the hepatocytes beyond necessity. In summary, it seems that TGF-beta 1 is a negative regulator of hepatocytes proliferation and in this way restricts the volume of the liver [20].

Interestingly, after extreme hepatectomy (such as that removing up to 90 % of liver parenchyma, using the ALPPS technique), even if an adequate liver volume can be achieved in short time, in particular in old subjects with a liver remnant also altered by previous chemotherapy, patients show variable features of nodular regenerative hyperplasia [21, 22] (NRH)-like alterations, with cell plates that are markedly thickened, up to 4–5 cell thick, without concomitant vascular regeneration and collagen deposition, responsible for impaired liver function. Therefore, the normal architecture of the liver has less or no chance to be reproduced in the regenerative effort, thus impairing patient recovery during the delicate early phases of liver regeneration. It can be hypothesized that in this case, an imbalance in the proper function of TGF-beta 1 could play a role [20].

In addition to TGF-beta, glucagons and glucocorticoid also play a role as inhibitory factors in liver regeneration. On the contrary, eicosanoids, nitric oxide, prostaglandin E2 (PGE2), insulin, and estrogen have all shown to facilitate hepatic regeneration [6].

Anyway, it is the dual activation of stimulators and repressors that makes liver regeneration a precisely regulated process that never goes beyond its predicted end point. In other words, it is the equilibrium between stimulators and inhibitors expressed after PH that may explain why liver regeneration is a tightly regulated growth process [2]. However, hepatocytes need to be "primed" before they can fully respond to growth factors such as HGF, TGF-alpha, and EGF [2, 16]. Priming requires the cytokines TNF and IL-6 in addition to other agents that prevent cytotoxicity. ROS and glutathione content can determine whether the TNF effect on hepatocytes is proliferative or apoptotic.

According to Fausto [2], at least four transcription factors, NFkB, STAT3 (which are strongly induced by TNF), AP-1, and C/EBP-beta, play major roles in the initiation of liver regeneration. In addition, extensive remodeling of the hepatic extracellular matrix occurs shortly after PH. Progression through the cell cycle beyond the initiation phase requires growth factors. The expression of cyclin D1 probably establishes the stage at which replication becomes growth factor independent and autonomous [2].

Several conditions are known to suppress hepatic regeneration and cause clinical problems. Biliary obstruction, diabetes, chronic ethanol consumption, nutritional status, male gender, and infections all limit liver regeneration. Controlling these factors, whenever possible, is crucial to optimize liver hypertrophy [6].

Biliary obstruction decreases regenerative capacity both in PVE and PH. High total bilirubin concentration at the time of PVE reduces the extent of hypertrophy in the non-embolized lobe. Proposed mechanisms include: (1) restricted portal venous flow, (2) altered expression of regeneration-associated factors, and (3) impaired enterohepatic circulation. Biliary obstruction rapidly decreases portal venous flow. Portosystemic shunting is associated with acute cholestasis and may also decrease the portal venous flow velocity. Furthermore, chronic biliary obstruction induces hepatic fibrosis and increase total perfusion resistance in the portal venous system. Hepatic fibrosis is a crucial mechanism, occurring in the liver after chronic viral infection; exposure to drugs, toxicant, and xenobiotics; and chronic metabolic alterations, also including steatosis, nonalcoholic fatty liver disease (NAFLD), and steatohepatitis (NASH) associated with obesity and diabetes, and it plays a key role in most of pathophysiologic alterations leading to chronic liver disease, but also to benign and malignant liver tumors.

In addition to hemodynamic changes, cholestasis modulates molecular events, with suppression of c-myc and C/EBP-alpha and C/EBP-beta and altered production of HGF, EGF, and IL-6, so reducing the regenerative capacity. Biliary obstruction also impairs enterohepatic circulation. Lack of bile in the intestine not only has a negative effect on the enteric immune system, but also negatively affects the regenerative capacity [23–25]. Interestingly, external bile drainage for obstructive jaundice markedly suppresses liver regeneration after PH. Therefore, internal biliary drainage is preferable to external drainage in patients with biliary obstruction scheduled for PVE [23, 24].

Insulin and Diabetes Insulin is one of the most important hepatotrophic factors in portal venous blood. The binding protein of insulin-like growth factor (IGF), a molecule similar to insulin, also rises significantly after PH. Therefore, impaired secretion of insulin and IGF in diabetic patients prevents liver regeneration following PH. This is reflected by decreased synthesis of RNA, DNA, and protein on the first postoperative day [6].

It has been suggested that diabetes mellitus is a risk factor for reducing the magnitude of hypertrophy in the non-embolized lobe. Insulin gene transfer via the spleen enhances liver regeneration without causing liver damage and improves nutritional status after hepatectomy in diabetic rats.

Interestingly, dogs subjected to 70 % hepatectomy, combined with pancreatectomy, had delayed recovery of hepatic function and more limited regenerative capacity than dogs who underwent hepatectomy alone [26]. The reduction in liver regeneration was proportional to the extent of the pancreatectomy, and the reduction was more dramatic when more than 90 % of the pancreas was resected. These results demonstrate that the pancreas plays a crucial role in hepatic regeneration, at least partly through the release of insulin [27].

These observations are crucial for a better knowledge of the role of diabetes, obesity, alteration in the glucose or galactose metabolism or in glycogenosynthesis, or changes related with the occurrence of maturity-onset diabetes of the young type 3 (MODY 3). Mutations of the gene responsible for this inherited disease (hepatocyte nuclear factor 1 (HNF1)-alpha) are frequently associated with the development of hepatic adenomas and/or other benign tumors or liver alterations. Analogously, patients with Beckwith–Wiedemann syndrome, due to alterations of the locus 11p15, that leads to overactivity of the IGF2 gene, have hemihypertrophy, hepatomegaly, but benign and malignant tumors including hepatoblastoma (see also Chap. 3).

Ethanol markedly inhibits IL-6 induced STAT3 phosphorylation, one of the key signals in the regenerative process in isolated hepatocytes. Both acute and chronic ethanol exposure inhibit hepatocyte proliferation induced by insulin and EGF [6].

Hepatic regeneration is metabolically intensive and requires a large amount of energy. Malnutrition is associated with high postoperative mortality and reduced regeneration following PH. Supplementation of glutamine, one of the sources of DNA and protein synthesis, promotes liver regeneration. Essential fatty acids, components of the cell membrane, and precursors of several functional mediators also play a role in hepatic regeneration. Oral feeding also seems of importance. Rats given enteral nutrition showed much better weight gain after 70 % hepatectomy than those given isocaloric nutrition parenterally. This may be due to differences in portal venous flow with enteral and parenteral feeding. Liver regeneration after PH is not altered in patients with NASH or in a model of NASH induced by a methionine–choline-deficient diet. These results imply that "overnutrition," in contrast to malnutrition, has a minor effect on regenerative capacity [6, 28].

Sex hormones also modulate hepatic regeneration. Following 70 % hepatectomy, plasma estrogen concentrations increase, whereas testosterone concentrations decrease in male animals. Furthermore, translocations of estrogens and its receptor complex have been observed following hepatectomy. These findings suggest that women may have an advantage over men terms of regeneration after a major reduction in liver volume [29–31]. Imamura et al. reported that male gender is one of the negative factors in hepatic regeneration following PVE [32]. Shan et al. reported that hepatic regeneration after PH was greater in women than in men [33].

These gender-related differential behavior in regeneration after PH but also other types of stresses to the liver may also account for the increased incidence of some benign tumor (hemangiomas, HA, FNH), in the female gender both because of a specific activity of estrogens and female hormones and also because of different secretions not only of hormones, but also cytokines, adipokines, or fat tissue-related factors and/or other factors, which are related to the female gender and that could be differentially activated as a response to a whatever liver stress or injury.

Aging In livers of old animals, the proliferative response is attenuated via a mechanism mediated by c-myc promoter blocking [6].

Infection Concerning the role of infection on liver regeneration, evidence exists only in animal models, and further clinical studies are required. However, it seems that, whereas viral infections such as BBV, HCV, and cytomegalovirus inhibit hepatic regeneration (maybe via the inhibition of cell cycle-dependent molecules), bacteremia-induced inflammation prior to PH or lipopolysaccharide stimulation enhances liver regeneration, by inducing upregulation not only of pro-inflammatory cytokines, such as IL-6 and TNF-alpha, but also of HGF mRNA [6].

Ischemia/reperfusion and vascular alterations.

After intrahepatic vasculitis from certain drugs (azathioprine, thioguanine, antiretroviral agents, or oxaliplatin) or autoimmune diseases or postsinusoidal obstructive conditions such as congestive cardiomyopathy or Budd–Chiari syndrome, a condition termed nodular regenerative hyperplasia (NHR) [21, 22] may develop, which is characterized by a widespread benign transformation of the hepatic parenchyma into small regenerative nodules. Steiner [22] in 1959 first coined the term, emphasizing that hepatocyte hyperplasia or regeneration took place in the absence of fibrous tissue proliferation resulting in a nodular liver simulating cirrhosis.

NHR can develop in all age groups but more commonly affects older individual. NRH comprises 27 % of all cases of non-cirrhotic portal hypertension in Europe and about 14 % in Japan. Autopsy studies indicate an overall incidence, ranging between 0.72 and 2.6 %. However, the majority of patients with milder forms of NRH presumably remain unidentified. Terms such as "hepatocellular adenomatosis" or "adenomatous hyperplasia" have previously been used. Histopathologic examination demonstrates diffuse micronodular transformation.

A wide range of congenital or acquired vascular changes involving both splanchnic and systemic circulation may impact on liver microcirculation, determining local alterations [34] that, at variable extents, can be involved in the occurrence or progression of benign liver tumors, namely, hemangiomas or FNH. They include, among others: portal vein agenesis or Abernethy syndrome, hereditary hemorrhagic telangiectasia, Kasabach–Merritt syndrome, peliosis hepatis, and ataxia telangiectasia (see also Chap. 3).

Recently, anecdotal evidence has been published on the proposed sequence from hemangioma to FNH, probably starting with thrombosis of the hemangioma, followed by involution of the lesion and subsequent occurrence of a hyperplastic regenerative reaction [35].

Ischemia/reperfusion (I/R) injury is a pathophysiologic process whereby hypoxic organ damage is accentuated following return of blood flow and oxygen delivery [36, 37]. Transient episodes of ischemia are encountered during solid organ transplantation, trauma, hypovolemic shock, and elective liver resection, when inflow occlusion or total vascular exclusion is used to minimize blood loss.

I/R injury is the underlying cause of graft dysfunction in marginal organs that exhibit poor tolerance to I/R. Some of these include the use of organs from older donors and grafts such as small-for-size or steatotic livers. They have been increasingly used due to the persistent shortage of organs. The use of steatotic livers for transplantation is associated with an increased risk of primary nonfunction or dysfunction after surgery.

Animal models of cold (4 °C) and warm (37 °C) hepatic I/R have been used for a better knowledge of the pathophysiology of hepatic I/R injury. However, comparison of the results of animal studies and their extrapolation to human being is feasible but with crucial limitations, due to substantial differences in anatomic, pathologic, and experimental conditions.

The lack of oxygen in hepatocytes during ischemia causes ATP depletion and alterations in H+, Na+, and Ca2+ homeostasis that activate hydrolytic enzymes and impair cell volume regulation leading to the swelling of sinusoidal endothelial cells (SECs) and Kupffer cells (KCs). This fact, together with the imbalance between nitric oxide (NO) and endothelin production, contributes to the narrowing of the sinusoidal lumen and thus to microcirculatory dysfunction. Capillary narrowing also contributes to hepatic neutrophil accumulation. Concomitantly, the activation of KC releases reactive oxygen species (ROS) and pro-inflammatory cytokines, including tumor necrosis factor alpha (TNF-alpha) and interleukin-1 (IL1). Similar to their production in KCs, ROS can derive from mitochondria and the xanthine dehydrogenase/xanthine oxidase (XDH/XOD) pathway in activated SEC and hepatocytes. Cytokines release through the induction of adhesion molecules (intercellular cell adhesion molecule and vascular cell adhesion molecule) and chemokines promote neutrophil activation and accumulation, thereby contributing to the progression of parenchymal injury by releasing ROS and proteases. In addition, IL-1 and TNF-alpha recruit and activate CD4+ T lymphocytes, which produce granulocyte–macrophage colony-stimulating factor, interferon gamma, and TNF-beta. These cytokines amplify KC activation and TBF-alpha and IL-1 secretion and promote neutrophil recruitment and adherence into the liver sinusoids. Platelet-activating factor can prime neutrophils for superoxide generation, whereas leukotriene B4 contributes to the amplification of the neutrophil response [37].

The extent to which the initial cellular injury contributes to propagation of the inflammatory response and further tissue damage is not yet well elucidated. A key link between the initial damage to cells and the activation of inflammatory signaling involves endogenous danger signals from ischemic cells. In particular, high-mobility group box 1 (HMGB1) that is released from the necrotic cells has been suggested as a regulator for the inflammation that is seen following acute tissue damage. Some of the effects of HMGB1 result from its interaction with the individual members of the toll-like receptor (TLR) family TLR2 and TLR4. Interaction of HMGB1 with TLR4 provides a critical link between tissue damage and activation of the innate immune response [36].

Factors influencing I/R include: (a) duration of the hepatic ischemia, (b) the extent of hepatic ischemia, and (c) the type of liver. A long ischemic period is a predicting factor for future graft function. Liver grafts preserved for more than 10 h are at high risk. Cold ischemia for 24 h induces very low survival. The mechanisms of hepatic I/R injury are also different. For instance, concerning the importance of XDH /XOD versus mitochondria, XDH/XOD plays a crucial role in hepatic I/R injury only when significant conversion of XDH to XOD occurs (80–90 % of XOD), such as after 16 h of cold ischemia. However, this ROS generation system is not so crucial for shorter ischemic periods (<6 h). Thus, even after prolonged ischemia and high conversion of XDH to XOD, these enzymes may only play a minor role compared to mitochondria. Similarly, in assessing the relative contribution of intracellular vs. vascular oxidant stress to hepatic I/R injury, oxidative stress in hepatocytes and the stimulatory state of KC after I/R depend on the duration of ischemia and may also differ between ischemia at 4 °C and that at 37 °C. The extent of hepatic ischemia and the type of liver submitted to I/R is also greatly relevant [37].

In fact, the mechanisms involved in hepatic I/R injury are different depending on the type of liver, namely, non-steatotic (non-S) versus steatotic (S) livers. In addition to the impairment of microcirculation, mitochondrial ROS generation dramatically increases during reperfusion in S livers. Results obtained under warm hepatic ischemia indicate that apoptosis is the predominant form of hepatocyte death in the ischemic non-S liver, whereas S livers develop massive necrosis after a massive insult. Decreased ATP production and dysfunction of regulators of apoptosis, such as Bcl-2, Bcl-xL, and Bax, have been proposed to explain the failure of apoptosis in S liver. Concerning the renin–angiotensin system, the non-S livers exhibited higher angiotensin II levels, whereas S grafts exhibited higher Ang [1–7] levels. Moreover, reduced retinol binding protein 4 and increased peroxisome proliferator-activated receptor (PPAR) gamma levels were observed in S vs. non-S livers. The vulnerability of S livers subjected to warm ischemia is also associated with increased adiponectin, oxidative stress, and IL-1 levels and a reduced ability to generate IL-10 and PPAR-alpha. The method used to induce steatosis is also of importance. Both dietary high fat and alcohol exposure induced the production of superoxide dismutase (SOD) catalase insensitive ROS, which may be involved in the mechanism of S liver failure after OLT. The total amount of these findings underlines the extreme variability of the various pathways and of their relative role in a given pathologic entity [37].

Conclusion

Ischemia/reperfusion, vascular alterations in the hepatic microcirculation, and liver regeneration are complex pathophysiologic phenomena that have been extensively studied both in humans and in experimental animals. They could also serve as models for hepatic injury, recovery from injury, and restoration of the liver mass. In various ways and at a variable extent, they can also be responsible for the occurrence, progression, or spontaneous regression of some types of benign liver tumors or impact on their natural history.

References

1. Fausto N, Webber EM et al (1994) Liver regeneration. In: Arias I, Boyer J, Fausto N (eds) The liver biology and pathobiology. Raven Press, New York, pp 1059–1084
2. Fausto N (2000) Liver regeneration. J Hepatol 32:19–31
3. Michalopoulos GK, DeFrances MC (1997) Liver regeneration. Science 276:60–66
4. Francavilla A, Zeng Q, Polimeno L (1994) Small for size liver transplanted into larger recipient. A model of hepatic regeneration. Hepatology 19:210–216

5. Higgins GM, Anderson RM (1931) Experimental pathology of the liver I. Restoration of the liver of the white rat following partial surgical removal. Arch Pathol 12:186–202
6. Yokoyama Y, Nagino M, Nimura Y (2007) Mechanisms of hepatic regeneration following portal vein embolization and partial hepatectomy: a review. World J Surg 31:367–374
7. Makuuchi M, Takayasu K, Takuma T et al (1984) Preoperative transcatheter embolization of the portal venous branch for patients receiving extended lobectomy due to the bile duct carcinoma. J Jpn Soc Clin Surg 45:14–20
8. Nagino M, Kanai M, Morioka A et al (2000) Portal and arterial embolization before extensive liver resection in patients with markedly poor functional reserve. J Vasc Interv Radiol 11:1063–1068
9. Lautt WW (1985) Mechanism and role of intrinsic regulation of hepatic arterial blood flow: hepatic arterial buffer response. Am J Physiol 249(5 Pt 1):G549–G556
10. Lautt WW, Legare DJ, d'Almeida MS (1985) Adenosine as putative regulator of hepatic arterial flow (the buffer response). Am J Physiol 248(3 Pt 2):H331–H338
11. Rochelleau B, Ethier C, Houle R et al (1999) Hepatic artery buffer response following left portal vein ligation: its role in tissue liver homeostasis. Am J Physiol 277(5 Pt 1):G1000–G1007
12. Schnitzbauer AA, Lang SA, Goessmann H et al (2012) Right portal vein ligation combined with in situ splitting induces rapid left lateral liver lobe hypertrophy enabling 2-staged extended right hepatic resection in small-for-size settings. Ann Surg 255:405–414
13. Schadde E, Ardiles V, Robles-Campos R et al (2014) Early survival and safety of ALPPS-first report of the international ALPPS registry. Ann Surg 260:829–836
14. Fausto N, Laird AD, Webber EM (1995) Role of growth factors and cytokines in hepatic regeneration. FASEB J 9:1527–1536
15. Hsu J-C, Bravo R, Taub R (1992) Interactions among LRF-a Jun B, c Jun, and c-Fos define a regulatory program in the G1 phase of liver regeneration. Mol Cell Biol 12:4654–4665
16. Webber EM, Godowski PJ, Fausto N (1994) In vivo response of hepatocytes to growth factors requires an initial priming stimulus. Hepatology 19:489–497
17. Webber EM, Bruix J, Pierce RH, Fausto N (1998) Tumor necrosis factor primes hepatocytes for DNA replication in the rat. Hepatology 28:1226–1234
18. Uemura T, Miyazaki M, Hirai R et al (2000) Different expression of positive and negative regulators of hepatocyte growth in growing and shrinking hepatic lobes after portal branch ligation in rats. Int J Mol Med 5:173–179
19. Mizuno S, Nimura Y, Suzuki H et al (1996) Portal vein branch occlusion induces cell proliferation of cholestatic rat liver. J Surg Res 60:249–257
20. Ueda S, Yamanoi A, Hishikawa Y et al (2003) Transforming growth factor beta 1 released from the spleen exerts a growth inhibitory effect on liver regeneration in rats. Lab Invest 83:1595–1603
21. Hartleb M, Gutkowski K, Milkiewicz P (2011) Nodular regenerative hyperplasia: evolving concepts on underdiagnosed cause of portal hypertension. World J Gastroenterol 17: 1400–1409
22. Steiner PE (1959) Nodular regenerative hyperplasia of the liver. Am J Pathol 35:943–953
23. Suzuki H, Iyomasa S, Nimura Y et al (1994) Internal biliary drainage, unlike external drainage, does not suppress the regeneration of cholestatic rat liver after partial hepatectomy. Hepatology 20:1318–1322
24. Tracy TF Jr, Bailey PV, Goerke ME et al (1991) Cholestasis without cirrhosis alters regulatory liver gene expression and inhibits hepatic regeneration. Surgery 110:176–182; discussion 182–183
25. Abe T, Arai T, Ogawa A et al (2004) Kupffer cell-derived interleukin 10 is responsible for impaired bacterial clearance in bile duct-ligated mice. Hepatology 40:414–423
26. Starzl TE, Porter KA, Kashiwagi N (1975) Portal hepatotrophic factors, diabetes mellitus and acute liver atrophy, hypertrophy and regeneration. Surg Gynecol Obstet 141:843–858
27. Kawarada Y, Sanda M, Kawamura K et al (1991) Simultaneous extensive resection of the liver and the pancreas in dogs. Gastroenterol Jpn 26:747–756

28. Hussein O, Szvalb S, Van den Akker-Berman LM et al (2002) Liver regeneration is not altered in patients with non alcoholic steatohepatitis (NASH) when compared to chronic hepatitis C infection with similar grade of inflammation. Dig Dis Sci 47:1926–1931
29. Francavilla A, Polimeno L, Di Leo A et al (1989) The effect of estrogen and tamoxifen on hepatocyte proliferation in vivo and in vitro. Hepatology 9:614–620
30. Francavilla A, Gavaler JS, Makowka L et al (1989) Estradiol and testosterone levels in patients undergoing partial hepatectomy. A possible signal for hepatic regeneration? Dig Dis Sci 34:818–822
31. Eagon PK, Porter LE, Francavilla A et al (1985) Estrogen and androgen receptors in the liver: their role in liver disease and re generation. Semin Liver Dis 5:59–69
32. Imamura H, Shimada R, Kubota M et al (1999) Preoperative portal vein embolization: an audit of 84 patients. Hepatology 29:1099–1105
33. Shan YS, Hsieh YH, Sy ED et al (2005) The influence of spleen size on liver regeneration after major hepatectomy in normal and early cirrhotic liver. Liver Int 25:96–100
34. Selzner M, Camargo CA, Clavien PA (1999) Ischemia impairs liver regeneration after major tissue loss in rodents. Hepatology 30:469–475
35. Turowski C, Feist H, Alzen G et al (2009) Conversion of a neonatal hepatic hemangioma to focal nodular hyperplasia. Pathol Int 59:251–254
36. Tsung A, Sahai R, Tanaka H et al (2005) The nuclear factor HMGB 1 mediates hepatic injury after murine liver ischemia-reperfusion. J Exp Med 201:1135–1143
37. Mendez-Braz M, Elias-Mirò M, Jimenez-Castro MB et al (2012) The current state of knowledge of hepatic ischemia –reperfusion injury based on its study in experimental models. J Biomed Biotech article ID 298657. http://dx.doi.org/10.1155/2012/298657

Part II

Imaging

Imaging Modalities

5

Francesco De Cobelli, Gabriele Ironi, Paolo Marra,
Antonio Esposito, and Alessandro Del Maschio

Detecting and characterizing focal liver lesions is one of the most controversial challenges in imaging today, as the differential diagnosis is wide.

Imaging diagnostics of the liver are hampered by the fact that 20–50 % of the population exhibits benign focal liver lesions, mostly cysts and hemangiomas, lowering the pretest probability of identifying malignant instances [1]. In addition, MRI, CT, and ultrasound provide increasing spatial resolution, improving the likelihood of disclosing very small changes with uncertain significance.

Duc to the complexity of liver focal disease, imaging evaluation must follow the investigation of patient clinical background with particular attention given to concomitant findings such as specific laboratory abnormalities, history of infections or toxic exposure, and underlying systemic diseases or known malignancies. Taking into account the broad prevalence and incidence of focal liver lesions, clinical imaging and differential diagnosis should primarily focus on the most common entities and thereafter consider the more rare entities. Due to the high prevalence of benign tumors, imaging of the liver is challenging in terms of distinguishing benign liver lesions, which in most instances can be left alone, from malign neoplasms requiring therapy. By far the most common entity is hemangioma with a prevalence of 2–20 % [1, 2] in general population, followed far behind by focal nodular hyperplasia (FNH) and liver adenoma, which is a rather rare entity. From a practical point of view, a confident diagnosis of hemangioma and FNH resolves 90 % of all focal benign liver lesions [3]. However, liver adenoma has to be excluded, although being benign, since it is often a candidate for surgical resection due to the risk of bleeding and malignant transformation.

Cross-sectional imaging modalities, such as US, CT, and MR imaging, are used in most centers to assess liver abnormalities. These modalities, often used in various combinations, have fundamental differences in data acquisition and hence differences in the type of physical characteristics of tissues that they scan.

F. De Cobelli (✉) • G. Ironi • P. Marra • A. Esposito • A. Del Maschio
Department of Radiology, San Raffaele Hospital, Via Olgettina, 60, 20132 Milan, Italy
e-mail: decobelli.francesco@hsr.it; Ironi.gabriele@hsr.it; Marra.paolo@hsr.it

L. Aldrighetti et al. (eds.), *Benign Tumors of the Liver*,
DOI 10.1007/978-3-319-12985-3_5

5.1 Ultrasound

Ultrasound (US) is usually the initial imaging modality for the assessment of upper abdomen including the liver. Because of the high incidence of benign liver abnormalities in the general population, the initial US for many patients is not the final diagnostic tool but the beginning of an extensive work-up that can evolve into many directions (US-guided biopsy, CT or MR imaging). The main advantages of hepatic sonography include its ability to guide biopsy, its ability to characterize common benign lesions (cysts, hemangiomas), and its safety and low cost (both from biological and social point of view). Limits include its inability to image the entire liver in some patients and lower accuracy compared to CT and MR in the detection and characterization of focal liver lesions.

The ability of US to detect a focal lesion depends on its size, location, echogenicity, and mass effect. Small echogenic lesions are easily detectable, while large isoechoic masses are more difficult to diagnose. Mass effect is more important for the diagnosis of large isoechoic lesions, and it may appear as deviation or invasion of intrahepatic vasculature, bulges on liver margins, or displacement of extrahepatic structures. The characterization of focal liver lesions and thus the specificity of US rely on grayscale and Doppler appearances [4].

The liver is best evaluated using a probe with a center frequency ranging from 2 to 5 MHz; higher-frequency transducers may be used to image superficial abnormalities of the liver surface. The left lobe is optimally scanned through a subxyphoid approach with the patient in supine decubitus, while the right lobe can be approached either subcostally or intercostally. Intercostal scanning should be performed in a supine position either during quiet respiration or breathhold on expiration to allow visualization of the superior regions of the liver and subphrenic area. The subcostal approach is best performed with the patient in the left lateral decubitus position in deep inspiration allowing insonation of the majority of the right lobe.

The first US level of liver evaluation is the traditional standard *brightness mode (B-mode)* a grayscale examination in which no Doppler is used.

The second level superimposes a *color Doppler* interrogation on the region of interest. This level produces an image that shows blood flow in vessels: color pixels are integrated into the conventional B-mode grayscale images. Color Doppler displays blood flow toward the transducer as red and blood flow away from the transducer as blue. The intensity of color encoding enables the examiner to distinguish between slow flow and fast flow. Additional benefits include direct visualization of turbulent flow by a mixture of the two colors (phenomena seen in arteriovenous malformations). The amount of color pixels in a lesion correlates with the degree of vascularization. Additionally, color coding of vessels allows guided placement of cursors for spectral Doppler imaging [5].

The third level superimposes a small interrogation region, called "sample volume," over a vessel of interest. Ideally, the sample volume should be placed in the midportion of the lumen, rather than toward the periphery, for optimal estimation of laminar flow. Targeted interrogation of the vessel produces a *spectral Doppler* waveform that is displayed at the bottom of the screen, while the color Doppler image is at the top. Every spectral waveform has morphologic features that provide information regarding direction, velocity, and acceleration. Directional information is determined on the basis of whether the waveform lies above or below the baseline; velocity information is determined on the basis of distance from the baseline at any given point of the curve; and acceleration information is obtained from the slope of the curve, with changes in acceleration being marked by waveform peaks, or inflection points. These inflection points (acceleration changes) generate characteristic audible sounds at Doppler US [5].

Conventional color Doppler and spectral Doppler are not always able to image the vascularity of small lesions because in some cases signals are under level of detection. This may be partially correct with the use of power Doppler and contrast agents.

Power Doppler imaging displays the integrated Doppler signal power and displays tumor vascularity in an angiogram-like appearance. Due to better noise differentiation, this technique demonstrates small tumor vessels more precisely. However, power Doppler does not encode flow direction.

Tissue harmonic imaging is now an important part of liver US evaluation because it provides extra information, altering management and revealing lesions not seen on conventional B-mode [6, 7]. Tissue harmonic imaging is a grayscale imaging technique that uses the information from harmonic signals (multiples of the insonating frequency) generated by nonlinear propagation of a sound wave as it passes through the tissue. While conventional US transmits and receives at the same frequency, in tissue harmonic imaging, the receiver separates the harmonic signal from the fundamental echoes. This results in the use of only the returning harmonic signal with a dramatic reduction in artifacts.

Sonography can effectively guide biopsy allowing real-time visualization of the needle tip as it moves toward the lesion. This makes biopsy of small lesions and lesions in uncooperative patients easier. If a lesion can be imaged, biopsy is generally more efficient and cost effective using sonographic guidance, even when initially detected with some other modalities [8].

The introduction of US contrast agents has had a remarkable impact on liver sonography, and they are being increasingly used for the evaluation of focal liver lesions. *Contrast-enhanced US* (*CEUS*) allows masses to be interrogated for the degree and distribution of enhancement during the early phases and the washout of contrast during the later phases. Unlike Doppler US, which can only image the macrocirculation, CEUS allows assessing of both macro- and microcirculation of lesions. Modern US contrast agents are gas microbubble contained within a stabilizing lipid shell. Microbubbles are less than 10 μm in diameter and are safe and effective ultrasound scatterers because of the large impedance difference between the surrounding fluid (e.g., blood) and the encapsulated gas. When given intravenously, microbubbles produce marked enhancement of the US signal for several minutes, in gray scale and Doppler mode. The interactions of microbubbles with US beam are complex [4]. When a microbubble is exposed to an oscillating acoustic signal, it undergoes alternate expansion and contraction. At low acoustic power, these alternate expansions and contractions are equal and symmetrical, and the frequency of scattered signal is unaltered. As the acoustic power increases, more complex nonlinear interactions occur as the expansion and contraction phases become unequal because the microbubbles resist compression more strongly than expansion. This nonlinear resonant behavior is associated with the production of harmonic signals at multiples (or fractions) of the insonating frequency and can be imaged with harmonic imaging techniques. At still higher powers, highly nonlinear behavior is associated with microbubble disruption. This disruptive phase can be imaged using color Doppler mode or in grayscale. Microbubble disruption is seen as a transient bright color or B-mode signal which persists only for a few frames after insonation of an individual area. Contrast-enhanced nonlinear imaging of focal liver lesions can be performed during the vascular phase assessing the dynamic enhancement pattern and the vascular morphology of the lesion. The signal enhancer is injected intravenously and is purely intravascular without the extracellular phase of CT and MR contrast agents. Its effect becomes almost immediately noticeable a few seconds after bolus injection and persists for 90 up to 180 s. Following injection, continuous scanning can be performed and, although the timing is dependent on the individual's cardiac function, it can be broadly divided into an arterial phase (approximately 10–25 s), portal venous phase (approximately 30–120 s), and a late phase (over 120 s) [9]. Due to high sensitivity of modern scanners, the supplied vials of contrast agent can be divided and administered as small boluses, each followed by a saline flush of 5–10 ml. This allows multiple injections to be used in the same session from one vial. The injections can be repeated after 5–10 min, allowing additional lesions to be analyzed [10]. Several studies have already demonstrated a dramatic improvement of diagnostic performance of CEUS in the detection and characterization of focal liver lesions when compared with baseline US, with reported sensitivity and specificity values approaching those of CT and MRI [11–17].

5.2 Computed Tomography

The broad availability of computed tomography (CT) and recent development and implementation of faster multi-row detector machines make this modality an excellent tool for the detection and characterization of focal liver lesions. CT is still the most commonly used modality for the evaluation of focal liver lesion after initial sonography.

The indication for CT evaluation of the liver include the detection and characterization of focal liver lesions, detection and characterization of diffuse liver disease, staging of an intrahepatic or extrahepatic malignancy, follow-up after treatment for an intrahepatic or extrahepatic malignancy, and image guidance for percutaneous drainage or biopsy. However, it should be noted that percutaneous biopsy of liver lesion is an uncommon indication for CT, since more than 90 % of these biopsies can be performed using ultrasound guidance.

Multidetector-row CT (MDCT) is a technological evolution that allows the simultaneous acquisition of multiple images during a single rotation of the X-ray tube. With MDCT the entire liver is rapidly imaged (in about 5 s) with thin collimation (1–3 mm) during a single breathhold. MDCT scanners allow acquisition of thin slices with isotropic voxel size. The advantages of thinner slices are less partial volume averaging and, more importantly, multiplanar reconstructions of superior quality (MPR) and true three-dimensional reconstructions. There have been controversial data in the literature about the role of thin-slice imaging for the detection and characterization of liver lesions. The benefits and limitations of varying slice thickness in small liver lesion diagnosis have been investigated: A 2- and 4-mm slice reconstruction provided improved diagnostic results for the assessment of small liver lesions sized 11 mm or less. Larger section of 6, 8, and 10 mm yielded significantly inferior detection rates as the partial volume effects become more significant at lower resolution. However 1-mm slices also turned out to be inferior because the benefit of higher resolution is counteracted by the marked decrease in signal-to-noise ratio at lowest beam collimation [18].

The use of thin slices produces a data set that can be manipulated and reviewed on a workstation to produce high-quality multiplanar reformations. Superior quality MPRs obtained in various planes (coronal, sagittal, or arbitrarily angulated sections) may improve the detection of small subcapsular lesions in the dome of the liver, show the feeding arteries and venous drainage of detected lesions, or help in the characterization of lesions by better evaluation of their enhancement patterns. Examples include peripheral nodules of enhancement of small hemangiomas or central scars in focal nodular hyperplasia [19–21]. Thus, the peripheral nodular enhancement of hepatic hemangiomas may be indeterminate at transverse CT alone, while in the sagittal or coronal planes, this nodular enhancement may be more clearly demonstrated, allowing a confident diagnosis of hemangioma. In addition, the anatomic coronal plane may even help surgeons for preoperative planning, through delineation of the relationship of the lesions with blood vessels and bile ducts [22].

The detection of liver lesions relies on creation of images that provide optimum liver-to-tumor contrast. The shorter scan times also allow the capture of distinct phases of contrast enhancement following the bolus administration of iodinated contrast material through a peripheral vein, typically in the arm. These phases provide important informations concerning the enhancement patterns and hence the possibility of characterization of focal liver lesions. Although unenhanced CT is not really a phase of enhancement, some lesions are readily apparent, especially those that are larger and/or more peripheral. Foley et al. [23] described the different phases of liver enhancement.

The first phase of enhancement that occurs following the intravenous contrast administration of iodinated contrast material is the early hepatic arterial phase, also termed the hepatic arterial phase [23]. This phase begins approximately 15 s after initiating the bolus and lasts for about 10–15 s. During the early arterial phase, there is vivid arterial enhancement only, with essentially no enhancement of hepatic parenchyma and portal system. Although this phase is advantageous for CT angiography, it is not useful for detecting hepatic tumors.

The next phase of enhancement is the late hepatic arterial phase, termed the portal venous inflow phase [23]. This phase begins approximately 30 s after initiating the bolus and lasts for about 15–20 s. During the late arterial phase, there are marked, although slightly less, arterial enhancement, early hepatic parenchymal enhancement, early portal venous enhancement, and no enhancement of the hepatic veins. This phase is best for detecting tumors that have a higher degree of vascularity, which tend to show vivid enhancement. By comparison, tumors that have lower degree of vascularity demonstrate little enhancement during this phase and are not well seen. For this reason, it is rarely advantageous to include the late arterial phase in patients with less vascular tumors.

The following phase of enhancement is the portal venous phase, which is termed the hepatic venous phase [23]. This phase begins approximately 60 s after initiating the bolus and lasts for about 45–60 s. During the venous phase there are less arterial enhancement, vivid hepatic parenchymal enhancement, vivid portal venous enhancement, and vivid hepatic venous enhancement. Tumors that have a lower degree of vascularity are well visualized as hypoattenuating masses during this phase. Tumors that have a higher degree of vascularity may have one of three different appearances during this phase [24–26]: they may continue to be hyperdense; they may be isoenhancing and disappear; or they may be hypoenhancing. Imaging the portal venous phase is important in all patients with suspected hepatic tumors, regardless of the degree of vascularity.

The last phase of enhancement is the equilibrium phase. This phase begins approximately 90–120 s after initiation of the bolus. During this phase, the contrast agent (which does not cross the cell membrane) undergoes equilibrium between the intravascular and the extravascular extracellular space. Liver lesions that have a large amount of extracellular fluid readily take up the contrast material and tend to disappear during this phase, unless they are large and/or necrotic. However some lesions demonstrate typical fill-in patterns (e.g., hemangioma).

In clinical practice, however, the number of phases that are usually acquired with CT is limited and often kept to a minimum, mainly because of concerns about radiation hazard. The issue of radiation is even more important in relatively young and otherwise healthy patients with an incidental liver lesion that needs characterization and follow-up. For the first characterization of a liver lesion, the unenhanced phase, the late arterial phase, and the portal venous phase are required. Delayed CT scans should be restricted to those cases where no conclusive perfusion pattern is exhibited in the dual-phase contrast series. Precontrast scan may be abandoned in a follow-up study in order to limit the radiation exposure.

Whereas large benign focal liver lesions exhibit typical patterns of morphology, attenuation, and perfusion, small lesions remain challenging even with MDCT, since the specific criteria for confident diagnosis become more ambiguous. Here, MR imaging provides more detailed information about tissue components and the availability of liver-specific contrast agents, adding further impact to this technique.

5.3 Magnetic Resonance

MR imaging can provide comprehensive and highly accurate diagnostic information concerning diffuse and focal liver abnormalities, obviating the need for other imaging modalities. While a confident diagnosis is usually made on the basis of ultrasound findings in cases of simple cysts and hemangiomas with typical hyperechoic appearance [27], lesions with nonspecific ultrasound features require further investigation [28]. In this scenario, MRI is establishing its role as a primary diagnostic technique with respect to spiral CT. Spiral CT, in fact, has limitations in achieving a reliable diagnosis of small incidental lesions [28, 29]. In contrast, MRI can offer improved capability in lesion detection and characterization based on the information provided by the analysis of lesion signal intensity on baseline sequences and contrast enhancement patterns in dynamic studies and eventually based on the use of liver-specific agents.

MR imaging can visualize several tissues and anatomic components of the liver separately based on:

- T1-weighted imaging (including chemical shift imaging for the detection of small amounts of fat and intracellular fat): provides most lesion detection sensitivity [30].
- T2-weighted imaging: allows distinction between solid and nonsolid liver lesions based on fluid content.
- Diffusion-weighted imaging (improvement of lesion detection and characterization): is a measure of the ability of water molecule protons to diffuse freely within intra- and extracellular environments. Diffusion-weighted imaging therefore reflects cellular density of a lesion: lesions with lowest apparent diffusion coefficient (ADC) are more likely to be malignant. [31].
- Dynamic pre- and post-contrast T1-weighted imaging: shows the enhancement patterns of liver lesions.
- T1-weighted imaging in the hepatic excretion phase of hepatocyte-specific contrast agents.

These imaging properties allow highly detailed evaluation of diffuse and focal liver abnormalities.

Gadolinium-based contrast agents have become an essential part of a liver MRI examination in a number of circumstances. Intravenous MR contrast agents can be divided into extracellular (ECA) and hepatocyte-specific agents [32].

ECA are hydrophilic, small-molecular-weight gadolinium chelates that, following intravenous injection, are rapidly distributed from the vascular compartment to the interstitial spaces and then excreted via the urinary system, similar to CT agents. They show a paramagnetic effect, and hence, they reduce T1 relaxivity increasing signal intensity on T1-weighted images. ECA provide information on vascularization and perfusion similar to that of iodinated contrast agents for CT. A dynamic contrast-enhanced study of the liver is performed with a timing scheme that enables selective imaging during the late hepatic arterial phase (approximately 28 s after bolus injection), the portal venous phase (approximately 70 s after injection), and the delayed phase of enhancement (approximately 2–7 min after injection). In the hepatic arterial-dominant phase, contrast enhancement is observed in the hepatic artery and portal vein, and not in the hepatic veins. Hepatic parenchyma is mildly enhanced. During this phase, hypervascular liver pathologies are depicted and characterized. During portal venous phase, contrast enhancement in the hepatic veins is observed and hepatic parenchyma is nearly maximally enhanced. Maximal vascular opacification is observed in this phase. Assessment of hypovascular liver pathologies and washout of hypervascular pathologies also occur in this phase. During delayed phase of enhancement, hepatic parenchymal enhancement persists. This phase provides additional information further to characterize focal hepatic lesions, by demonstrating their late-phase temporal handling of contrast. Hemangiomas reveal progressive enhancement and persistent enhancement is observed in small-sized hemangiomas; washout of hypervascular metastases and HCC is also apparent during this phase [33].

HAS are paramagnetic compounds that have dual elimination, with a portion of the dose distributed extracellularly and eliminated by the kidneys; the remainder is taken up by hepatocytes and excreted into the bile. HAS produce strong and sustained enhancement of liver parenchyma on T1-weighted images. Because of the selective increase in the signal intensity of normal hepatocytes compared with focal tumors, contrast-to-noise ratio between lesions and healthy liver is usually increased, and lesion detectability is improved on T1-weighted images [34].

Two gadolinium-based hepatocyte-specific contrast agents are commercially available at present: gadoxetic acid, which is marketed under the name of Eovist in the United States and Primovist elsewhere worldwide (Bayer Schering Pharma, Berlin, Germany), and gadobenate dimeglumine marked under the name of MultiHance (Bracco, Milan, Italy). HAS combine the properties of extracellular gadolinium chelates, allowing hepatic arterial and portal venous phase imaging, with delayed hepatocyte uptake and partial excretion into the biliary system. This combination of hepatocyte uptake and biliary excretion results in the additional so-called hepatocellular phase.

An important difference between the two agents is that 50 % of the administered dose of gadoxetic acid, but only 5 % of the gadobenate dimeglumine dose, is excreted via the hepatobiliary system in a healthy person; the remainder is excreted by the kidneys. Because of its greater hepatic uptake, gadoxetic acid results in more intense hepatocellular phase enhancement than gadobenate dimeglumine [35, 36] and is cleared from the body more rapidly (elimination half-lives: 1 h for gadoxetic acid and 1–2 h for gadobenate dimeglumine). In addition, hepatobiliary phase images are acquired 20 min after Primovist injection (with persistent enhancement for more than 2 h), compared to 45–120 min after MultiHance injection.

In the hepatocellular phase, normal liver parenchyma appears uniformly bright on T1-weighted images because of the accumulation of HAS. Focal liver lesions that contain normal hepatocytes connected to functioning bile ducts accumulate HAS and therefore enhance in the hepatocellular phase. If any part of this axis is disrupted, hepatocellular phase enhancement is impaired or absent. Hence, hepatocellular phase imaging provides unique information about the structure and function of liver lesions by demonstrating the presence (or absence) of functioning hepatocytes.

5.4 Comparison of Modalities

Incidental detection of liver lesion is common due to the increased use of cross-sectional imaging modalities and the high prevalence of benign liver lesions.

In such cases, US is regularly the initial examination. Cysts and cystic liver lesions are easier to detect than solid liver lesions at US. Noncystic liver lesions in an otherwise normal liver may have similar echogenicity to each other and to the background liver and may be difficult to detect and characterize at US. Compared with conventional B-mode grayscale US, significant advantages arise from the additional use of color Doppler and power modes with respect to tumor vascularity [37]. However, despite recent improvements in color Doppler sonographic equipment, conventional color Doppler is still limited by its lack of sensitivity in the detection of flow in intranodular microvessels or flow in deeply located liver lesions, and the examination procedures is hampered by motion artifacts. Nevertheless, developments in ultrasound contrast agents provide increasing competition to MDCT and MR [37].

The use of US technique is limited by the fact that it is an operator dependent imaging modality. US ability to detect liver lesions and to identify them as benign is therefore mostly based on operator's experience. This consideration has a big impact in the work-up of liver lesions, as a less expert operator could require more imaging techniques to confirm the nature of a lesion.

Furthermore, a good quality US examination must take into account attention to several factors, such as machine set-up and operator's ability to manipulate all aspects of US equipment in order to obtain optimal images.

CT and MR imaging provide reproducible image quality with better anatomic detail and topographic display. A biopsy is often unnecessary if the liver lesion has a classical appearance on CT or MR imaging.

The fundamental limitation of CT is its lack of intrinsic soft tissue contrast; for detection and characterization, CT mainly relies on high spatial resolution and vascularity of liver lesions. Whereas large tumors exhibit typical patterns of morphology, attenuation, and perfusion, small lesions (<2 cm) still remain challenging since the specific criteria for confident diagnosis become more ambiguous. At CT, distinction between a small benign liver lesion and a metastasis or a small HCC can be difficult. Finally, MDCT generates a significant radiation dose to the patient. Thus, the number of necessary scans as well as the application of thin slices should be strictly checked for each patient with respect to the individual clinical question and history of the patient.

MR imaging provides a more comprehensive work-up of focal and diffuse liver diseases. This is based on the unique properties of MR imaging that has a combination of high intrinsic soft tissue contrast of the liver and liver lesions and high sensitivity for the presence or absence of intravenous nonspecific contrast (gadolinium) and liver-specific contrast media. Because MR imaging lacks the hazard of ionizing radiation, most centers perform a multiphasic gadolinium-enhanced examination as a standard part of their work-up of liver diseases. In such cases, MR imaging can provide essential and very specific tissue characteristics of the lesion and the surrounding liver (cirrhosis versus noncirrhosis) and hence can considerably narrow down the differential diagnosis to only one or two entities or even provide a very specific diagnosis. MR imaging is the standard of reference for the evaluation of focal liver lesions, and it plays a pivotal role as a comprehensive approach for the work-up of patients with suspected or known liver abnormalities.

References

1. Karhunen PJ (1986) Benign hepatic tumours and tumour like conditions in men. J Clin Pathol 39(2):183–188
2. Ishak KG, Rabin L (1975) Benign tumors of the liver. Med Clin North Am 59(4):995–1013
3. Valette PJ, Pilleul F, Crombe-Ternamian A (2003) MDCT of benign liver tumors and metastases. Eur Radiol 13(Suppl 5):M31–M41
4. Harvey CJ, Albrecht T (2001) Ultrasound of focal liver lesions. Eur Radiol 11(9):1578–1593
5. McNaughton DA, Abu-Yousef MM (2011) Doppler US of the liver made simple. Radiographics 31(1):161–188. doi:10.1148/rg.311105093
6. Shapiro RS, Wagreich J, Parsons RB, Stancato-Pasik A, Yeh HC, Lao R (1998) Tissue harmonic imaging sonography: evaluation of image quality compared with conventional sonography. AJR Am J Roentgenol 171(5):1203–1206. doi:10.2214/ajr.171.5.9798848
7. Hann LE, Bach AM, Cramer LD, Siegel D, Yoo HH, Garcia R (1999) Hepatic sonography: comparison of tissue harmonic and standard sonography techniques. AJR Am J Roentgenol 173(1):201–206. doi:10.2214/ajr.173.1.10397127
8. Tchelepi H, Ralls PW (2004) Ultrasound of focal liver masses. Ultrasound Q 20(4):155–169
9. Bolondi L, Correas JM, Lencioni R, Weskott HP, Piscaglia F (2007) New perspectives for the use of contrast-enhanced liver ultrasound in clinical practice. Dig Liver Dis 39(2):187–195. doi:10.1016/j.dld.2006.08.008
10. Sutherland T, Temple F, Lee WK, Hennessy O (2011) Evaluation of focal hepatic lesions with ultrasound contrast agents. J Clin Ultrasound 39(7):399–407. doi:10.1002/jcu.20847
11. Bartolotta TV, Taibbi A, Midiri M, Lagalla R (2009) Focal liver lesions: contrast-enhanced ultrasound. Abdom Imaging 34(2):193–209. doi:10.1007/s00261-008-9378-6
12. Quaia E, Calliada F, Bertolotto M, Rossi S, Garioni L, Rosa L et al (2004) Characterization of focal liver lesions with contrast-specific US modes and a sulfur hexafluoride-filled microbubble contrast agent: diagnostic performance and confidence. Radiology 232(2):420–430. doi:10.1148/radiol.2322031401
13. Solbiati L, Tonolini M, Cova L, Goldberg SN (2001) The role of contrast-enhanced ultrasound in the detection of focal liver lesions. Eur Radiol 11(Suppl 3):E15–E26. doi:10.1007/s003300100003
14. Catala V, Nicolau C, Vilana R, Pages M, Bianchi L, Sanchez M et al (2007) Characterization of focal liver lesions: comparative study of contrast-enhanced ultrasound versus spiral computed tomography. Eur Radiol 17(4):1066–1073. doi:10.1007/s00330-006-0444-6
15. Li R, Guo Y, Hua X, He Y, Ding J, Guo A et al (2007) Characterization of focal liver lesions: comparison of pulse-inversion harmonic contrast-enhanced sonography with contrast-enhanced CT. J Clin Ultrasound 35(3):109–117. doi:10.1002/jcu.20310
16. Quaia E, D'Onofrio M, Palumbo A, Rossi S, Bruni S, Cova M (2006) Comparison of contrast-enhanced ultrasonography versus baseline ultrasound and contrast-enhanced computed

tomography in metastatic disease of the liver: diagnostic performance and confidence. Eur Radiol 16(7):1599–1609. doi:10.1007/s00330-006-0192-7

17. Larsen LP, Rosenkilde M, Christensen H, Bang N, Bolvig L, Christiansen T et al (2007) The value of contrast enhanced ultrasonography in detection of liver metastases from colorectal cancer: a prospective double-blinded study. Eur J Radiol 62(2):302–307. doi:10.1016/j.ejrad.2006.11.033
18. Kopp AF, Heuschmid M, Claussen CD (2002) Multidetector helical CT of the liver for tumor detection and characterization. Eur Radiol 12(4):745–752. doi:10.1007/s00330-001-1177-1
19. Brancatelli G, Federle MP, Katyal S, Kapoor V (2002) Hemodynamic characterization of focal nodular hyperplasia using three-dimensional volume-rendered multidetector CT angiography. AJR Am J Roentgenol 179(1):81–85. doi:10.2214/ajr.179.1.1790081
20. Kamel IR, Georgiades C, Fishman EK (2003) Incremental value of advanced image processing of multislice computed tomography data in the evaluation of hypervascular liver lesions. J Comput Assist Tomogr 27(4):652–656
21. Kamel IR, Lawler LP, Fishman EK (2004) Comprehensive analysis of hypervascular liver lesions using 16-MDCT and advanced image processing. AJR Am J Roentgenol 183(2):443–452. doi:10.2214/ajr.183.2.1830443
22. Sahani D, Saini S, Pena C, Nichols S, Prasad SR, Hahn PF et al (2002) Using multidetector CT for preoperative vascular evaluation of liver neoplasms: technique and results. AJR Am J Roentgenol 179(1):53–59. doi:10.2214/ajr.179.1.1790053
23. Foley WD, Mallisee TA, Hohenwalter MD, Wilson CR, Quiroz FA, Taylor AJ (2000) Multiphase hepatic CT with a multirow detector CT scanner. AJR Am J Roentgenol 175(3):679–685. doi:10.2214/ajr.175.3.1750679
24. Paulson EK, McDermott VG, Keogan MT, DeLong DM, Frederick MG, Nelson RC (1998) Carcinoid metastases to the liver: role of triple-phase helical CT. Radiology 206(1):143–150. doi:10.1148/radiology.206.1.9423664
25. Frederick MG, Paulson EK, Nelson RC (1997) Helical CT for detecting focal liver lesions in patients with breast carcinoma: comparison of noncontrast phase, hepatic arterial phase, and portal venous phase. J Comput Assist Tomogr 21(2):229–235
26. Sheafor DH, Frederick MG, Paulson EK, Keogan MT, DeLong DM, Nelson RC (1999) Comparison of unenhanced, hepatic arterial-dominant, and portal venous-dominant phase helical CT for the detection of liver metastases in women with breast carcinoma. AJR Am J Roentgenol 172(4):961–968. doi:10.2214/ajr.172.4.10587129
27. Leifer DM, Middleton WD, Teefey SA, Menias CO, Leahy JR (2000) Follow-up of patients at low risk for hepatic malignancy with a characteristic hemangioma at US. Radiology 214(1):167–172. doi:10.1148/radiology.214.1.r00ja09167
28. Vilgrain V, Boulos L, Vullierme MP, Denys A, Terris B, Menu Y (2000) Imaging of atypical hemangiomas of the liver with pathologic correlation. Radiographics 20(2):379–397. doi:10.1148/radiographics.20.2.g00mc01379
29. Kim T, Federle MP, Baron RL, Peterson MS, Kawamori Y (2001) Discrimination of small hepatic hemangiomas from hypervascular malignant tumors smaller than 3 cm with three-phase helical CT. Radiology 219(3):699–706. doi:10.1148/radiology.219.3.r01jn45699
30. Semelka RC, Martin DR, Balci C, Lance T (2001) Focal liver lesions: comparison of dual-phase CT and multisequence multiplanar MR imaging including dynamic gadolinium enhancement. J Magn Reson Imaging 13(3):397–401
31. Miller FH, Hammond N, Siddiqi AJ, Shroff S, Khatri G, Wang Y et al (2010) Utility of diffusion-weighted MRI in distinguishing benign and malignant hepatic lesions. J Magn Reson Imaging 32(1):138–147. doi:10.1002/jmri.22235
32. Bhargava P, Vaidya S, Kolokythas O, Katz DS, Dighe M (2011) Hepatic vascular shunts: embryology and imaging appearances. Br J Radiol 84(1008):1142–1152. doi:10.1259/bjr/82649468
33. Semelka RC, Helmberger TK (2001) Contrast agents for MR imaging of the liver. Radiology 218(1):27–38. doi:10.1148/radiology.218.1.r01ja2427
34. Petersein J, Spinazzi A, Giovagnoni A, Soyer P, Terrier F, Lencioni R et al (2000) Focal liver lesions: evaluation of the efficacy of gadobenate dimeglumine in MR imaging–a multicenter phase III clinical study. Radiology 215(3):727–736. doi:10.1148/radiology.215.3.r00jn14727

35. Filippone A, Blakeborough A, Breuer J, Grazioli L, Gschwend S, Hammerstingl R et al (2010) Enhancement of liver parenchyma after injection of hepatocyte-specific MRI contrast media: a comparison of gadoxetic acid and gadobenate dimeglumine. J Magn Reson Imaging 31(2):356–364. doi:10.1002/jmri.22054
36. Goodwin MD, Dobson JE, Sirlin CB, Lim BG, Stella DL (2011) Diagnostic challenges and pitfalls in MR imaging with hepatocyte-specific contrast agents. Radiographics 31(6):1547–1568. doi:10.1148/rg.316115528
37. Klein D, Jenett M, Gassel HJ, Sandstede J, Hahn D (2004) Quantitative dynamic contrast-enhanced sonography of hepatic tumors. Eur Radiol 14(6):1082–1091. doi:10.1007/s00330-004-2299-z

Systematics of Imaging Morphology

6

Francesco De Cobelli, Paolo Marra, Gabriele Ironi, Antonio Esposito, and Alessandro Del Maschio

6.1 Non-hepatocellular Lesions

6.1.1 Hemangioma

The most common benign hepatic tumor with a reported prevalence of up to 20 % is hemangioma (Figs. 6.1 and 6.2), occurring at any age with a female predominance [1, 2]. The vast majority is incidentally found in asymptomatic subjects by ultrasound, but patients with large lesions may present with abdominal pain or mass effect symptoms that should be investigated with panoramic imaging modalities such as MR or CT, able to detect and provide accurate information about rare complications such as intratumoral hemorrhage and rupture. Cavernous hemangiomas are well circumscribed and vary from less than 1 cm to over 30 cm in size. Ten to twenty percent are multiple and often associated with focal nodular hyperplasia [1].

- At *ultrasound*, hemangiomas are usually shown as well-defined, oval-shaped homogeneous hyperechoic lesions with or without posterior acoustic enhancement, even though these features are not always found together [3, 4]. Furthermore, different variations of the usual images are seen in large lesions because of thrombosis, fibrosis, hemorrhage, or calcifications, resulting in a heterogeneous or sometimes hypoechoic appearance that may require further investigation with MR or CT [4]. Power/color Doppler US is not so useful because of the extremely low flow velocities and the small size of vascular structures inside hemangiomas [3], while *CEUS* may show the typical peripheral nodular contrast medium enhancement and the iris-diaphragm phenomenon [5].

F. De Cobelli (✉) • P. Marra • G. Ironi • A. Esposito • A. Del Maschio
Department of Radiology, San Raffaele Hospital, Via Olgettina, 60, 20132 Milan, Italy
e-mail: decobelli.francesco@hsr.it; marra.paolo@hsr.it; ironi.gabriele@hsr.it

L. Aldrighetti et al. (eds.), *Benign Tumors of the Liver*,
DOI 10.1007/978-3-319-12985-3_6

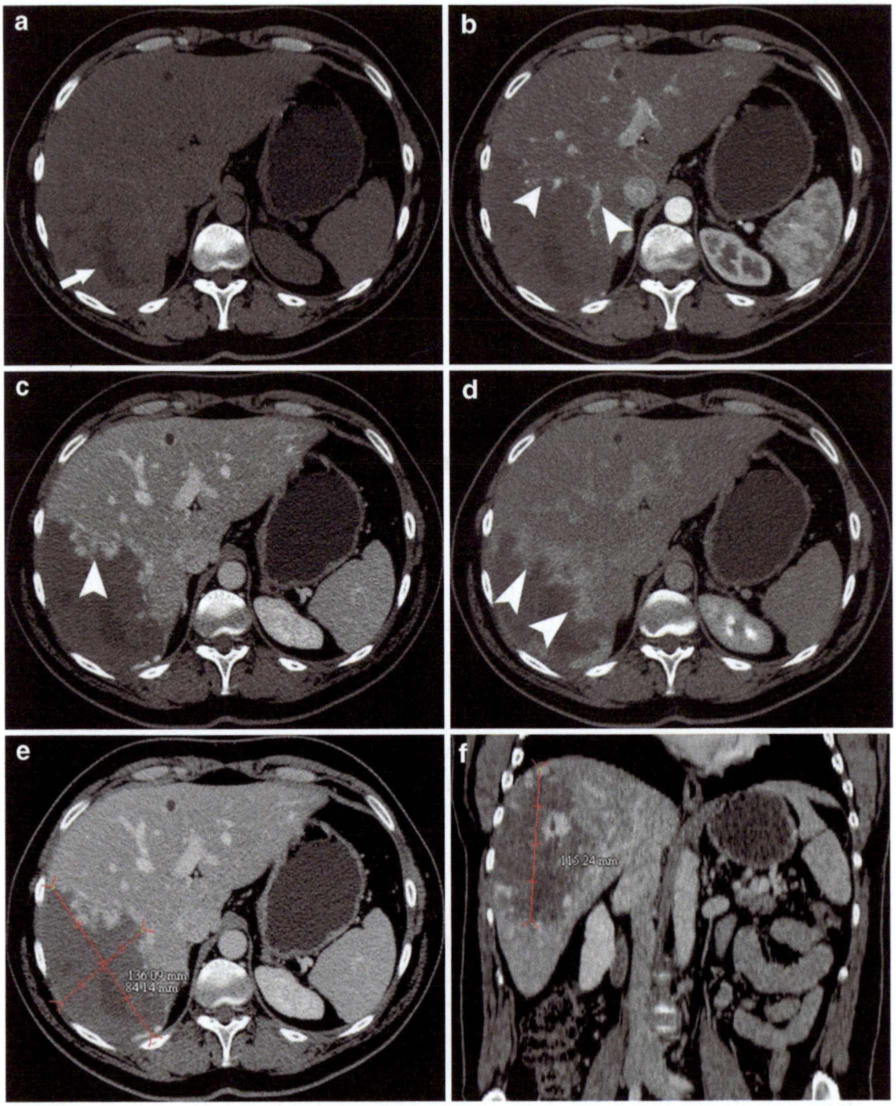

Fig. 6.1 A young asymptomatic man with giant cavernous hemangioma. On unenhanced CT scan, (**a**) the lesion is hypodense with well-defined lobulated margins. This large tumor shows a central non-enhanced area corresponding to the cystic cavity, probably necrotic (*arrow*). During the arterial phase, (**b**) there is a hyperdense peripheral nodular enhancement that progresses centrally during the portal and equilibrium phases (*arrowhead*, **c**, **d**). Axial and MPR coronal images (**e**, **f**) are useful to quantify the exact extension of the tumor. Due to the posterior location of the hemangioma (protected from abdominal trauma), no surgical resection was proposed

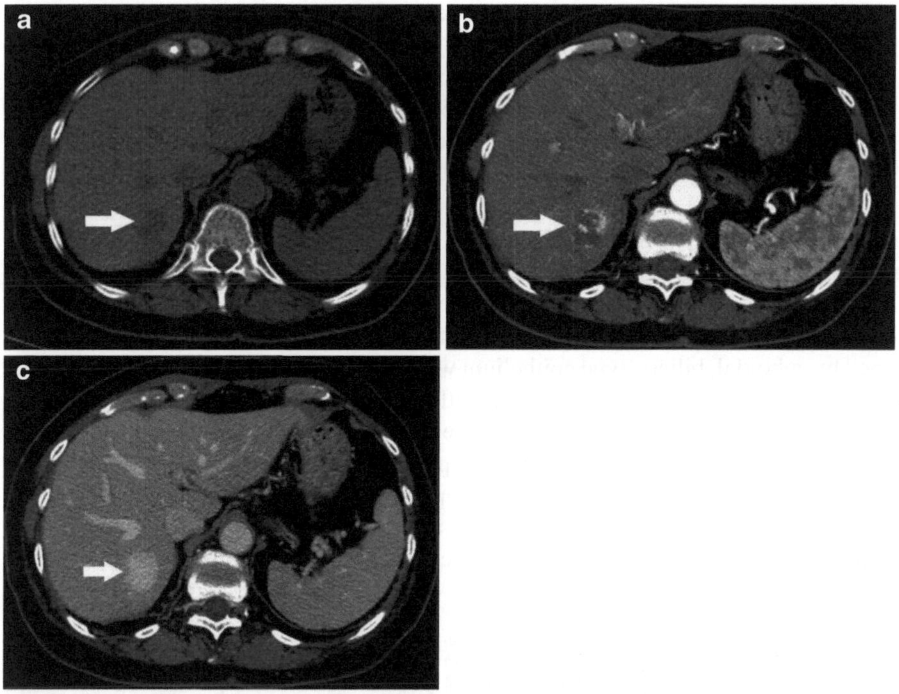

Fig. 6.2 A typical cavernous hemangioma incidentally discovered in a middle-aged man. On unenhanced CT scan, (**a**) the oval-shaped lesion (*arrow*) is homogeneously hypodense with well-define margins. In the dynamic study, this benign tumor presents the typical peripheral globular enhancement in the arterial phase (*arrow*, **b**) and gets completely filled in with the contrast media in the portal-venous phase (*arrow*, **c**). The patient underwent US follow-up

- At *MRI*, the high blood/water content gives the hemangiomas a typical hypointense appearance on T1w sequences and a marked hyperintensity on T2w sequences. DCE-MRI usually shows a slow perfusion pattern with early peripheral globular enhancement that proceeds centripetally. Indeed small hemangiomas may completely and homogeneously enhance in the early arterial phase, while large hemangiomas are progressively filled in with gadolinium, leading to a persistent homogeneous hyperintensity in the delayed phase. Fibrotic or thrombotic components and calcifications inside the hemangioma result as hypointense areas on T2w images, also confirmed by focal intratumor hypointensity on post-gadolinium T1w sequences [6].
- On *CT*, hemangiomas are sharply defined masses that are usually hypoattenuating compared with the adjacent hepatic parenchyma, if normal (i.e., nonsteatotic), on unenhanced images [7]. On unenhanced images, the vascular components of hemangiomas have the same attenuation value as the blood within blood vessels; intratumor thrombosis or fibrosis is hypoattenuating while calcium is hyperattenuating. The enhancement pattern is the same seen at MRI; the identification of globular enhancement that is isodense to the aorta is characteristic of hemangiomas [8].
- Concerning follow-up of benign liver tumors we couldn't find consensus guidelines in the literature. However we completely agree with the recently published

guidelines suggested by the American College of Gastroenterology [9]. According to these guidelines follow-up imaging is not required in classical asymptomatic hemangioma. On the other hand, rapid growth of a hemangioma has been reported, justifying radiologic follow-up of patients with large lesions, particularly those in a subcapsular location.

6.1.2 Simple Hepatic Cyst

Simple cysts are (Fig. 6.3) congenital lesions affecting 2–7 % of the population. They can be single or multiple and consist of usually small-sized (10 mm) serous contents lined by cuboidal, biliary-type epithelium with no communication with the bile ducts. Simple cysts tend to occur more frequently in the right hepatic lobe and are more prevalent in women; also complex cysts are more frequent in women [4]. Adult-onset cysts may be classified as nonparasitic, parasitic (echinococcus), or hemorrhagic (spontaneous/post-traumatic). Multiple hepatic cysts should be differentiated from autosomal dominant polycystic liver disease (APCKD) and von Hippel-Lindau syndrome [2]. Most patients are asymptomatic and the diagnosis is incidental.

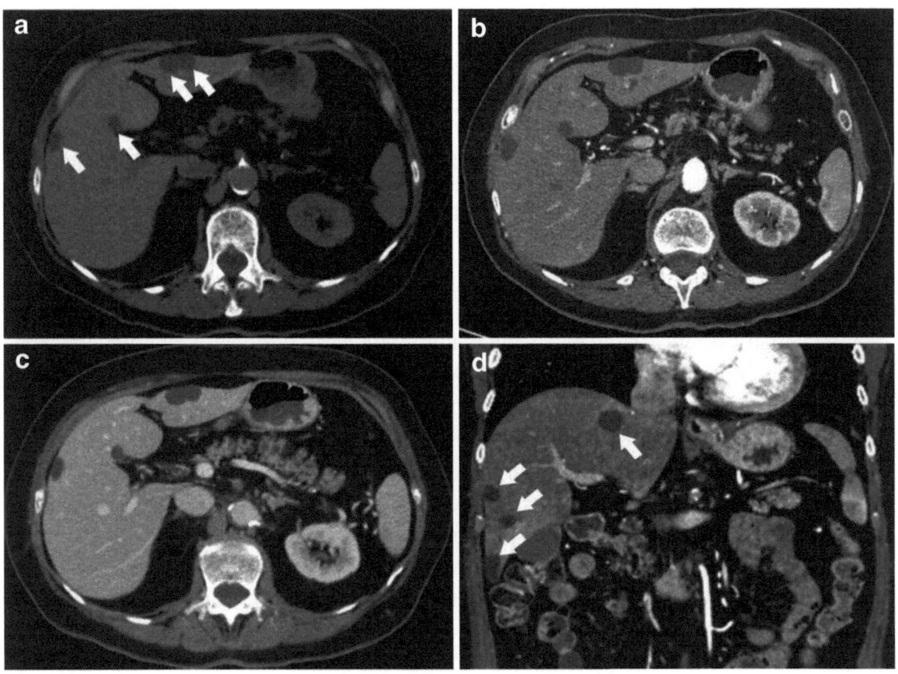

Fig. 6.3 Multiple simple hepatic cysts. The lesions were incidentally discovered during a CT angiogram in a middle-aged woman with abdominal angina due to mesenteric ischemia. They are located both at the right and left lobes (*arrows*) and present fluid density both on pre-contrast CT (**a**) and on contrast-enhanced CT (**b**, arterial phase; **c**, portal-venous phase; **d**, coronal arterial phase) with no significant enhancement of the walls; no evident septations or calcifications are seen, confirming the benign nature of these very common lesions

Simple cysts should be differentiated from unilocular biliary cystadenoma, as this entity has premalignant potential, and cystic metastases [8]. Features that suggest malignancy include internal mural nodules, coarse calcifications, and irregularities in the wall [10]; moreover cystadenomas are usually multilocular [1]. Ciliated hepatic foregut cysts are located along the convex external surface of the liver, bulge the liver contour, and are usually intersegmental in location. Foregut cysts usually possess a definable enhancing wall [2].

- At *ultrasound* hepatic cysts appear as anechoic fluid-filled spaces without clear walls and with posterior acoustic enhancement [4].
- Features of cysts at *MRI* include T2 hyperintensity with uniform smooth round, ovoid, or slightly lobulated margins and low signal on T1w sequences with no enhancement on early and late post-gadolinium images. Variations in the appearance of cysts occur and include septations, lobulation, and elevated T1 signal due to protein or blood products, sometimes with a fluid-fluid level. Fluid-containing lesions such as cysts and hemangiomas can be easily detected and distinguished from solid benign and malignant lesions using *DWI*; however, this differential diagnosis can be performed also with conventional MRI [8].
- On *CT* hepatic cysts appear as homogeneous and hypoattenuating (water density <20 HU) lesions on basal scan, with no enhancement of their walls or content after intravenous administration of contrast material. They have typically well-defined borders without perceptible walls [8].

6.1.3 Biliary Cystadenoma

Cystadenoma is the most commonly encountered primary cystic neoplasms of the liver, usually found incidentally on abdominal imaging. Cystadenomas can be differentiated from simple cysts based on the appearance at US or recurrence after surgery. At *US* they appear as hypoechoic lesions with irregular walls, septations, and coarse calcifications, features not present in simple cysts [8]. On *CT* and at *MRI*, cystadenomas may present some contrast enhancement of the wall or septations [1, 10]. As cystadenoma may potentially have a malignant degeneration evolving to cystadenocarcinoma, it is typically surgically resected requiring liver resection (indeed, when treated through unroofing like simple cysts, recurrence rates are high); imaging is not able to differentiate benign from malignant lesions, and biopsy is usually not indicated since unreliable [8]. Hepatic cystadenomas should be differentiated from cystic metastases, large simple or complicated hepatic cysts, complex abscesses, echinococcal cysts, and intrahepatic bilomas or hematomas.

6.1.4 Angiomyolipoma

Angiomyolipoma is a rare benign, unencapsulated mesenchymal tumor that is composed of varying proportions of three elements: smooth muscle cells, thick-walled blood vessels, and mature adipose tissue [1]. US, CT, and MRI typically demonstrate the fat component and prominent central vessels. At *US*, angiomyolipoma may be highly echogenic and indistinguishable from a hemangioma, unless it presents sound attenuation, speed propagation artifacts, or refraction artifacts [11]. On *CT* it has been reported to consist of two parts: a peripheral angiomyomatous component with soft tissue attenuation and a fatty hypoattenuating component [11]. *MRI* characteristics vary depending on the proportion of intratumoral fat: frequently, angiomyolipoma has a high fat content, with high signal intensity on T1-weighted images and a significant drop in signal intensity on fat-suppressed images, while areas of microscopic fat infiltration demonstrate diffuse loss of signal on out-of-phase sequences [6, 11]. On T2-weighted sequences, hepatic angiomyolipoma is homogeneously or heterogeneously hyperintense [1]. On contrast-enhanced CT and MR studies, it usually demonstrates early intense contrast enhancement that peaks later than that of a hepatocellular carcinoma [11, 12].

6.2 Hepatocellular Lesions

6.2.1 Focal Nodular Hyperplasia (FNH)

Focal nodular hyperplasia (FNH) is the second most common benign hepatic lesion following hemangioma; it is typical in young females, usually asymptomatic [13]. FNH (Figs. 6.4 and 6.5) consists of unencapsulated hepatocyte nodules circumscribed by fibrous septa (containing mononuclear inflammatory cells) that coalesce into a central or eccentric vascular structure resembling a stellate scar [1]; however, a central scar may not be visualized in up to 50 % of cases, particularly in lesions less than 3 cm in diameter [1, 14]. Approximately 20 % are multiple and association with cavernous hemangiomas is frequent [1]. Bile ductules are present at the junction of the fibrous septa and hepatocytes; however, they do not connect to the intrahepatic bile ducts [1]. Hemorrhage is very uncommon and malignant degeneration is not reported [15].

Fig. 6.4 A young woman with asymptomatic focal nodular hyperplasia. The lesion was incidentally detected at US (*arrows*, **a**, **b**) where it appears as a well-defined isoechoic nodule surrounded by a hypoechoic halo, probably representing the compressed surrounding hepatic parenchyma. To better characterize the nodule, the patient underwent CE-MRI with hepatocyte-specific contrast agent (Gd-BOPTA). Unenhanced axial T2-weighted and STIR images (**c**, **d**) reveal a slightly hyperintense liver lesion in the right liver lobe (*arrow*); the tumor is slightly hypointense on T1-weighted images (*arrow*, **e**) with no significant dropout of the MR signal on "opposite-phase" acquisitions (*arrow*, **f**). An intense and homogeneous enhancement is seen during the arterial phase (*arrow*, **g**, basal; *arrow*, **h**, arterial) after contrast administration, with no significant washout in the portal-venous and equilibrium phases. In these phases, the tumor returns isointense to the surrounding gradually enhancing parenchyma (**i**, **j**). Late hepatobiliary T1-weighted images (**k**), also acquired with fat saturation technique (**l**), confirm the benign nature of the lesion, composed of functioning hepatocytes that uptake and normally dismiss the hepatocyte-specific contrast agent. In this case, the typical central scar is just detectable as a hypointense component in the hepatobiliary phase imaging (*arrowhead*). Contrast-enhanced MR provided solid criteria for the diagnosis of FNH and neither biopsy nor surgical resection was indicated; this patient underwent just a periodical US follow-up

- At *US* FNH is typically isoechoic to liver parenchyma, often with a hypoechoic halo or lobulated contours [16]. The color and power Doppler often shows a characteristic "spoke-wheel" pattern of internal vascularity, characterized by a central feeding artery with a centrifugal stellate branching [11, 14]. When the central scar is visible (in about 20 % of cases), it is hyperechoic [16]. On *CEUS* FNH enhances at the very arterial phase and becomes homogeneously isoechoic after 30 s in the vast majority of the cases [5, 16].

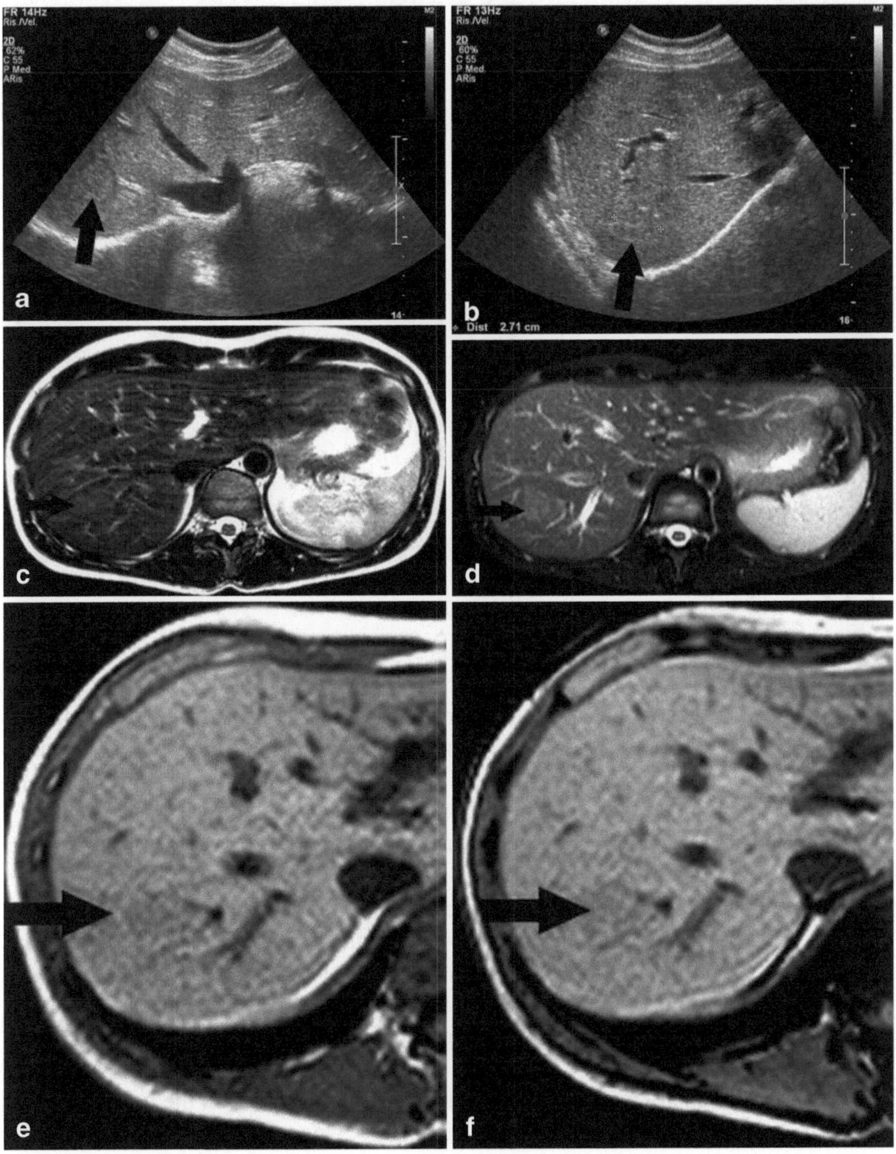

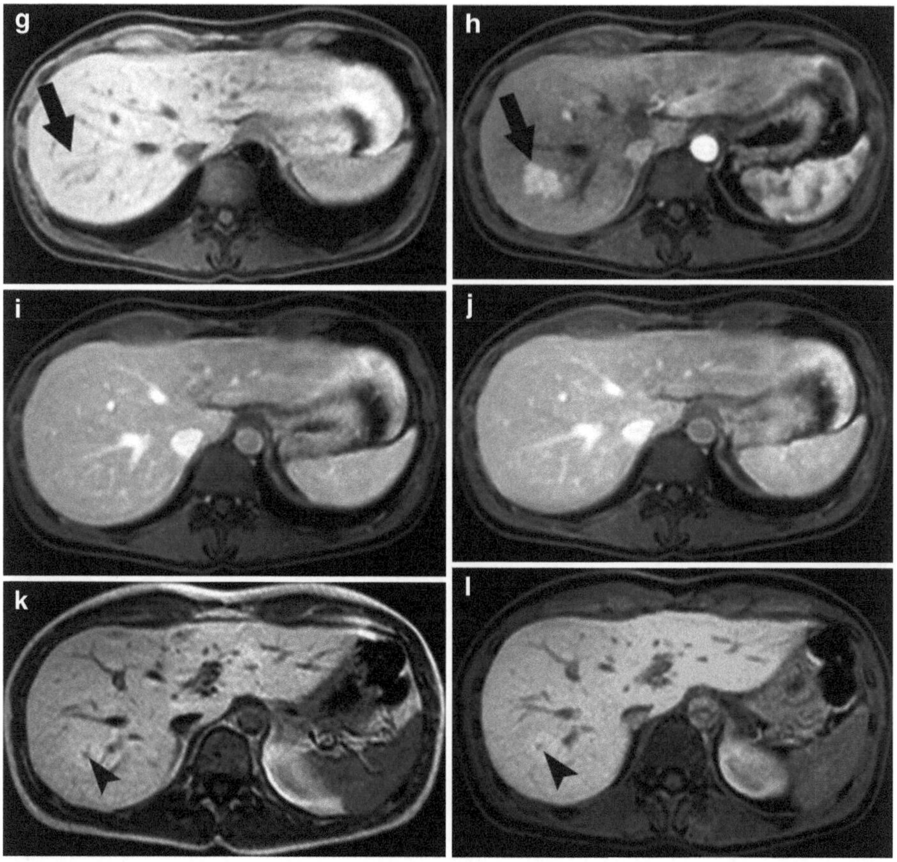

Fig. 6.4 (continued)

- Typical findings at *MRI* include iso- or hypointensity on T1-weighted sequences (90–100 % of cases) and slight hyperintensity or isointensity on T2-weighted sequences (99–100 % of cases) with homogeneous signal intensity. The central scar is bright on T2-weighted images, due to the presence of vascular channels, bile ductules, and myxomatous tissue; furthermore, delayed contrast enhancement of the scar is a characteristic feature, due to the progressive accumulation of contrast material in the fibrotic tissue. After the administration of intravenous gadolinium, FNH demonstrates intense and homogeneous contrast enhancement progressively fading in the portal-venous and delayed phases. Prominent peripheral draining veins or a dominant draining vein may be observed surrounding the lesion on equilibrium phase images. Hepatocyte-specific contrast agents are helpful in the diagnosis of FNH and in particular in the differential diagnosis with hepatic adenoma. In fact liver-specific MR contrast materials result in homogeneous hyperintensity in comparison to the surrounding liver on the hepatospecific phase, due to the presence of functioning hepatocytes and biliary ductules. On the contrary, the scar appears hypointense in the hepatobiliary phase [6, 7, 14, 16, 17].

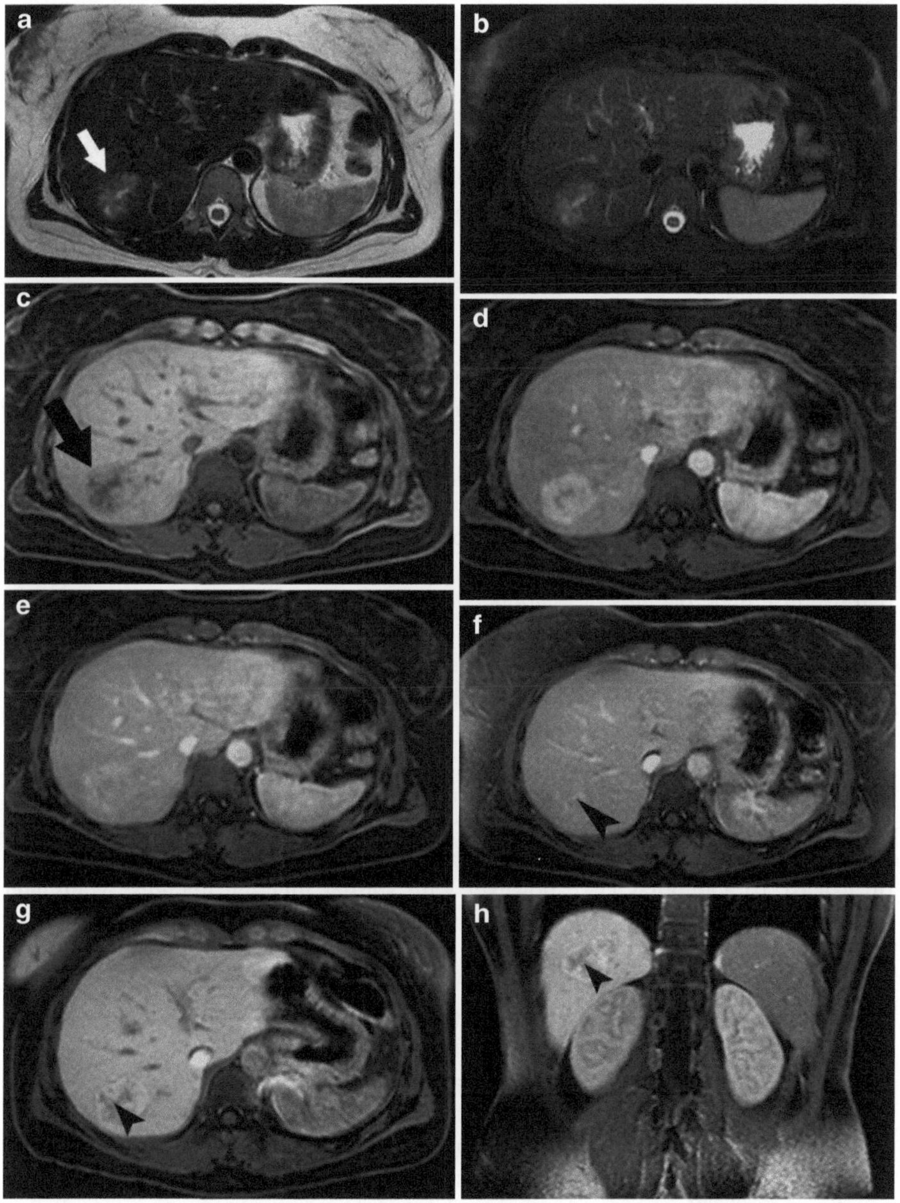

Fig. 6.5 A typical FNH with prominent central scar in a young woman. The incidentally discovered mass is slightly hyperintense on T2-weighted imaging with and without fat signal suppression (*white arrow*, **a**, **b**) with a more hyperintense star-shaped central scar. On the dynamic study with a hepatocyte-specific contrast agent, the (*black arrow* in the basal T1w image, **c**) tumor presents avid enhancement (**d**) that homogenizes to that of the normal liver in the portal-venous phase (**e**). The scar, initially hypointense on T1-weighted images with fat suppression (**c**), gets progressively filled in with the contrast agent and becomes hyperintense (*arrowhead*, **f**) about 5 min after its administration, probably due to the slow accumulation of gadolinium in the hypovascular interstitium. On the hepatobiliary phase, (**g**, **h**) the lesion results heterogeneously hyperintense with a hypointense central scar (*arrowhead*). The woman underwent periodic US surveillance

- On *CT* scans, FNH is a focal iso- or hypoattenuating mass. When present, the central scar is hypoattenuating too. Contrast-enhanced CT shows a rapid arterial enhancement in most cases (95–100 %), while at the portal-venous phase the lesion is either iso- or slightly hyperattenuating relative to a normal liver [8].
- According to the ACG guidelines [9], follow-up imaging is not required in subjects with a firm diagnosis of asymptomatic FNH. However, we believe that follow-up is prudent in patients with large or subcapsular lesions.

6.2.2 Hepatic Adenoma

Hepatic adenomas (Fig. 6.6) are rare benign tumors of well-differentiated hepatocytes lacking bile ducts or portal tracts; most of them are solitary and typically occur in female patients [17]. These hepatic lesions are characterized by dilated sinusoids and prominent arteries with poor connective tissue support, features that predispose to bleeding complications [1, 6]. Adenomatous cells may be variably filled with glycogen and fat, giving MRI a superior diagnostic performance due to contrast resolution and tissue distinction capability compared with CT [11]. Oral contraceptive use in female patients or anabolic steroid use in male patients is associated to hepatic adenomas development or to rapid modifications in their size, often causing acute bleeding [4, 18]. Hepatic adenomas are classified histologically in four subtypes: HNF1-α inactivated and telangiectatic/inflammatory represent the vast majority, while β-catenin-mutated and unclassified adenomas are very uncommon; each subtype may present peculiar, even not specific, morphologic aspects. For example, HNF1-α-inactivated adenomas have a prevalent fat composition, while telangiectatic/inflammatory adenomas are characterized by a strong vascularization [16]. Hepatic adenomatosis is probably a separate condition characterized by the presence of at least 10 adenomas [19], however with similar imaging features. Malignant degeneration to hepatocellular carcinoma accounts for about 5 % of adenomas [20].

- At *ultrasound* hepatic adenomas correspond to very homogeneous hyperechoic lesions due to fat content, with central or peripheral Doppler signal [3, 16]; Doppler signal is usually absent in HNF1-α-inactivated adenomas and is more characteristic of telangiectatic/inflammatory adenomas that present stronger vascularization and may mimic the presence of central arteries complicating the differential diagnosis with FNH. However, this subtype of hepatic adenomas presents specific findings at *CEUS*, such as arterial hypervascularity with centripetal filling, linear vascularities, peripheral rim of sustained enhancement, and central washout in the late venous phase [16].
- At *MRI* they are generally well circumscribed, without contour lobulation, and have variable degrees of hemorrhage, necrosis, fat, and, rarely, calcification [17]. Adenomas are hyperintense to isointense on T1-weighted images and slightly hyperintense on T2-weighted images [17]. The striking finding is a diffuse and homogeneous signal dropout on opposed-phase T1-weighted sequences due to the presence of microscopic fat, which is detectable in about a half of hepatic

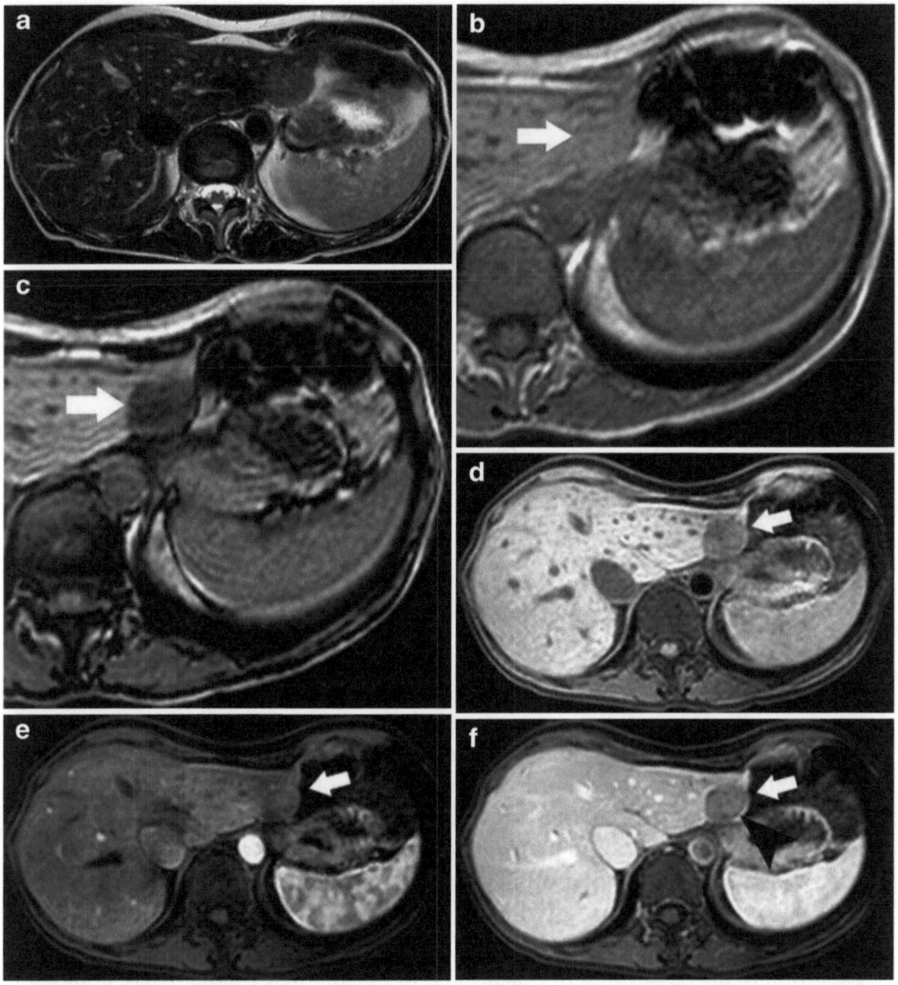

Fig. 6.6 Hepatic adenoma in an adult woman. The tumor is easily detectable on unenhanced T2-weighted images (*black arrow*, **a**) as a slightly hyperintense exophytic mass of the left lobe. The lesion shows a hyperintense signal on the "in-phase" T1-weighted images (*white arrow*, **b**) with a marked dropout of the MR signal on the corresponding "out-of-phase" images (*white arrow*, **c**), due to the presence of intracellular fat, a typical feature of HNF1-α-inactivated benign adenomas. On the pre-contrast T1w fat-suppresed image, the lesion (*arrow*, **d**) is hypointense and during the arterial phase (**e**) it demonstrates moderate and heterogeneous enhancement with a kind of pseudocapsule in the portal-venous and equilibrium phases (*arrows*, **f**, **g**). In these phases, the lesion appears mainly hypointense compared to the liver. On delayed-phase T1-weighted and T1-weighted fat-suppressed images (**h**, **i**), the lesion remains hypointense (*black arrow*), being composed of hepatocytes lacking connection to portal tracts and bile ducts. The lesion was detected during imaging follow-up in a patient that underwent a previous hepatic resection for an adenoma located in the V segment; in this case, no surgical resection was suggested and the patient continued periodic imaging monitoring

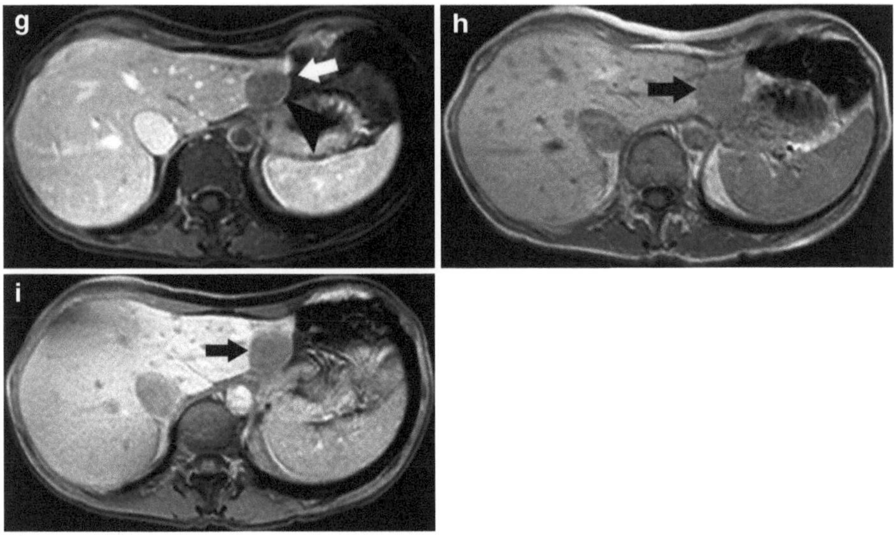

Fig. 6.6 (continued)

adenomas [21] and in 93 % of HNF1-α-inactivated adenomas [16]. Dynamic imaging with extracellular contrast agent demonstrates moderate enhancement on arterial phase images; the adenoma may show washout and enhancement similar to that of surrounding liver parenchyma on portal-venous and delayed-phase images, with or without a delayed-enhancing pseudocapsule [17, 22]. The lack of bile ducts and portal tracts of adenomas gives them a typical hypointense aspect on hepatobiliary phase imaging with hepatocyte-specific contrast agents [23]. However, peripheral or faint diffuse enhancement has been reported in some cases due to some hepatocytes maintaining the capability of uptake and excretion in the hepatobiliary phase [17]. In hepatic MR exams where contrast is contraindicated, *DWI* may increase the detection rate of focal liver lesions and diagnostic confidence in the differential diagnosis, even if benign lesions such as adenomas and focal nodular hyperplasia may have restricted diffusion with overlapping values to regenerative nodules, dysplastic nodules, HCC, and metastases [24]. However, an actual cutoff ADC value to distinguish benign tumors from malignancies in patients with solid lesions is not achievable due to interindividual and platform variability [25].

- On unenhanced *CT* scans, strong hypoattenuation is typical of fat-containing adenomas, while the presence of arterial enhancement and washout in the dynamic study is extremely variable. Telangiectatic/inflammatory adenomas are hypoattenuating and often heterogeneous, with hyperattenuating areas in relation to recent bleeding. The characteristic lesion behavior of this specific type of adenoma on multiphasic examination is a strong arterial enhancement (93 %) and a persistent enhancement in the delayed phase (96 %) [16].

- As recently published in the ACG guidelines [9], asymptomatic hepatocellular adenoma < 5 cm should be managed conservatively through CT or MRI at 6 to 12 months intervals; the duration of monitoring is based on growth pattern and stability of lesion over time. On the contrary, asymptomatic hepatocellular adenoma > 5 cm requires surgical or non surgical intervention as there is a risk of rupture or malignancy. In addition to this, hepatocellular adenomas of the β-catenin subtype should be considered for early referral for resection as malignant transformation is seen most frequently in this subtype, occurring in up to 5–10 % of cases [9].

6.2.3 Regenerative Nodules/Nodular Regenerative Hyperplasia

Regenerative nodules typically arise in livers with chronic disease and may have malignant potential, being considered one of the steps of hepatocarcinogenesis. Indeed these lesions are frequently detected during US screening for HCC and require further investigation with contrast-enhanced multiphasic CT or DCE-MRI [15]. On pre-contrast *MRI* acquisitions, regenerative nodules are homogeneous and appear isointense on T1-weighted images and iso- to hypointense on T2-weighted sequences depending on the presence or absence of glycogen and iron deposits in the nodules. They also appear hypointense compared to the surrounding parenchyma which presents high T2 signal intensity due to inflammation. Regenerative nodules normally accumulate MR liver-specific contrast agents. Hyperintense areas inside hypointense nodules may suggest the presence of high-grade dysplasia or hepatocellular carcinoma with the so-called nodule-in-nodule appearance [15, 6]. Non-enhanced *CT* detects regenerative nodules when they are surrounded by hypodense fibrotic bands or when they accumulate iron; siderotic regenerative nodules are typically hyperattenuating to the liver on non-enhanced CT and are isoattenuating to the liver after contrast injection [26]. On dynamic studies with *US*, *CT*, and *MR* examinations, regenerative nodules are usually hypovascular as they have portal blood supply; hypervascularity may suggest degeneration to malignancy [26]. *Diffusion-weighted imaging* seems to improve the detection rate of focal liver lesions also in the cirrhotic liver; however, there is no evidence yet that DWI and the derived ADC (apparent diffusion coefficient) values may be used to differentiate benign regenerative nodules from dysplastic nodules and hepatocellular carcinomas [27].

Nodular regenerative hyperplasia is an uncommon benign hepatic entity characterized by the presence of multiple diffuse regenerative nodules. This condition is associated with various diseases such as Budd-Chiari syndrome, myeloproliferative syndromes, lymphoproliferative syndromes, and collagen vascular disorders and with drugs such as immunosuppressive or antineoplastic medications [4].

References

1. Lewis RB, Lattin GE Jr, Makhlouf HR, Levy AD (2010) Tumors of the liver and intrahepatic bile ducts: radiologic-pathologic correlation. Magn Reson Imaging Clin N Am 18(3):587–609. doi:10.1016/j.mric.2010.08.010, xii
2. Semelka RC, Martin DR, Balci NC (2005) Focal lesions in normal liver. J Gastroenterol Hepatol 20(10):1478–1487. doi:10.1111/j.1440-1746.2005.03854.x
3. Bartolotta TV, Taibbi A, Midiri M, Lagalla R (2009) Focal liver lesions: contrast-enhanced ultrasound. Abdom Imaging 34(2):193–209. doi:10.1007/s00261-008-9378-6
4. Bonder A, Afdhal N (2012) Evaluation of liver lesions. Clin Liver Dis 16(2):271–283. doi:10.1016/j.cld.2012.03.001
5. Dietrich CF, Sharma M, Gibson RN, Schreiber-Dietrich D, Jenssen C (2013) Fortuitously discovered liver lesions. World J Gastroenterol 19(21):3173–3188. doi:10.3748/wjg.v19.i21.3173
6. Bartolozzi C, Cioni D, Donati F, Lencioni R (2001) Focal liver lesions: MR imaging-pathologic correlation. Eur Radiol 11(8):1374–1388
7. Heiken JP (2007) Distinguishing benign from malignant liver tumours. Cancer Imaging 7(Spec No A):S1–S14. doi:10.1102/1470-7330.2007.9084
8. Semelka RC (2005) Hepatic imaging. Radiol Clin North Am 43(5):xi. doi:10.1016/j.rcl.2005.07.006
9. Marrero JA, Ahn J, Reddy KR (2014) ACG Clinical Guideline: The Diagnosis and Management of Focal Liver Lesions, Am J Gastroenterol. 109(9):1328–1347. doi:10.1038/ajg.2014.213
10. Alobaidi M, Shirkhoda A (2004) Malignant cystic and necrotic liver lesions: a pattern approach to discrimination. Curr Probl Diagn Radiol 33(6):254–268. doi:10.1067/j.cpradiol.2004.08.002
11. Prasad SR, Wang H, Rosas H, Menias CO, Narra VR, Middleton WD et al (2005) Fat-containing lesions of the liver: radiologic-pathologic correlation. Radiographics 25(2):321–331. doi:10.1148/rg.252045083
12. Valls C, Iannacconne R, Alba E, Murakami T, Hori M, Passariello R et al (2006) Fat in the liver: diagnosis and characterization. Eur Radiol 16(10):2292–2308. doi:10.1007/s00330-006-0146-0
13. van den Bos IC, Hussain SM, de Man RA, Zondervan PE, Ijzermans JN, Preda A et al (2008) Magnetic resonance imaging of liver lesions: exceptions and atypical lesions. Curr Probl Diagn Radiol 37(3):95–103. doi:10.1067/j.cpradiol.2007.07.002
14. Marin D, Brancatelli G, Federle MP, Lagalla R, Catalano C, Passariello R et al (2008) Focal nodular hyperplasia: typical and atypical MRI findings with emphasis on the use of contrast media. Clin Radiol 63(5):577–585. doi:10.1016/j.crad.2007.06.011
15. Op de Beeck B, Luypaert R, Dujardin M, Osteaux M (1999) Benign liver lesions: differentiation by magnetic resonance. Eur J Radiol 32(1):52–60
16. Ronot M, Vilgrain V (2014) Imaging of benign hepatocellular lesions: current concepts and recent updates. Clin Res Hepatol Gastroenterol 38(6):681–8. doi:10.1016/j.clinre.2014.01.014
17. Campos JT, Sirlin CB, Choi JY (2012) Focal hepatic lesions in Gd-EOB-DTPA enhanced MRI: the atlas. Insights Imaging 3(5):451–474. doi:10.1007/s13244-012-0179-7
18. Goodwin MD, Dobson JE, Sirlin CB, Lim BG, Stella DL (2011) Diagnostic challenges and pitfalls in MR imaging with hepatocyte-specific contrast agents. Radiographics 31(6):1547–1568. doi:10.1148/rg.316115528
19. Flejou JF, Barge J, Menu Y, Degott C, Bismuth H, Potet F et al (1985) Liver adenomatosis. An entity distinct from liver adenoma? Gastroenterology 89(5):1132–1138
20. Cogley JR, Miller FH (2014) MR imaging of benign focal liver lesions. Radiol Clin North Am 52(4):657–682. doi:10.1016/j.rcl.2014.02.005
21. Martin DR, Danrad R, Hussain SM (2005) MR imaging of the liver. Radiol Clin North Am 43(5):861–886. doi:10.1016/j.rcl.2005.05.001, viii

22. Khosa F, Khan AN, Eisenberg RL (2011) Hypervascular liver lesions on MRI. Am J Roentgenol 197(2):W204–W220. doi:10.2214/ajr.10.5382
23. Hwang HS, Kim SH, Jeon TY, Choi D, Lee WJ, Lim HK (2009) Hypointense hepatic lesions depicted on gadobenate dimeglumine-enhanced three-hour delayed hepatobiliary-phase MR imaging: differentiation between benignancy and malignancy. Korean J Radiol 10(3):294–302. doi:10.3348/kjr.2009.10.3.294
24. Miller FH, Hammond N, Siddiqi AJ, Shroff S, Khatri G, Wang Y et al (2010) Utility of diffusion-weighted MRI in distinguishing benign and malignant hepatic lesions. J Magn Reson Imaging 32(1):138–147. doi:10.1002/jmri.22235
25. Sasaki M, Yamada K, Watanabe Y, Matsui M, Ida M, Fujiwara S et al (2008) Variability in absolute apparent diffusion coefficient values across different platforms may be substantial: a multivendor, multi-institutional comparison study. Radiology 249(2):624–630. doi:10.1148/radiol.2492071681
26. Brancatelli G, Federle MP, Ambrosini R, Lagalla R, Carriero A, Midiri M et al (2007) Cirrhosis: CT and MR imaging evaluation. Eur J Radiol 61(1):57–69. doi:10.1016/j.ejrad.2006.11.003
27. Lee JM, Choi BI (2011) Hepatocellular nodules in liver cirrhosis: MR evaluation. Abdom Imaging 36(3):282–289. doi:10.1007/s00261-011-9692-2

Differential Diagnosis of Benign Liver Tumors

7

Francesco De Cobelli, Paolo Marra, Gabriele Ironi, Antonio Esposito, and Alessandro Del Maschio

7.1 Principles of Differential Diagnosis

As the availability of imaging modalities such as US, MRI, and CT has grown in recent years, the incidental detection of liver lesions has increased consequently. Indeed, the diagnosis of a liver mass usually occurs in asymptomatic patients and does not require any treatment. In most cases the correct diagnosis of a benign liver lesion is achieved noninvasively, on the basis of epidemiology, anamnestic data, clinical background, and imaging features. Rarely a biopsy or a surgical procedure is necessary, especially when a lesion shows a nontypical imaging pattern and the patient presents with chronic liver disease or a known malignancy.

7.1.1 Age and Sex: Congenital and Acquired Liver Lesions

Liver masses in children are often of vascular origin such as infantile hepatic hemangioma (IHH), rapidly involuting congenital hemangioma (RICH), and noninvoluting congenital hemangioma [1]. In most cases, these are congenital lesions that tend to spontaneously regress, while rarely they present as large liver tumors with cardiac function impairment due to important arteriovenous shunting [9]. When such complications are not present, a US follow-up may be sufficient. Another benign lesion that can be detected in children is mesenchymal hamartoma which has a cystic or multicystic appearance [9]. Hepatic adenoma is a rare diagnosis in the pediatric population; when present, it may suggest underlying pathologies such as glycogen storage disease or Fanconi anemia. Imaging features of adenoma in children do not significantly differ from those found in adults [9]. When dealing

F. De Cobelli (✉) • P. Marra • G. Ironi • A. Esposito • A. Del Maschio
Department of Radiology, San Raffaele Hospital, Via Olgettina, 60, 20132 Milan, Italy
e-mail: decobelli.francesco@hsr.it; Marra.paolo@hsr.it; Ironi.gabriele@hsr.it

L. Aldrighetti et al. (eds.), *Benign Tumors of the Liver*,
DOI 10.1007/978-3-319-12985-3_7

with children, it is particularly important to rule out the presence of hepatoblastoma, hepatocellular carcinoma, or other malignancies that may infiltrate the liver from the surrounding structure (e.g., the kidney).

When dealing with young women, the most commonly encountered liver lesions, in addition to hemangiomas, are focal nodular hyperplasia and hepatic adenomas. The last are known to be associated to oral contraceptive assumption. The condition in which hepatic adenomas are 10 or more is called adenomatosis, and its relationship with oral contraceptive therapy has been demonstrated too [13]. In most cases, an initial diagnosis with US should be confirmed with MRI for a better characterization of the tumor, while follow-up can be carried out with US; CT should be avoided due to the issue of ionizing radiations.

Hepatic cysts are commonly found at any age with a prevalence of about 2–7 % in the population. A particular congenital condition is the autosomal dominant polycystic disease which is a familial disorder associated to multiple hepatic and renal cysts, often with chronic renal failure [6].

7.1.2 Clinical Background

Before diagnosis, it is fundamental to take into account the clinical background of the patient. A first distinction regards the presence of a normal or a cirrhotic liver. Cirrhosis is caused by congenital or acquired conditions that cause continuous cycles of hepatocyte death and regeneration: in this pathological context, liver structure may become nodular, and it may be difficult to distinguish benign lesions from regenerative nodules and hepatocellular carcinomas. Causes of cirrhosis are hemochromatosis, glycogen storage disorders, biliary atresia, infantile cholestasis, hepatitis, hereditary tyrosinemia, α1-antitrypsin deficiency, porphyria cutanea tarda, Wilson disease, and chronic alcohol consumption [9, 10]. Infections or systemic inflammatory diseases cause liver abscesses and granulomas that usually show typical aspects at liver imaging: provenance and eating habits of patients may suggest an eventual parasitic infection.

Clinical parameters such as inflammatory markers, cholestasis, and liver necrosis markers should be always evaluated.

7.1.3 Clinical Presentation

Liver lesions are usually detected as incidental findings in patients undergoing evaluation for unrelated symptoms. Rarely, large lesions may cause pain in the abdomen or right upper quadrant secondary to stretching of the liver capsule. Compression symptoms from left lobe lesions, such as early satiety, are uncommon. Clinical signs may include hepatomegaly, fever of unknown origin, abnormal liver function tests, and jaundice [2, 6].

7.1.4 Oncologic Patients

Oncologic patients represent a particular diagnostic dilemma because in these subjects a detected liver lesion with atypical aspect should be considered malignant until proven otherwise (Fig. 7.1). The liver indeed is the most common target of metastatic disease, and accurate detection and characterization of FLLs is prognostically fundamental as it can help to identify patients who are most likely to benefit from liver surgery. As many FLLs in these patients are benign, a precise and preferably noninvasive method to distinguish them from malignant metastatic nodules is needed [11]. However, the lower sensitivity of ultrasound in the detection of focal liver malignancies compared to CT and MR should be considered when dealing with patients with high probability of liver metastatic disease [17]. Furthermore the US detection of a previously unknown lesion in oncologic patients, even with benign features, gives rise to the suspicion of metastatic disease that may need further investigation or restaging with contrast-enhanced CT or MR.

7.2 Benign Lesions That May Mimic Liver Neoplasm

7.2.1 Liver Abscess

Liver abscesses (Fig. 7.2) present as single or multiple lesions of variable sizes, even coalescing. Imaging is fundamental for diagnosis and may eventually guide percutaneous drainage. The use of intravenous contrast is vital since hepatic abscesses have a typical appearance. On multiphasic *CT*, they consist in centrally hypodense (due to purulent necrosis) lesions frequently associated to peripheral enhancing rims; the core is usually hypovascular. Thin-section imaging during the portal-venous phase can optimize detection of small lesions and air bubbles [15]. Fungal abscesses typically manifest as microabscesses that involve the liver, spleen, and occasionally kidneys. They are usually multiple, small (2–20 mm), round, and hypodense with or without peripheral enhancement. A peripheral hypodense zone representing edema may be seen, along with septations and fluid-debris levels [15].

US offers a prompt evaluation of the probable abdominal source of infection (cholecystitis, appendicitis, or diverticulitis) and the biliary tract [6]. At *US* liver abscesses are usually solid lesion with variable echogenicity acutely, but with maturation, pus formation, necrosis, and liquefaction, they tend to become hypoechoic with distinct margins [17]; in case of gas-producing organisms, US shows intense echogenicity with posterior reverberations [5]. At *color Doppler sonography*, liver abscesses are centrally avascular, usually with some peripheral flow corresponding to areas of contrast enhancement at CEUS [4].

At *MRI* liver abscesses present central low T1w signal and intermediate to slightly hyperintense heterogeneous T2w signal; the abscess wall enhances on the

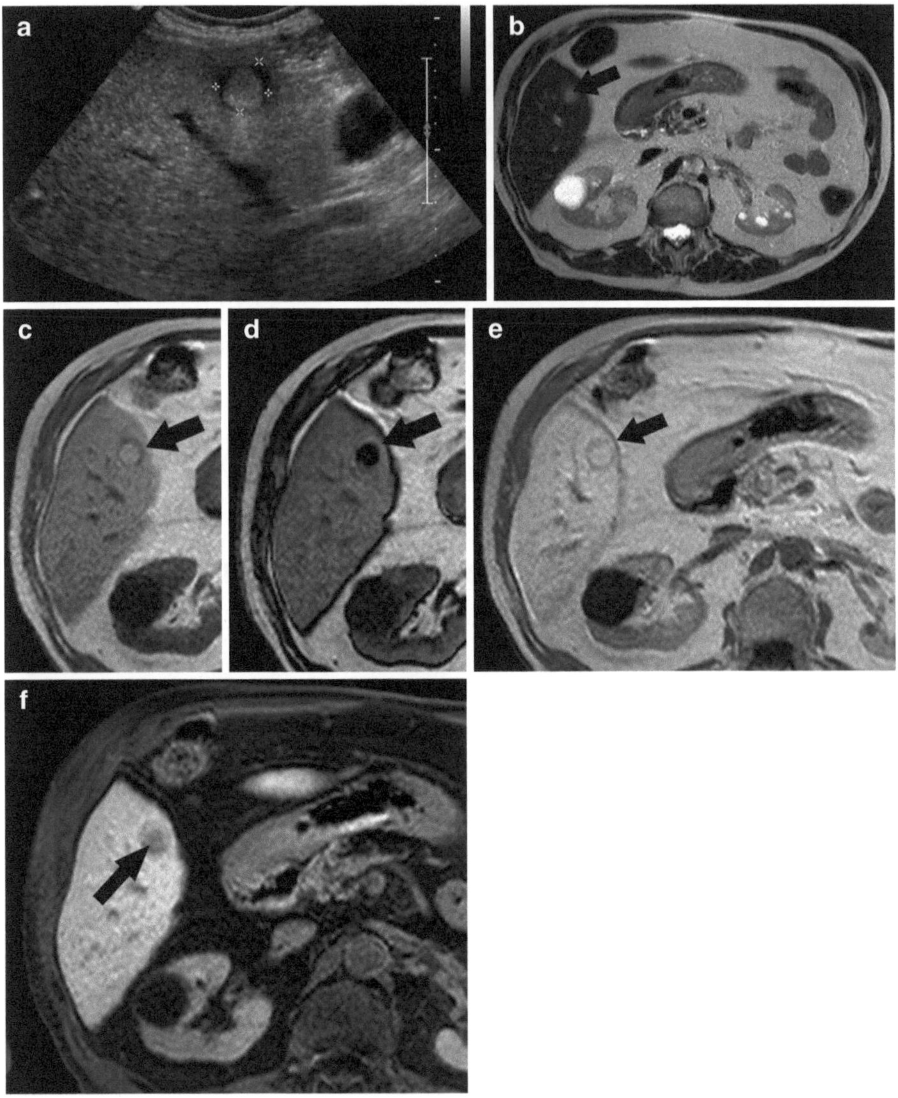

Fig. 7.1 Atypical hepatocellular carcinoma in a patient with chronic liver disease and a previous hepatic resection for HCC. At US screening, an isoechoic nodule with an hypoechoic halo (**a**) was detected, and the patient was referred for MRI with hepatocyte-specific contrast agent (Gd-EOB-DTPA) to characterize the lesion. On T2-weighted images, (**b**) the nodule is slightly hyperintense with blurred margins (*black arrow*), probably due to peritumor edema; on chemical shift imaging, the lesion presents a dropout of the signal in the opposite-phase sequences (**c**, in phase; **d**, out of phase), as being predominantly composed of intracellular fat. At the dynamic study (not shown), the tumor is hypovascular. On hepatobiliary phase T1-weighted images without fat suppression, the lesion is isointense (*black arrow*, **e**) simulating the presence of functional hepatocytes; however, the fat-saturated sequence (**f**) reveals marked hypointensity of the nodule, consistent with fat infiltration and loss of hepatocellular function. In relation to a nontypical imaging pattern and to the clinical history, the patient was referred to fine-needle biopsy of the lesion that resulted a moderately differentiated HCC at histology

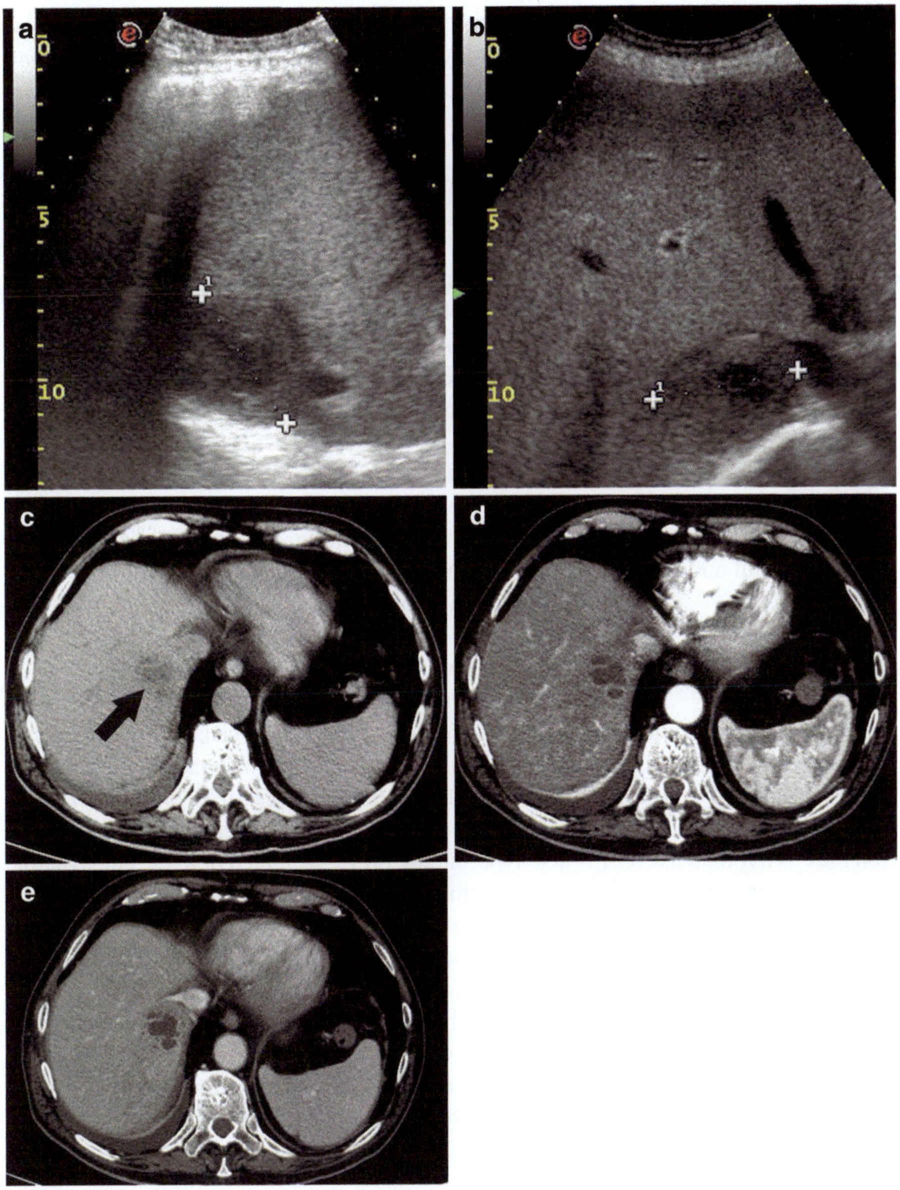

Fig. 7.2 A 72-year-old man with a hepatic pyogenic abscess. The patient was examined with liver ultrasound for abdominal pain in the upper right quadrant. A heterogeneous hypoechoic lesion with ill-defined margins and hypoechoic core was noted (**a**, **b**). A contrast-enhanced CT scan was requested to better investigate the lesion and to rule out the presence of source of infection or malignancies. On an unenhanced CT scan, (**c**) the lesion is heterogeneously hypodense (*black arrow*); a peripheral rim enhancement is seen on the arterial and portal phase images (respectively **d** and **e**) after administration of contrast media. At the dynamic study, the lesion shows also the typical "cluster sign," consistent with abscess; no source of infection (e.g., diverticulitis, cholecystitis) was found. Due to the small dimensions of the lesions, no percutaneous drainage was indicated and the patient assumed antibiotic therapy with complete remission of symptoms

arterial phase and generally intensifies on the interstitial phase on postcontrast T1w sequences. Perilesional enhancement may be seen due to hyperemic inflammatory reaction in the adjacent liver [16]. Fungal abscesses appear as low signal foci on gadolinium-enhanced T1 images, characterized by minimal appreciable rim enhancement. The absence of granulation tissue in the capsule is most likely related to the neutropenia of immunocompromised patients [15].

Echinococcal abscesses (hydatid cysts) present as spherical cystic lesions, with fibrous rims and well-defined margins. Typically, there is little tissue reaction, unless the cyst breaks and leaks fluid that can induce a marked inflammatory reaction: heterogeneous high T2 and low T1 signal is due to internal proteinaceous fluids. The enhancing wall, seen on postcontrast T1w images, is usually thin. Coarse calcifications of the wall are present in 50 % of cases and are better identified with *CT*. Daughter cysts or septations are found in approximately 75 % of patients [12].

Tuberculosis is globally the most common cause of infectious hepatic granulomas that present with variable signal intensity on basal T1w and T2w sequences and minimal enhancement. Lesions tend to involve the portal triad and are associated to enlarged portal and retroperitoneal lymph nodes [16].

7.2.2 Other Inflammatory Masses

Focal hypereosinophilic infiltration is a focal hepatic lesion caused by eosinophil-related tissue damage, associated with various conditions such as parasitic infections, allergic reactions, hypereosinophilic syndrome, and tumors. It is characterized by indistinct margin and a nonspherical shape. At MRI a focal hypereosinophilic infiltration mass is hypointense on T1- and hyperintense on T2-weighted images. The dynamic imaging is characterized by poor enhancement on the arterial phase with homogeneous enhancement on portal-venous phase images. A predominant hypointensity characterizes the hepatobiliary phase of liver-specific contrast agents at MRI [8].

Inflammatory pseudotumor (Fig. 7.3) is a very rare entity characterized by an inflammatory infiltrate usually of undetermined nature, composed of plasma cells, histiocytes, and fibrosis [3, 4]. It presents with nonspecific clinical symptoms (fever, weight loss, and leukocytosis) or may be detected incidentally. Due to its rarity and its atypical imaging features, a percutaneous biopsy should be performed to rule out the presence of malignancy.

7.3 Miscellanea

7.3.1 Post-traumatic Lesions

Surgery and trauma are the two most common causes of intrahepatic bleeding. On *CT*, the appearance of an intrahepatic hemorrhage changes progressively with time. In an acute or subacute setting, hemorrhage has a higher attenuation value than pure fluid due to the presence of aggregated fibrin components. In chronic cases, a hematoma has an attenuation identical to that of pure fluid. Because of the paramagnetic

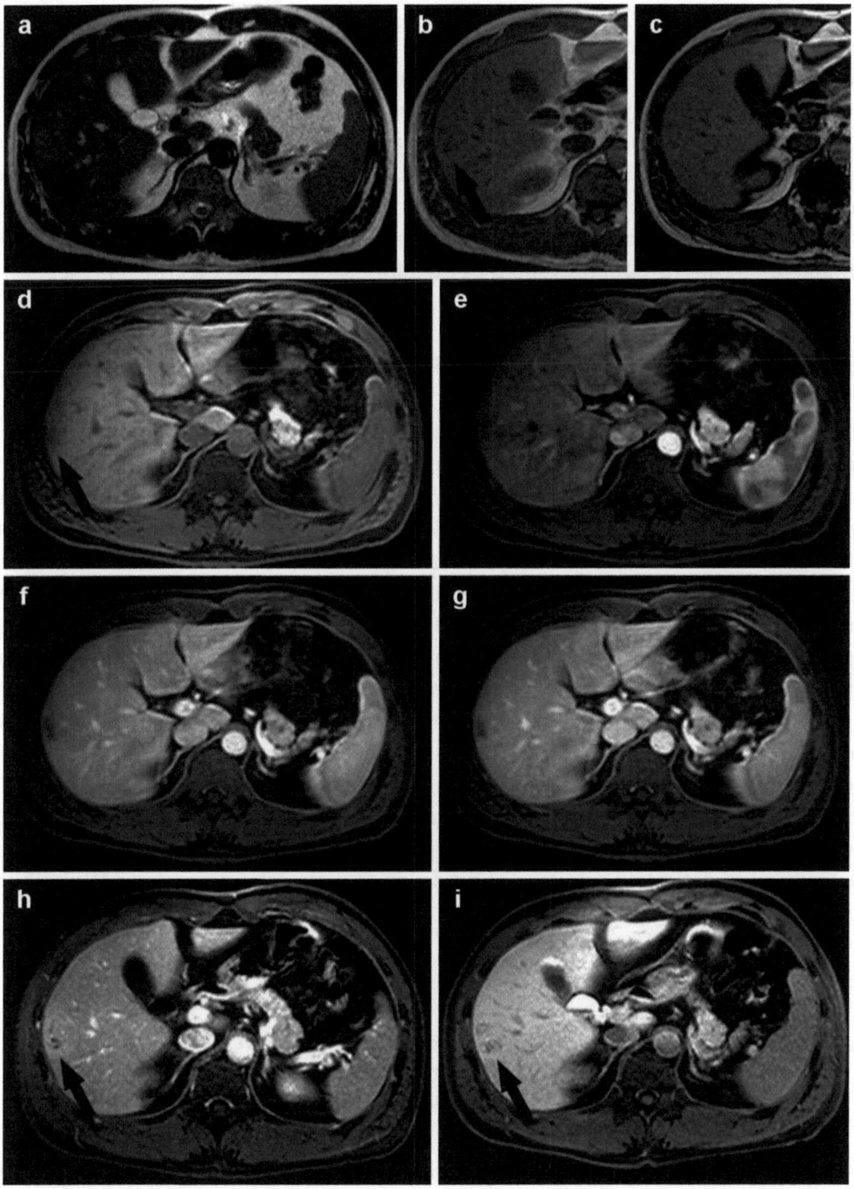

Fig. 7.3 Inflammatory pseudotumor in a young Asian male. On the pre-contrast T2-weighted image, (**a**) a slightly hyperintense lesion in the right lobe is visible (*black arrow*). On both the corresponding pre-contrast T1-weighted in-phase (*arrow*, **b**) and out-of-phase (**c**) images, the lesion is hypointense with no signal variation due to chemical shift artifact. The tumor is hardly seen on basal T1w images (*black arrow*, **d**); some early peripheral enhancement (**e**) is seen after bolus injection of contrast agent, reflecting the cellular components and inflammatory changes within the lesion. However, the lesion shows poor vascularity with slow accumulation of contrast agent (during portal and venous phases, respectively **f** and **g**) in probably fibrotic components that become hyperintense in T1 fat-suppressed images (*arrow*, **h**) acquired 5 min post-contrast injection. Hepatobiliary phase imaging (**i**) reveals a hypointense area representing the absence of functioning hepatocytes within the lesion (*arrow*). The patient underwent percutaneous fine-needle biopsy that confirmed the diagnosis of inflammatory pseudotumor

effect of methemoglobin, *MRI* is even more suitable than CT for the detection and characterization of hemorrhage. A subacute hematoma appears as a heterogeneous mass with pathognomonic high signal intensity on T1-weighted images and intermediate signal intensity on T2-weighted images [12].

Bilomas result from rupture of the biliary system, which can be spontaneous, traumatic, or iatrogenic. Extravasation of bile into the liver parenchyma generates an intense inflammatory reaction, thereby inducing formation of a well-defined pseudocapsule. At both CT and MR imaging, a biloma usually appears as a well-defined or slightly irregular cystic mass without septa or calcifications [12].

7.3.2 Focal Steatosis and Focal Fatty Sparing Areas

Focal (Fig. 7.4) or multifocal (Fig. 7.5) steatosis is a common finding that can present with a pseudotumor hyperechoic appearance at *US*, hypodense on *CT*; however, its distribution is quite typical with involvement of periportal and periligamentous spaces, subcapsular areas, and gallbladder fossa [18]. On the contrary, focal fatty sparing areas in a steatotic liver appear as a hypoechoic lesion at *US*, usually with a distribution pattern similar to that of focal fatty infiltration. The topography of these lesions seems to be related to aberrant portal or venous drainage, thus justifying the similar distribution pattern of these apparently opposed conditions [18]. Other conditions in which hepatic steatosis may be observed with atypical distribution and require particular attention are the omental packing (usually posttraumatic or post-surgical) and the presence of (maybe unsuspected) metastases that alters peritumor blood flow. On *CT* the diagnosis of focal steatosis or focal fatty sparing is easy: the accumulation of fat in the liver proportionally decreases x-ray attenuation. However, the most accurate technique to correctly characterize focal steatosis or focal fatty sparing and to definitely rule out the presence of metastatic disease is *MRI* with the chemical shift imaging technique, based on the acquisition of in-phase and opposed-phase T1-weighted images [18].

7.3.3 Fibropolycystic Liver Disease (Congenital Hepatic Fibrosis, Autosomal Dominant Polycystic Disease, Bile Duct Hamartoma, Caroli Disease, Choledochal Cyst)

Patients with congenital hepatic fibrosis at *MRI* and on *CT* typically show features suggestive for liver morphologic changes and portal hypertension such as hypertrophy of the left lateral segment, hypertrophy of the left medial segment, atrophy of the right lobe, varices, splenomegaly, associated ductal plate malformations, and renal abnormalities [7]. Congenital hepatic fibrosis encompasses a spectrum of related lesions that are caused by abnormal embryologic development of the ductal plates and may be variably associated to biliary hamartomas, multiple hepatic cysts,

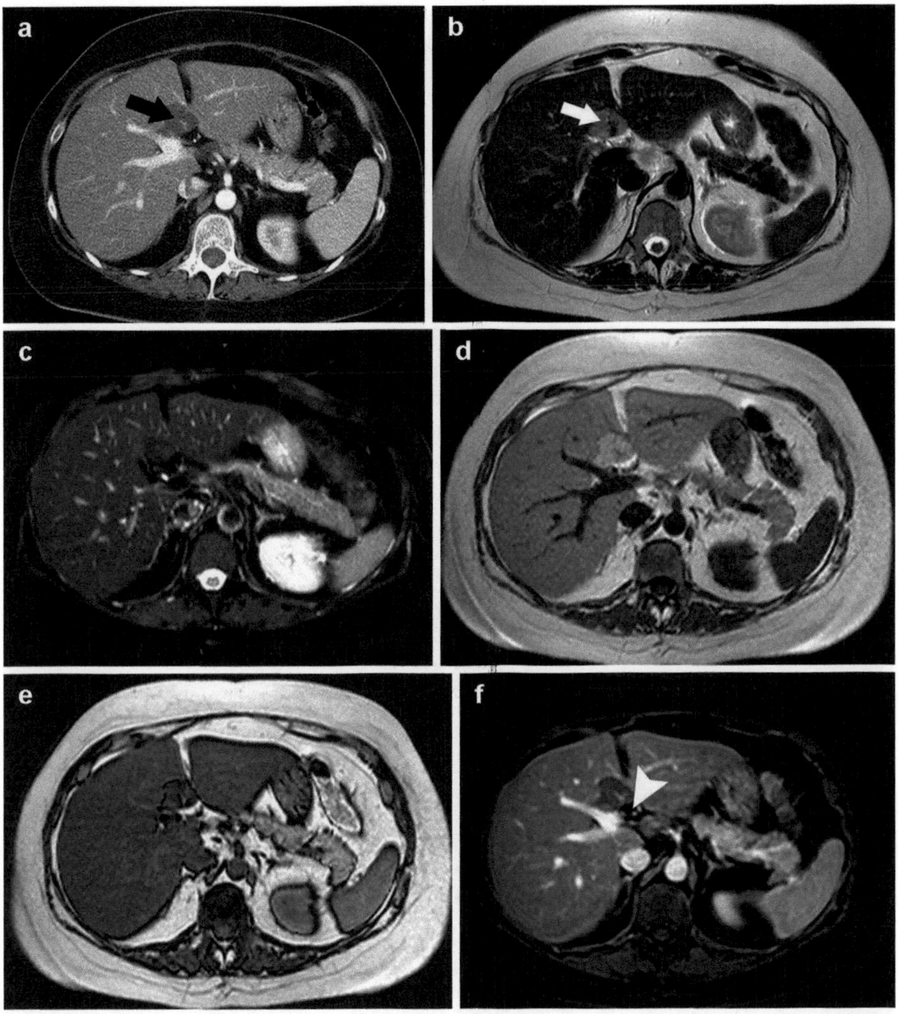

Fig. 7.4 Focal steatosis with typical location at the IV segment. On contrast-enhanced CT (**a**) a hypodense lesion (*black arrow*) was noted in a subcapsular region of the medial margin of the IV segment, adjacent to the portal vein. This finding was further investigated with an MRI study that shows a slightly hyperintense mass (*white arrow*) on T2-weighted images (**b**). The decay of the signal on both T2w fat-saturated (**c**) and T1w out-of-phase images (**e**, compared to the relative in-phase images, **d**) is consistent with a prevalent fat composition of the mass. On gadolinium-enhanced fat-suppressed T1w images (**f**) the lesion presents no enhancement with normal liver vessels coursing within (*arrowhead*). Based on imaging appearance, the presence of a tumor is safely excluded considering the typical location of the lesion (porta hepatis), the absence of mass effect, and the presence of vessels coursing within the mass [18]

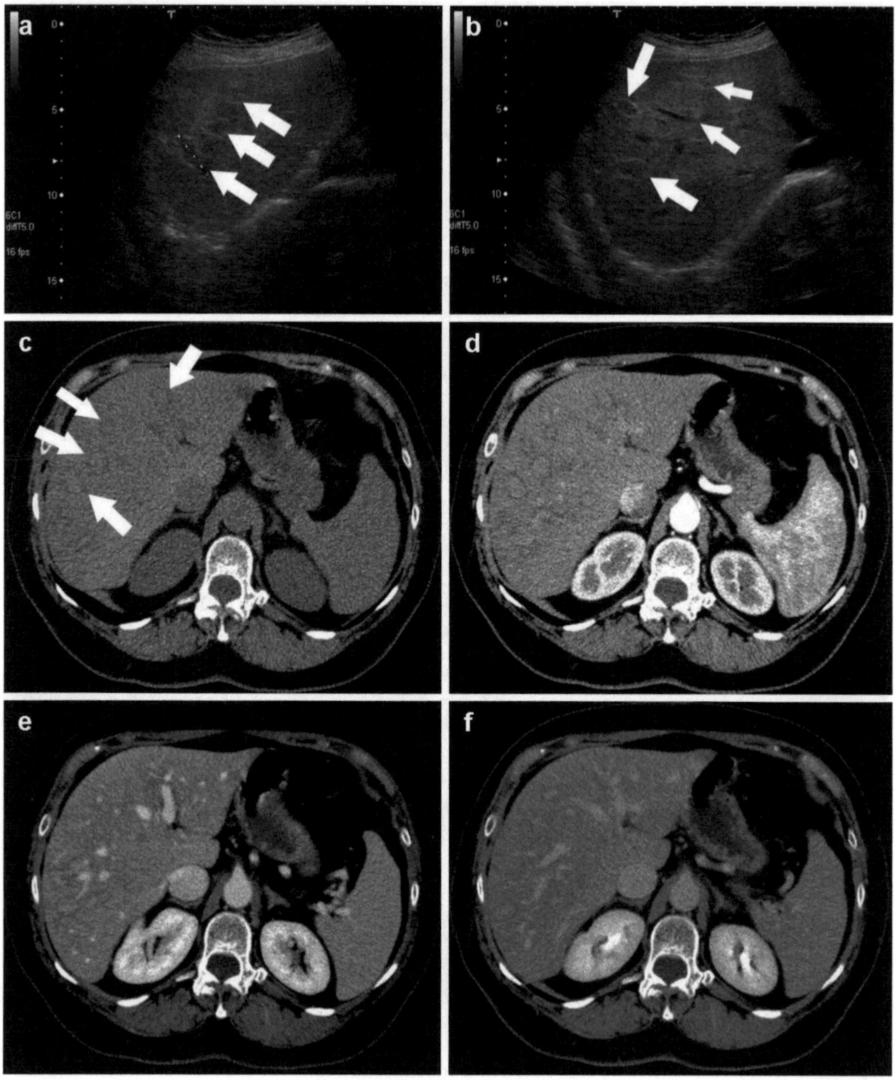

Fig. 7.5 Multifocal steatosis mimicking metastatic liver disease in a patient with breast cancer. At oncologic follow-up with abdominal ultrasound, the liver presented multiple hypoechoic nodules with hyperechoic halo (*white arrows*, **a**, **b**). This patient was further investigated with contrast-enhanced CT that confirmed the presence of isodense nodules surrounded by isodense rim (*arrows*, **c**, basal scan) with an enhancement pattern similar to that of the normal liver (**d**, arterial phase; **e**, portal-venous phase; **f**, equilibrium phase). In the suspicion of a metastatic disease, a fine-needle biopsy was taken with a definitive histological diagnosis of steatosis. The patient underwent periodical US monitoring

and dilatation of intra- or extrahepatic biliary ducts, lesions that may mimic cystic liver neoplasms or metastatic disease. Specific imaging features related to these pathologies, whose complete discussion is beyond the aim of this chapter, allow the correct diagnosis ruling out the presence of oncologic disease. Biliary hamartomas usually manifest as multiple cysts that are nearly uniform in size and measure up to 15 mm in diameter, while the autosomal dominant polycystic disease is dominated by an enlarged and diffusely cystic liver. In Caroli disease, cystic or fusiform dilatation of the intrahepatic ducts is seen, usually with the so-called central dot sign that consists in a portal vein branch protruding into the lumen of a dilated bile duct. Finally choledochal cyst manifests as a fusiform or cystic dilatation of the extrahepatic bile duct [7, 14, 19].

7.4 Differential Diagnosis with Summary Table

7.4.1 Cyst-Like Lesions

Cystic lesions are predominantly benign in nature; features that suggest a malignant potential, requiring further investigation or a strict follow-up, are the presence of internal mural nodules, coarse calcifications, and irregularities of the wall.

7.4.2 Hypovascular Lesions

Hypovascular lesions are usually considered benign until the patient has a past history of cancer. Commonly encountered hypovascular solid lesions in the normal liver include areas of focal fatty sparing and necrotic (inflammatory) nodules that should be differentiated from cholangiocarcinoma. In oncologic patients, hypovascular nodules are highly suggestive for metastatic disease.

7.4.3 Hypervascular Lesions

The differential diagnosis of hypervascular hepatic lesions in the normal liver is usually among hemangioma, focal nodular hyperplasia, adenoma, and hypervascular metastasis (usually from neuroendocrine tumors). In the presence of chronic liver disease, vascular shunts, regenerative nodules, and dysplastic nodules may be hypervascular and should be differentiated from hepatocellular carcinoma.

The table summarizes key imaging feature of the most commonly encountered benign liver tumors and tumorlike conditions

Imaging peculiarities of the most commonly detected benign liver tumors and tumorlike conditions	
	Specific imaging features at US, CT, and MR
Hepatocellular	
Focal nodular hyperplasia	Central feeding artery with a centrifugal stellate branching; central scar of vessels, bile ducts, and myxomatous tissue; avid arterial enhancement without significant washout; iso- to hyperintensity in the hepatobiliary phase at MRI with hepatocyte-specific contrast agents
Hepatic adenoma	Variable degrees of hemorrhage, necrosis, and calcification; about 50 % present with high amounts of intracellular fat that causes a significant signal dropout in "out-of-phase" T1w images; variable contrast enhancement without significant washout; sometimes equilibrium-phase enhancing pseudocapsule; hypointensity in the hepatobiliary phase at MRI with hepatocyte-specific contrast agents
Regenerative nodules	Variable content of glycogen or iron causing, respectively, T1w hyperintensity and T2w hypointensity; signal intensity should be homogeneous; hypovascular at the dynamic study; they normally accumulate hepatocyte-specific contrast agents resulting to iso- to hyperintensity in the hepatobiliary phase at MRI
Non-hepatocellular	
Hemangioma	Blood containing lesion (T2w hyperintensity at MRI, hypodensity on CT); peripheral nodular contrast enhancement proceeding centripetally with no washout; no hepatocyte-specific contrast agents uptake
Hepatic cyst	Homogeneously fluid-filled cavity with no contrast enhancement; rarely septations, lobulation, and fluid-fluid levels (due to protein or blood products)
Biliary cystadenoma	Irregular walls, septations, and coarse calcifications; contrast enhancement of the walls and septations
Angiomyolipoma	Imaging appearance depends on the proportional content of smooth muscle cells, thick-walled blood vessels, and mature adipose tissue; signal dropout on T1w "opposed-phase" or fat-saturated MR images due to micro- or macroscopic fat infiltration; progressive contrast enhancement with no washout
Tumorlike conditions	
Abscess	Imaging appearance depends on the degree of maturation (solid, necrotic fluid-filled, and cystic); single or multiple lesions often coalescing; avascular core with variable enhancing rim; septations (cluster sign) and fluid-debris levels; peripheral edema and contrast enhancement due to the inflammatory reaction in the surrounding liver
Focal steatosis Focal fatty sparing	Typical location: periportal and periligamentous spaces, subcapsular areas and gallbladder fossa, omental packing; absence of mass effect and the presence of vessels coursing within the mass; focal steatosis presents dropout of the signal in T1w "out-of-phase" images while focal fatty sparing areas show no such signal loss

References

1. Adeyiga AO, Lee EY, Eisenberg RL (2012) Focal hepatic masses in pediatric patients. AJR Am J Roentgenol 199(4):W422–W440. doi:10.2214/AJR.11.7581
2. Assy N (2009) Characteristics of common solid liver lesions and recommendations for diagnostic workup. World J Gastroenterol 15(26):3217. doi:10.3748/wjg.15.3217
3. Assy N, Nasser G, Djibre A, Beniashvili Z, Elias S, Zidan J (2009) Characteristics of common solid liver lesions and recommendations for diagnostic workup. World J Gastroenterol 15(26):3217–3227
4. Bartolotta TV, Taibbi A, Midiri M, Lagalla R (2009) Focal liver lesions: contrast-enhanced ultrasound. Abdom Imaging 34(2):193–209. doi:10.1007/s00261-008-9378-6
5. Benedetti NJ, Desser TS, Jeffrey RB (2008) Imaging of hepatic infections. Ultrasound Q 24(4):267–278. doi:10.1097/RUQ.0b013e31818e5981
6. Bonder A, Afdhal N (2012) Evaluation of liver lesions. Clin Liver Dis 16(2):271–283. doi:10.1016/j.cld.2012.03.001
7. Brancatelli G, Federle MP, Vilgrain V, Vullierme MP, Marin D, Lagalla R (2005) Fibropolycystic liver disease: CT and MR imaging findings. Radiographics 25(3):659–670. doi:10.1148/rg.253045114
8. Campos JT, Sirlin CB, Choi JY (2012) Focal hepatic lesions in Gd-EOB-DTPA enhanced MRI: the atlas. Insights Imaging 3(5):451–474. doi:10.1007/s13244-012-0179-7
9. Faingold R, Albuquerque PA, Carpineta L (2011) Hepatobiliary tumors. Radiol Clin North Am 49(4):679–687. doi:10.1016/j.rcl.2011.05.002, vi
10. Lewis RB, Lattin GE Jr, Makhlouf HR, Levy AD (2010) Tumors of the liver and intrahepatic bile ducts: radiologic-pathologic correlation. Magn Reson Imaging Clin N Am 18(3):587–609. doi:10.1016/j.mric.2010.08.010, xii
11. Morana G, Cugini C, Mucelli RP (2008) Small liver lesions in oncologic patients: characterization with CT, MRI and contrast-enhanced US. Cancer Imaging 8(Spec No A):S132–S135. doi:10.1102/1470-7330.2008.9020
12. Mortele KJ, Ros PR (2001) Cystic focal liver lesions in the adult: differential CT and MR imaging features. Radiographics 21(4):895–910. doi:10.1148/radiographics.21.4.g01jl16895
13. Ronot M, Vilgrain V (2014) Imaging of benign hepatocellular lesions: current concepts and recent updates. Clin Res Hepatol Gastroenterol 38(6):681–688. doi:10.1016/j.clinre.2014.01.014
14. Santiago I, Loureiro R, Curvo-Semedo L, Marques C, Tardaguila F, Matos C, Caseiro-Alves F (2012) Congenital cystic lesions of the biliary tree. AJR Am J Roentgenol 198(4):825–835. doi:10.2214/AJR.11.7294
15. Semelka RC (2005) Hepatic imaging. Radiol Clin North Am 43(5):xi. doi:10.1016/j.rcl.2005.07.006
16. Semelka RC, Martin DR, Balci NC (2005) Focal lesions in normal liver. J Gastroenterol Hepatol 20(10):1478–1487. doi:10.1111/j.1440-1746.2005.03854.x
17. Shin DS, Jeffrey RB, Desser TS (2010) Pearls and pitfalls in hepatic ultrasonography. Ultrasound Q 26(1):17–25. doi:10.1097/RUQ.0b013e3181ce1537
18. Valls C, Iannacconne R, Alba E, Murakami T, Hori M, Passariello R, Vilgrain V (2006) Fat in the liver: diagnosis and characterization. Eur Radiol 16(10):2292–2308. doi:10.1007/s00330-006-0146-0
19. Venkatanarasimha N, Thomas R, Armstrong EM, Shirley JF, Fox BM, Jackson SA (2011) Imaging features of ductal plate malformations in adults. Clin Radiol 66(11):1086–1093. doi:10.1016/j.crad.2011.05.008

Part III

Systematic Review of Benign Liver Tumors

Cysts and Polycystic Liver Disease

8

Antonio Giuliani, Sergio Aloia, Enrico Crolla, Loredana Sodano, Aldo Rocca, and Fulvio Calise

8.1 Introduction

Cystic and polycystic lesions within the liver have been reported to occur in up to 5 % of the population [1]. These lesions can present with general or specific symptoms, depending of the nature and the size of the lesions, or they can be silent and discovered accidentally. These diseases can be classified in two principal groups: parasitic and nonparasitic hepatic cysts. The latter are the most frequent and consist of a heterogeneous group of disorders, which differ in etiology, prevalence, and symptoms.

Differential diagnosis of hepatic cysts includes infectious (hydatid cyst, amebic, and pyogenic abscesses) and noninfectious (simple cyst, polycystic liver disease (PCLD), cystadenoma, intrahepatic pseudocysts secondary to pancreatitis, liver hematomas, biliomas, ciliated hepatic foregut cyst).

Most of them are found incidentally on imaging studies and tend to have a benign course, but a minority may cause symptoms but rarely can be associated with serious morbidity and mortality.

Sometimes, these lesions are not easily differentiated at initial presentation or by imaging studies, and management can become challenging [2]. Symptoms can be various; in the worst cases symptoms can be accompanied with an occupation of space syndrome that in PCLD can lead to liver transplantation for abdominal organ and big vessel compression.

With improving diagnostic techniques and minimally invasive technology, the management of hepatic cystic and polycystic disease continues to evolve, and laparoscopic surgery has a prominent diagnostic and therapeutic role.

A. Giuliani, MD, PhD (✉) • S. Aloia • E. Crolla • L. Sodano • A. Rocca • F. Calise
Department of Transplantation, Unit of Hepatobiliary Surgery and Liver Transplant, Cardarelli Hospital, Via A. Cardarelli, 9, Naples 80130, Italy
e-mail: giuldoc@hotmail.com; sergio.aloia@hotmail.it; enrico.crolla@gmail.com; loredanasodana@hotmail.it; aldorocca@hotmail.it; fulvio.calise@aocardarelli.it

L. Aldrighetti et al. (eds.), *Benign Tumors of the Liver*,
DOI 10.1007/978-3-319-12985-3_8

Table 8.1 Classification of cystic and polycystic liver disease

Infectious		Noninfectious	
Parasitic	Nonparasitic	Simple cyst	Partial cystic component
Hydatic cyst	Pyogenic liver abscesses	PCLD	Intrahepatic pseudocysts
Amebic abscess		Peribiliary cyst	Bilomas
			Post-traumatic hematoma

At the time of diagnosis, it is important to exclude cystadenoma and cystadenocarcinoma in the differential diagnosis using CT scan or MRI, although simple cysts and PCLD are not associated with an increased risk of malignancy [3].

In Table 8.1 there is a classification of benign cystic and polycystic liver diseases.

Surgical treatment should only be reserved for really symptomatic patients because approximately 25 % of patients who undergo surgery for referred symptomatic benign liver lesions remain somehow symptomatic even after surgery [4].

8.2 Simple Cyst

Simple hepatic cyst is a biliary malformation, which, generally, does not have communication with the intrahepatic biliary tree. Most cysts measure less than 3 cm and are asymptomatic [2].

Microscopically, they are lined by a single layer of cuboid or columnar epithelial cells, resembling biliary epithelial cells. Its origin is derived from aberrant bile ducts that have lost communication with the biliary tree and continue to secrete intraluminal fluid [4].

The female-to-male ratio is 1.5:1, and prevalence is from 2.5 to 18 % at ultrasound studies with a more frequent incidence in adults over 50 years, although the number of clinically relevant cysts, however, remains low [4, 5]. The rate of single cysts is about 68–75 % [5, 6].

8.2.1 Pathogenesis and Epidemiology

Simple cysts contain a clear, bile-like fluid. Because bile duct epithelium covers the simple cyst inner lining, it is hypothesized that simple cysts arise during embryogenesis when intrahepatic ductules fail to connect with extrahepatic ducts [7–10]: these aberrant ductules eventually dilate to form simple cysts.

8.2.2 Symptoms

Less than 4 % of simple cysts are almost always asymptomatic, but larger cysts greater than 5 cm especially when they reach a size over 10–12 cm and, particularly, are located in the left or anterior segments may cause compression of the stomach

(Figs. 8.1 and 8.2) or modification of the abdominal profile with evident symptomatic manifestations [11, 12].

A not so rare complication is intracystic bleeding, generally due to an overwhelming size (over 15–20 cm). A surgical treatment is evidently indicated in this case.

Case Report 1

A simple cyst of segments 5–8 in a 35-year-old female patient with an acute pain on the upper right abdomen and loss of hemoglobin. CT scan (Figs. 8.3 and 8.4) showed a rapid volume increase in 25 days due to an intralesional hemorrhage. The patient was treated by laparoscopic fenestration with no recurrence after 4 years.

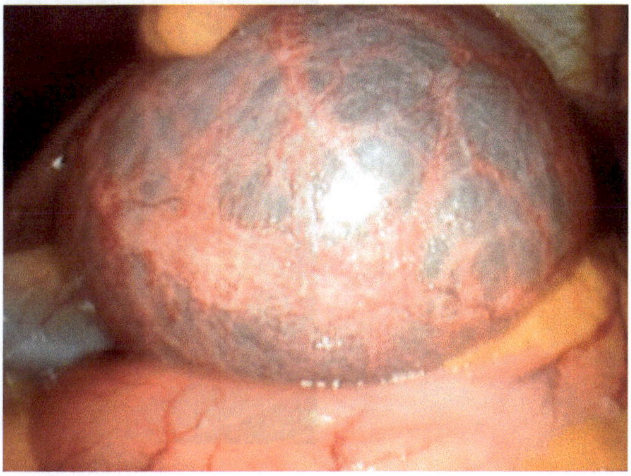

Fig. 8.1 Large simple cyst of the segment III with stomach compression

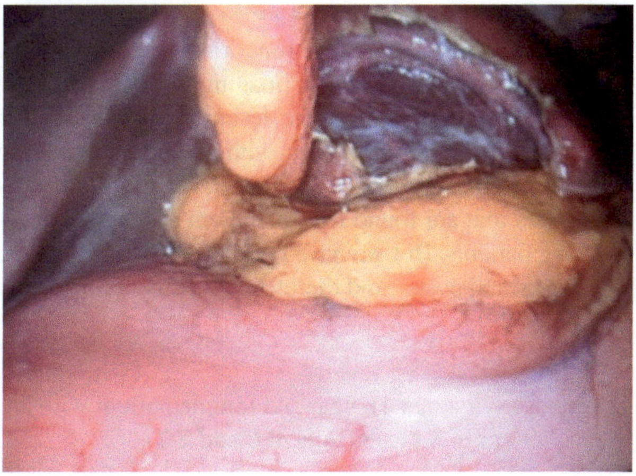

Fig. 8.2 After fenestration evidence of compression of the stomach

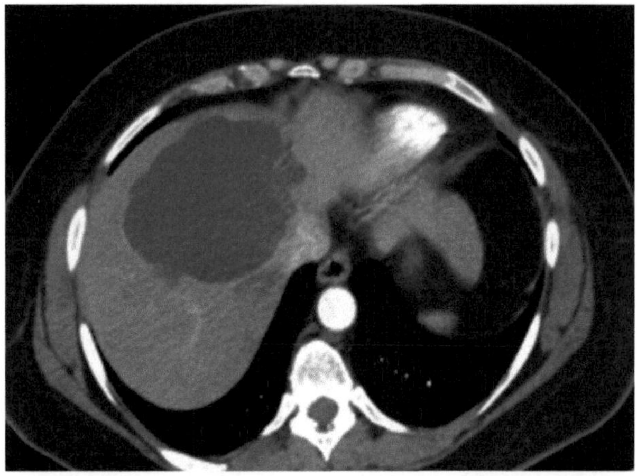

Fig. 8.3 First CT scan of case report 1

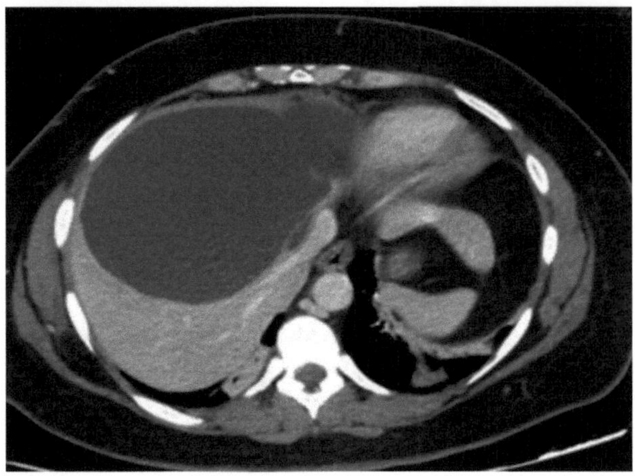

Fig. 8.4 CT scan of case report 1 at 25 days after first CT scan

8.2.3 Instrumental and Laboratory Diagnosis

Almost all patients have liver function tests within the normal range.

Ultrasound (US) is the best imaging modality to study simple cysts, which appear as a circular or oval, anechoic lesion with smooth borders and acoustic posterior enhancement and, in most cases, without internal septations [13] (Fig. 8.5). Also, ultrasound is strongly advised to monitor the evolution of these cysts: generally one time a year. Cysts that are found less than 3 cm at first diagnosis generally do not grow even in young patients. But we have been able to ascertain occasionally unexpected growth in size of small cysts. And therefore instrumental follow-up is generally advisable.

Case Report 2

A simple cyst in a 41-year-old female patient with an unexpected growth from 4 to 19 cm in 8 years (Figs. 8.6 and 8.7).

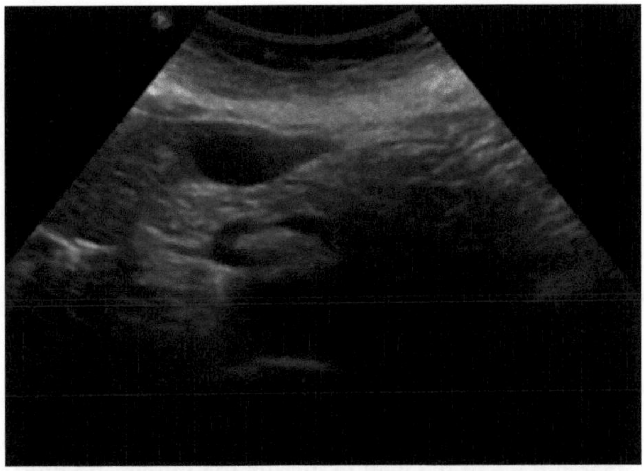

Fig. 8.5 Ultrasound image of a simple liver cyst of segment III (4 cm in diameter)

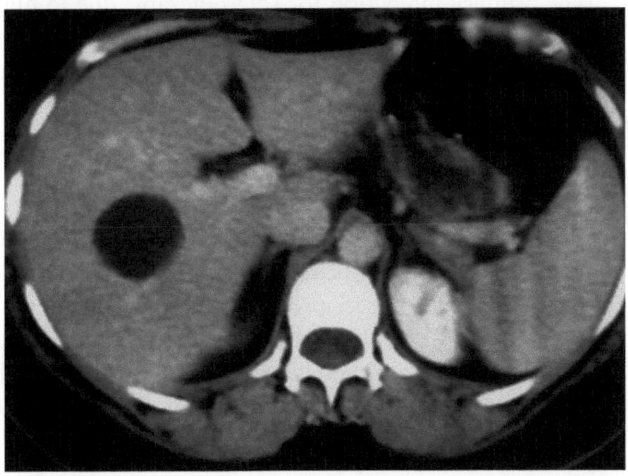

Fig. 8.6 Simple cyst of case report 2 at CT scan

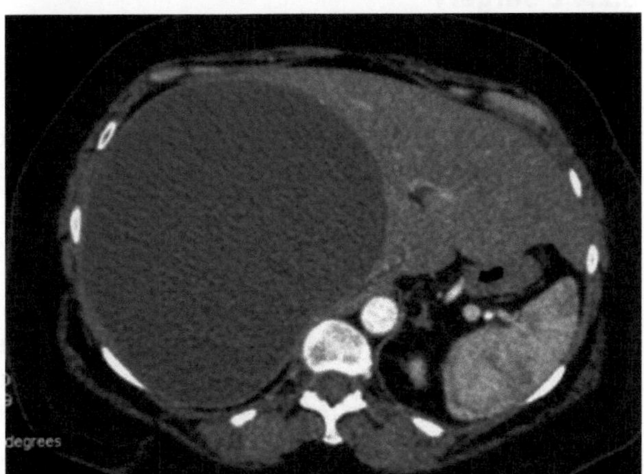

Fig. 8.7 Simple cyst of case report 2 at CT scan 8 years after Fig. 8.6

Further imaging studies, including computed tomography (CT scan) (Fig. 8.8) or magnetic resonance imaging (MRI) (Fig. 8.9), are not routinely required and show a nonseptated, round, and water-dense lesion. But in case of a surgical program due to a symptomatic disease, MRI is recommended to exclude communication with the biliary tree [14].

8.2.4 Treatment

Symptomatic patients require therapy, either sclerotherapy or surgical fenestration.

8.2.4.1 Sclerotherapy

This treatment consists of the percutaneous destruction of the epithelial lining of the inner surface of the wall to disrupt the intracystic fluid secretion.

The primary indication for sclerotherapy, due to high recurrence rates, is represented by those patients who are not eligible for surgery and general anesthesia [15].

A drainage catheter, under local anesthesia, is introduced under ultrasound guidance, followed by injection of water-soluble contrast to rule out communication with adjacent bile duct or peritoneal cavity; then a sclerosing agent (ethanol, minocycline hydrochloride, and ethanolamine oleate) is injected.

The risk of alcohol intoxication limits the amount of injection to 100–200 ml [16] than, the solution is aspirated and the catheter removed.

The size of the cyst does not play a role in the amount of sclerosing agent given because after the cyst collapses, the sclerosing agent will come into contact with the cyst inner wall. Contraindications of sclerotherapy include intracystic bleeding and fistula between the cyst and biliary tree or peritoneum. The optimal efficacy may be seen up to a year after sclerotherapy, and symptomatic recurrence rate is around 20 % after 4 months [2].

8.2.4.2 Surgery

Surgical treatment consists of fenestration (with open or laparoscopic approach) and an optional transposition of an omental patch.

Fenestration consists in the excision of the roof of the cyst in order to provide communication between the inner part of the cyst and the peritoneal cavity. Excision must attentively follow the border of the liver in order to take away the most part of the cyst.

Cysts located in segments VII and VIII have the higher recurrence rates due to anatomical position.

Morbidity is 0–15 % with no mortality and a reoperation rate of 9 % [17]. Possible, although rare, complications are hemorrhage and biliary injury.

Laparoscopy has become the procedure of choice for fenestration because it is associated with significant reduction in hospital stay, postoperative pain, and morbidity and decreased blood loss with a better quality of life in the first year after surgery, as we have been able to show in a previous study, with the possibility to avoid intraabdominal adhesions in case of repeated surgery with a lower rate of complications [18].

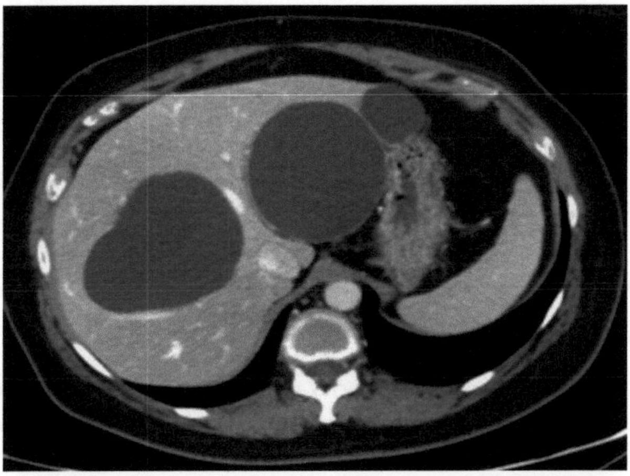

Fig. 8.8 Simple cysts at CT scan

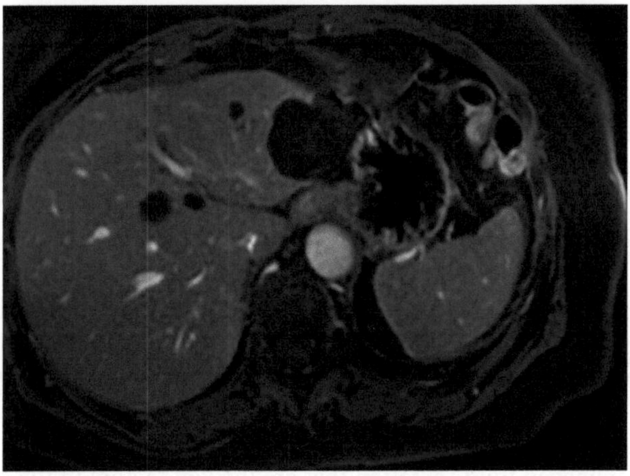

Fig. 8.9 Simple cysts at MRI

In our experience we performed laparoscopically from 1996 to August 2014 230 laparoscopic liver procedures of which 24 (10.4 %) were fenestration for symptomatic cysts with 0 % mortality and near to 0 % morbidity.

Totally we treated surgically 32 patients with simple cyst of which only 8 (25 %) were operated with an open approach where surgical procedures for benign simple cysts was only 3 % of all surgical liver procedures performed (32/1,029).

In the Italian Registry of Laparoscopic Liver Resection held by Aldrighetti on 1,677 laparoscopic liver resection, 43 (10.4 %) were performed for benign cystic disease including simple or complicated cysts, hydatid cysts, and cystadenomas [19].

Therefore, to limit recurrence rate, it is necessary to resect as much of the wall as possible to prevent closure of the remnant wall and re-accumulation of cyst fluid. Complete resection of the cyst is not necessary and is associated with higher complication rates.

Transposition of an omental patch to the cyst bed has been advocated as a means for lowering the recurrence rate, especially in posterolateral segments where early adhesion of the liver surface to either the diaphragm or abdominal wall may lead to refilling. These observations are however anecdotic and need to be confirmed by controlled studies.

At our knowledge there are no randomized prospective studies comparing fenestration and sclerotherapy.

8.3 Polycystic Liver Disease (PCLD)

Polycystic liver is arbitrarily defined when >20 hepatic cysts are present.

PCLD is a genetic disease responsible for the development of multiple hepatic cysts. It presents in two forms, with autosomal dominant polycystic kidney disease (AD-PKD) or only in an autosomal dominant polycystic liver disease (AL-PLD) [20].

8.3.1 Pathogenesis and Epidemiology

Both forms have an autosomal dominant transmission and similar clinical presentation. PCLD associated with ADPKD is linked with mutations in the *PKD1* (short arm of chromosome 16, encoding polycystin-1) or *PKD2* gene (chromosome 4, encoding polycystin-2), whereas isolated PCLD is associated with heterozygous mutation in *PRKC-SH* or *SEC63* genes [21–26].

How the gene mutations eventually lead to liver cyst formation has not been fully elucidated. Probably, a mutation in an individual intrahepatic bile duct epithelial cell results in a clonal expansion of the mutated cell, which loses communication with the intrahepatic bile ducts [27, 28].

There are some abnormalities in cholangiocyte proliferation and apoptosis and enhanced fluid secretion that are the key factors in the pathogenesis and in the progressive expansion of hepatic cysts in PCLD: *cholangiocyte proliferation*, *fluid secretion*, and *cyst expansion*.

Remodelling of the extracellular matrix surrounding the cysts by the activity of metalloproteases (highly elevated in liver cyst epithelia) is necessary for cyst expansion [29].

Hepatic cyst epithelium is sensitive to the proliferative effects of estrogens and IGF-1. Hereby, estrogens act not only directly but also by promoting the synthesis and release of growth factors from the cyst epithelium [30]. For this reason pregnancy, multiparity, and use of steroids further increase the risk for severe hepatic cystic disease.

The prevalence of isolated PCLD is estimated to be 1/100,000, while the prevalence of liver cysts in ADPKD is 58, 85, and 94 % in subgroups of age (respectively, 15–24, 25–34, and 35–46 year) [31].

Overall prevalence is the same in gender, but female population is associated with more severe liver disease.

8.3.2 Symptoms

Almost always, cysts are small and asymptomatic.

Moreover, in the majority of patients with ADPKD, PCLD is not normally the main cause of symptoms [28].

In a minority of patients (3 %), the expansion of liver cysts causes serious invalidating abdominal symptoms [32]. Data indicate that the annual growth of polycystic livers is about 0.9–3.2 % [32].

Symptoms normally begin in the third or fourth decade of life and are due to cyst growth. Presentation in childhood is therefore rare.

When present, symptoms are related mainly to the volume of the enlarged liver rather than to the volume of a specific cyst and include abdominal distension, dyspnea, epigastric pain, early satiety, vomiting, and shortness of breath [33].

Symptoms are exacerbated when there is compression of the portal vein, the inferior vena cava, or extrahepatic bile duct.

Some patients can suffer from malnutrition that is the main indication for liver transplantation.

Complications are infrequent and include bleeding, rupture, and infection of cysts [2].

The most severe complication is bacterial infection, especially in those who are under dialysis for ADPKD or in immunosuppressed patients after renal transplantation [2, 34]. The management consists of aspiration and drainage and antibiotic therapy. Cholestasis secondary to compression of adjacent biliary and portal hypertension secondary to portal or hepatic veins compression are rare.

Some patients may suffer from a rare complication as pruritus due to biliary obstruction even in the presence of normal laboratory tests [36].

Cerebrovascular pathology and cardiac-associated pathology (mitral valve prolapsed) occur respectively in 8 and 25 % of cases [37].

8.3.3 Instrumental and Laboratory Diagnosis

US shows multiple, fluid-filled, round or oval cysts with sharp margins being responsible for an extreme difficulty, by this tool, to identify vascular and biliary structures adjacent to the cysts. CT scan (Fig. 8.10) shows fluid attenuation with no contrast enhancement, while MRI demonstrates hyperintense on T2-weighted and hypointense on T1-weighted images [2] (Fig. 8.11). Both give a precise map of the liver and are mandatory to carry on a surgical approach.

A gastroscopy also may be useful to show a compression of the stomach or the duodenum causing early satiety, nausea, abdominal pain, and discomfort.

It is possible to stage the disease on CT scan findings according to Gigot's classification [35] (Table 8.2) and Qian's classification [34] (Table 8.3), while Schnelldorfer's classification differentiates patients who could benefit from resection compared with transplantation [38] (Table 8.4).

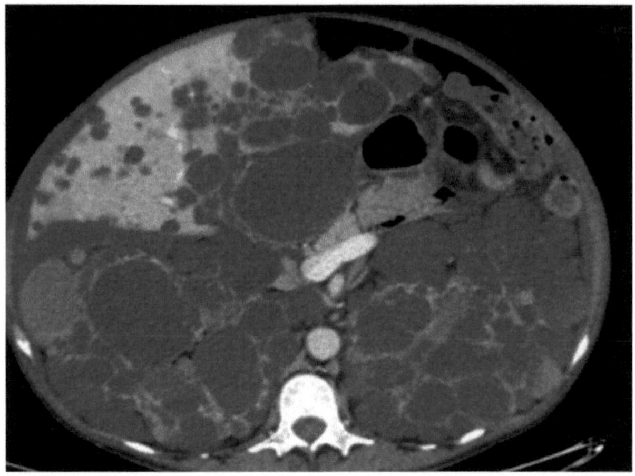

Fig. 8.10 APKD CT scan

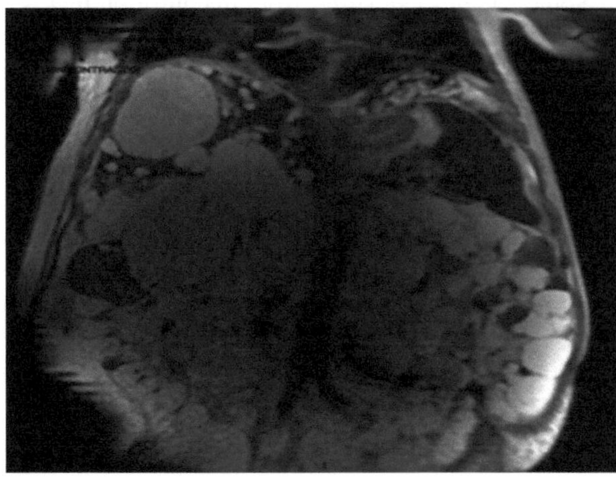

Fig. 8.11 APKD MRI (same case of Fig. 8.6)

8.3.4 Treatment

PCLD does not normally require a surgical treatment. When symptoms appear, the cystic and hepatic volumes require reduction.

8.3.4.1 Conservative Management

Medical management has been proposed in advanced PCLD with diffuse disease, but the efficacy of conservative management is still under investigation.

Two recent randomized controlled trials have demonstrated that lanreotide, a long-acting somatostatin analogue, was associated with a limited reduction of liver volume (at CT or MRI) in both types of PCLD [39–41].

Also, there are some limited experiences with the use of m-TOR inhibitors (sirolimus and everolimus) for treating PCLD with poor results, and this class of medication should not be recommended for clinical practice or outside of clinical trials

Table 8.2 Gigot's classification of PCLD

	CT findings	Treatment
Type I	Less than 10 large cysts	Laparoscopic fenestration
Type II	Diffuse involvement of liver parenchyma but with remaining large areas of non-cystic liver parenchyma	Laparoscopic fenestration
Type III	Massive, diffuse involvement of liver parenchyma with only a few areas of normal tissue between cysts	Contraindication to fenestration requiring resection or liver transplantation in symptomatic cases

Table 8.3 Qian's classification of PCLD

	CT findings
Grade 0	0 cysts
Grade I	1–10 cysts
Grade II	11–20 cysts
Grade III	More than 20 cysts
Grade IV	More than 20 cysts and symptomatic hepatomegaly

Table 8.4 Schnelldorfer's classification of PLCD

	Type A	Type B	Type C	Type D
Symptoms	Absent or mild	Moderate or severe	Severe (or moderate)	Severe (or moderate)
Cyst characteristics	Any	Limited no, large cysts	Any	Any
Areas of relative normal liver parenchyma	Any	>2 sectors	>1 sector	<1
Presence of portal vein or hepatic vein occlusion in the preserved hepatic sectors	Any	Absent	Absent	Present
Therapy	Observation/medical	Fenestration	Resection +/− fenestration	Transplantation

8.3.4.2 Sclerotherapy and Alternative Treatments

Sclerotherapy seems to be ineffective in the management of PCLD [2].

Transcatheter embolization has been recently proposed, targeting at decreasing arterial supply to the cyst. Although improvement of symptoms and significant reduction of liver size were observed in most of the patients, the limited experience in such a technically demanding procedure still questions the limitation to a widespread use [42].

However, both techniques have no role in the routine practice.

8.3.4.3 Surgery

Current surgical options include fenestration, liver resection, or liver transplantation.

Fenestration and liver resection, when feasible, should be performed by a laparoscopic approach although symptomatic relief is usually temporary, and repeat surgery is required for recurring symptoms in half of the patients [43].

However, the quality of life is better after laparoscopic approach [18] allowing less impact on patients, and an eventual liver transplantation is less difficult after laparoscopic surgery compared to the open surgical approach (Fig. 8.12).

Partial liver resection associated with fenestration of the remnant liver has been historically proposed, and, although highly successful in some patients, it is associated with high morbidity and mortality rates, and its indications are becoming more selective, while liver transplantations seem to be the only curative modality.

A potential source of complications in partial liver resection is the distortion of the intrahepatic vasculature and biliary tree which may lead to an increased risk of bleeding and biliary leakage.

Surgical resection should therefore be limited to patients when fenestration is not possible or to those ones who are not candidates for transplant.

Cyst fenestration and resection are both palliative methods, not curative; therefore, a laparoscopic approach is strongly recommended to relieve symptoms.

8.3.4.4 Liver Transplantation

Orthotopic liver transplantation (OLT) is the only curative and definitive option for PCLD.

OLT is indicated in patients with extremely disabling symptoms that lead to a seriously decreased quality of life. Malnutrition and nutritional deficiencies despite a normal liver synthetic capacity are to be considered in undertaking such a decision [44].

In the European Liver Transplant Registry, 734 patients received an OLT for symptomatic PCLD (from January 1988 to December 2009). The 5-year survival rate of 85 % for the indication of liver polycystosis is higher than the survival rate for other indications (72 %) [32, 45].

As patients have no chance of receiving an OLT by strict application of the Model for End-Stage Liver Disease (MELD), MELD exception criteria are used [46]. In this setting, the degree of malnutrition is assessed by a decreased mid-arm circumference in the nondominant arm (men < 23.8 cm; women < 23.1 cm); however, in case of PCLD, these cutoff values have never been validated. Shared criteria for including patients in a waiting list for LT are:

- A massive complicated polycystic liver likely to resolve after OLT
- Not a candidate for, or failed to respond to, non-transplant interventions for relief of symptoms
- Clinically significant manifestations of liver disease that can be attributed to massive polycystic liver: cachexia, ascites, portal hypertension, hepatic venous outflow obstruction, biliary obstruction, cholestasis, and recurrent cyst infection
- Severe malnutrition

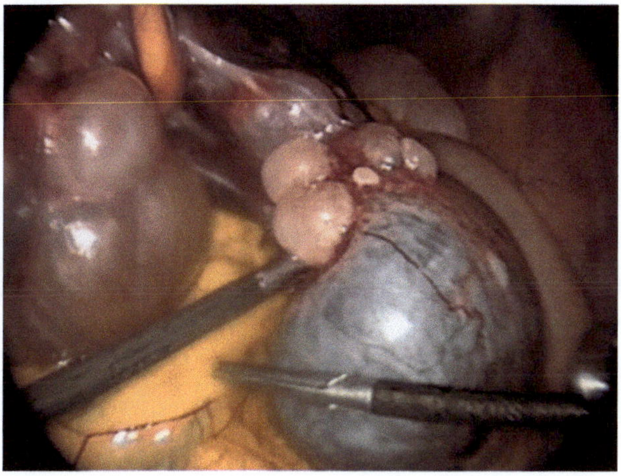

Fig. 8.12 Laparoscopic fenestration for PCLD

- Serum albumin <2.2 mg/dl
- Lean body mass, reflected by decreased mid-arm circumference, measured in the nondominant arm midway between the acromion and the olecranon processes: <23.1 cm in female patients and <23.8 cm in male patients

Patients who meet these criteria should be granted a MELD score exception: patients with and without renal insufficiency (glomerular filtration rate or creatinine clearance <30 ml/min) may receive a MELD score of 15 and 20, respectively. The score may be increased by an additional 3 points every 3 months upon reapplication [47].

Another criteria proposed by Van Kiempema [45] is an objective measurement of total liver volume with a minimum threshold although an arbitrary cutoff of 5,000 ml does not seem to be strictly related to the quality of life.

The most important problem encountered during OLT is the hepatectomy of the polycystic liver, mostly because of adhesions from previous surgical procedures. Extensive adhesions might preclude successful execution of the transplant procedure, and some authors are reluctant to treat polycystic liver patients who are potential OLT candidates by surgical liver volume-reducing procedures before OLT [48].

Moreover, some clinical trials indicate that somatostatin analogues when given for 6–12 months in patients with ADPKD and PCLD decrease total polycystic liver volume, attenuate polycystic kidney volume, and improve perception of health. However, the effect size (5 % decrease of total liver volume after 6–12 months) is probably too low to be of benefit for patients who are listed for transplantation [40].

Kirchner et al. [49] evaluated the outcome and quality of life in patients with polycystic livers after OLT or combined liver–kidney transplantation. Transplantation improved previous health status, symptoms, and quality of life to a level comparable with that of an age-matched general population. This improvement of the quality of life after transplantation supports the choice of OLT as a therapeutic option in PCLD.

A significant proportion (42 %) of the procedures consists of combined liver and kidney transplants. This combined transplantation should only be performed in patients with advanced renal insufficiency (i.e., clearance < 30 ml/min) [48, 50].

Combined liver–kidney transplantation results in poorer survival than OLT alone [45].

Case Report 3

A 61-year-old male patient with PCLD on ADPKD. From 1995 to 2011 he underwent 5 laparoscopic fenestrations for symptomatic PCLD and bilateral open nephrectomy. On April 2011 a combined liver–kidney transplantation was performed. Now he is in good health condition with an excellent quality of life.

Moreover, OLT should be weighed carefully in view of the organ shortage for treating a benign disease.

Therefore, in an era of organ shortage, other therapeutic options to reduce cyst volume need to be considered before listing patients for OLT, especially because liver function in patients with symptomatic PCLD is maintained. For this reason the laparoscopic approach has to be considered the best option when a surgical reduction of the cyst volume is needed.

References

1. Bakoyiannis A, Delis S, Triantopoulou C, Dervenis C (2013) Rare cystic liver lesions: a diagnostic and managing challenge. World J Gastroenterol 19:7603–7619
2. Macedo FI (2013) Current management of noninfectious hepatic cystic lesions: a review of the literature. World J Hepatol 5:462–469
3. Del Poggio P, Buonocore M (2008) Cystic tumors of the liver: a practical approach. World J Gastroenterol 14:3616–3620
4. Farges O, Aussilhou B (2012) Simple cysts and polycystic liver disease: surgical and non-surgical management. In: Jarnagin WR, Blumgart LH (eds) Blumgart's surgery of the liver, biliary tract and pancreas, 5th edn. Saunders, Philadelphia, pp 1066–1079
5. Shaked O, Siegelman ES, Olthoff EK, Reddy KR (2011) Biologic and clinical features of benign solid and cystic lesions of the liver. Clin Gastroenterol Hepatol 9:547–562
6. Carrim ZI, Murchison JT (2003) The prevalence of simple renal and hepatic cysts detected by spiral computed tomography. Clin Radiol 58:626–629
7. Lantinga MA, Gevers TJG, Drenth JPH (2013) Evaluation of hepatic cystic lesions. World J Gastroenterol 19:3543–3554
8. Choi BY, Nguyen MH (2005) The diagnosis and management of benign hepatic tumors. J Clin Gastroenterol 39:401–412
9. Sanfelippo PM, Beahrs OH, Weiland LH (1974) Cystic disease of the liver. Ann Surg 179:922–925
10. Jones WL, Mountain JC, Warren KW (1974) Symptomatic nonparasitic cysts of the liver. Br J Surg 61:118–123
11. Larssen TB, Rørvik J, Hoff SR, Horn A, Rosendahl K (2005) The occurrence of asymptomatic and symptomatic simple hepatic cysts. A prospective, hospital-based study. Clin Radiol 60:1026–1029

12. Taylor BR, Langer B (1997) Current surgical management of hepatic cyst disease. Adv Surg 31:127–148
13. Vachha B, Sun MR, Siewert B, Eisenberg RL (2011) Cystic lesions of the liver. AJR Am J Roentgenol 196:W355–W366
14. Yamada T, Furukawa K, Yokoi K, Mamada Y, Kanazawa Y, Tajiri T (2009) Liver cyst with biliary communication successfully treated with laparoscopic deroofing: a case report. J Nippon Med Sch 76:103–108
15. Treckmann JW, Paul A, Sgourakis G, Heuer M, Wandelt M, Sotiropoulos GC (2010) Surgical treatment of nonparasitic cysts of the liver: open versus laparoscopic treatment. Am J Surg 199:776–781
16. Yang CF, Liang HL, Pan HB, Lin YH, Mok KT, Lo GH, Lai KH (2006) Single-session prolonged alcohol-retention sclerotherapy for large hepatic cysts. AJR Am J Roentgenol 187:940–943
17. Loehe F, Globke B, Marnoto R, Bruns CJ, Graeb C, Winter H, Jauch KW, Angele MK (2010) Long-term results after surgical treatment of nonparasitic hepatic cysts. Am J Surg 200:23–31
18. Giuliani A, Migliaccio C, Ceriello A, Aragiusto G, La Manna G, Calise F (2014) Laparoscopic vs. open surgery for treating benign liver lesions: assessing quality of life in the first year after surgery. Updates Surg 66:127–133
19. Aldrighetti L, Cipriani F, Ratti F, Casciola L and Calise F on behalf of the Italian National Survey Group (2012) The Italian experience in minimally invasive surgery of the liver: a national survey. In: Calise F, Casciola L (eds) Minimally, surgery of the liver, Springer, Milan, pp 295–312
20. Tahvanainen P, Tahvanainen E, Reijonen H, Halme L, Kaariainen H, Hockrstedt K (2003) Polycystic liver disease is genetically heterogeneous: clinical and linkage studies in eight Finnish families. J Hepatol 38:39–43
21. Drenth JP, Martina JA, Te Morsche RH, Jansen JB, Bonifacino JS (2004) Molecular characterization of hepatocystin, the protein that is defective in autosomal dominant polycystic liver disease. Gastroenterol 126:1819–1827
22. Drenth JP, te Morsche RH, Smink R, Bonifacino JS, Jansen JB (2003) Germline mutations in PRKCSH are associated with autosomal dominant polycystic liver disease. Nat Genet 33:345–347
23. Li A, Davila S, Furu L, Qian Q, Tian X, Kamath PS, King BF, Torres VE, Somlo S (2003) Mutations in PRKCSH cause isolated autosomal dominant polycystic liver disease. Am J Hum Genet 72:691–703
24. Waanders E, Venselaar H, te Morsche RH, de Koning DB, Kamath PS, Torres VE, Somlo S, Drenth JP (2010) Secondary and tertiary structure modeling reveals effects of novel mutations in polycystic liver disease genes PRKCSH and SEC63. Clin Genet 78:47–56
25. Woodford LM, Grantham JJ, Bennett WM, Meyers CM, Walker DL, Bae K, Zhang QJ, Thompson PA, Miller JP, Harris PC (2007) Comprehensive molecular diagnostics in autosomal dominant polycystic kidney disease. J Am Soc Nephrol 18:2143–2160
26. Janssen MJ, Waanders E, Woudenberg J, Lefeber DJ, Drenth JP (2010) Congenital disorders of glycosylation in hepatology: the example of polycystic liver disease. J Hepatol 52:432–440
27. Everson GT, Taylor MR, Doctor RB (2004) Polycystic disease of the liver. Hepatology 40:774–782
28. Torres VE, Harris PC (2009) Autosomal dominant polycystic kidney disease: the last 3 years. Kidney Int 76:149–168
29. Murray SL, Grubman SA, Perrone RD, Perrone RD, Rojkind M, Moy E, Lee DW, Jefferson DM (1996) Matrix metalloproteinase activity in human intrahepatic biliary epithelial cell lines from patients with autosomal dominant polycystic kidney disease. Connect Tissue Res 33:249–256
30. Alvaro D, Gigliozzi A, Attili AF (2000) Regulation and deregulation of cholangiocyte proliferation. J Hepatol 33:333–340

31. Everson GT (1993) Hepatic cysts in autosomal dominant polycystic kidney disease. Am J Kidney Dis 22:520–525
32. Temmerman F, Missiaen L, Bammens B, Laleman W, Cassiman D, Verslype C, van Pelt J, Nevens F (2011) Systematic review: the pathophysiology and management of polycystic liver disease. Aliment Pharmacol Ther 34:702–713
33. Van Keimpema L, De Koning DB, Van Hoek B, Van Den Berg AP, Van Oijen MG, De Man RA, Nevens F, Drenth JP (2011) Patients with isolated polycystic liver disease referred to liver centres: clinical characterization of 137 cases. Liver Int 31:92–98
34. Qian Q, Li A, King BF, Kamath PS, Lager DJ, Huston J, Shub C, Davila S, Somlo S, Torres VE (2003) Clinical profile of autosomal dominant polycystic liver disease. Hepatology 37:164–171
35. Gigot JF, Jadoul P, Que F, Van Beers BE, Etienne J, Horsmans Y, Collard A, Geubel A, Pringot J, Kestens PJ (1997) Adult polycystic liver disease: is fenestration the most adequate operation for long-term management? Ann Surg 225:286–294
36. Johnson DK, Panchili S, Kolasseri S, Mavali RT (2014) Polycystic liver disease presenting as pruritus. Ann Gastroenterol 27:76–78
37. Pirson Y, Chauveau D, Torres V (2002) Management of cerebral aneurysms in autosomal dominant polycystic kidney disease. J Am Soc Nephrol 13:269–276
38. Schnelldorfer T, Torres VE, Zakaria S, Rosen CB, Nagorney DM (2009) Polycystic liver disease: a critical appraisal of hepatic resection, cyst fenestration, and liver transplantation. Ann Surg 250:112–118
39. Hogan MC, Masyuk TV, Page LJ, Kubly VJ, Bergstralh EJ, Li X, Kim B, King BF, Glockner J, Holmes DR, Rossetti S, Harris PC, LaRusso NF, Torres VE (2010) Randomized clinical trial of long-acting somatostatin for autosomal dominant polycystic kidney and liver disease. J Am Soc Nephrol 21:1052–1061
40. Hogan MC, Masyuk TV, Page L, Holmes DR, Li X, Bergstralh EJ, Irazabal MV, Kim B, King BF, Glockner JF, Larusso NF, Torres VE (2012) Somatostatin analog therapy for severe polycystic liver disease: results after 2 years. Nephrol Dial Transplant 27:3532–3539
41. Caroli A, Perico N, Perna A, Antiga L, Brambilla P, Pisani A, Visciano B, Imbriaco M, Messa P, Cerutti R, Dugo M, Cancian L, Buongiorno E, De Pascalis A, Gaspari F, Carrara F, Rubis N, Prandini S, Remuzzi A, Remuzzi G, Ruggenenti P, ALADIN Study Group (2013) Effect of longacting somatostatin analogue on kidney and cyst growth in autosomal dominant polycystic kidney disease (ALADIN): a randomised, placebo-controlled, multicentre trial. Lancet 382:1485–1495
42. Takei R, Ubara Y, Hoshino J, Higa Y, Suwabe T, Sogawa Y, Nomura K, Nakanishi S, Sawa N, Katori H, Takemoto F, Hara S, Takaichi K (2007) Percutaneous transcatheter hepaticartery embolization for liver cysts in autosomal dominant polycystic kidney disease. Am J Kidney Dis 49:744–752
43. Robinson TN, Stiegmann GV, Everson GT (2005) Laparoscopic palliation of polycystic liver disease. Surg Endosc 19:130–132
44. Stickel F, Inderbitzin D, Candinas D (2008) Role of nutrition in liver transplantation for end-stage chronic liver disease. Nutr Rev 66:47–54
45. van Keimpema L, Nevens F, Adam R, Porte RJ, Fikatas P, Becker T, Kirkegaard P, Metselaar HJ, Drent JPH, for the European Liver and Intestine Transplant Association (ELITA) (2011) Excellent survival after liver transplantation for isolated polycystic liver disease: an European Liver Transplant Registry study. Transplant Int 24:1239–1245
46. Freeman RB Jr, Gish RG, Harper A, Davis GL, Vierling J, Lieblein L, Klintmalm G, Blazek J, Hunter R, Punch J (2006) Model for end-stage liver disease (MELD) exception guidelines: results and recommendations from the MELD Exception Study Group and Conference (MESSAGE) for the approval of patients who need liver transplantation with diseases not considered by the standard MELD formula. Liver Transpl 12:S128–S136
47. Arrazola L, Moonka D, Gish RG, Everson GT (2006) Model for end-stage liver disease (MELD) exception for polycystic liver disease. Liver Transpl 12:S110–S111

48. Pirenne J, Aerts R, Yoong K, Gunson B, Koshiba T, Fourneau I, Mayer D, Buckels J, Mirza D, Roskams T, Elias E, Nevens F, Fevery J, McMaster P (2001) Liver transplantation for polycystic liver disease. Liver Transpl 7:238–245
49. Kirchner GI, Rifai K, Cantz T, Nashan B, Terkamp C, Becker T, Strassburg C, Barg-Hock H, Wagner S, Lück R, Klempnauer J, Manns MP (2006) Outcome and quality of life in patients with polycystic liver disease after liver or combined liver-kidney transplantation. Liver Transpl 12:1268
50. Rasmussen A, Davies HF, Jamieson NV, Evans DB, Calne RY (1995) Combined transplantation of liver and kidney from the same donor protects the kidney from rejection and improves kidney graft survival. Transplantation 59:919–921

Cystic Bile Duct Dilatations and Caroli's Disease

9

Felice Giuliante, Agostino Maria De Rose, and Gennaro Nuzzo

9.1 Epidemiology

Congenital bile duct dilatations (BDD) are rare medical conditions in Western countries but represent the second most common cause of congenital malformations after biliary atresia [1]. Todani and colleagues [2] in 1977 expanded the first classification proposed by Alonso-Lej and colleagues in 1959 [3] for choledochal cysts including the occurrence of intrahepatic and multiple cysts, in addition to 3 types of bile duct dilation. On the approximately 4,000 cases reported worldwide, 2,500–3,000 cases come from Japanese and Korean series [1]. In Southeast Asia the incidence is 1 in 1,000/1,750 live births, unlike in Europe and United States where this rate is from 10 to 1,000 times more rare, with an estimated incidence ranging from 1/15,000 to 1/200,000 live births [4, 5]. The reason for this Asian preponderance is still unclear. In these countries 25 % of BDD are diagnosed within the first year of life and 60 % during the first decade of life, and about 20 % go undiagnosed into adulthood, unlike in Western countries where half of the cases are diagnosed between the age of 30 and 45 years [1]. There is also an unexplained female preponderance, commonly reported as 4:1 or 3:1 [5].

BDD are classified according to the site (extra and/or intrahepatic), extent (segmental or complete), and shape (cystic or saccular, fusiform) of the biliary anomaly. Todani classification, widely accepted and used as a standard [2] (Fig. 9.1), defines *type I*, also known as choledochal cyst (IA cystic (Fig. 9.2), IB segmental (Fig. 9.3), IC fusiform shape (Fig. 9.4)), as dilatation of the common bile duct (CBD); *type II* as diverticulum of the supraduodenal CBD; and *type III* as dilatation of the intraduodenal portion of the CBD, also known as choledochocele (type A choledochocele,

F. Giuliante (✉) • A.M. De Rose • G. Nuzzo
Hepatobiliary Surgery Unit, Catholic University of the Sacred Heart – A. Gemelli Hospital, Largo A. Gemelli, 8, Rome 00168, Italy
e-mail: fgiuliante@rm.unicatt.it; agostinom.derose@virgilio.it; gennaro.nuzzo@rm.unicatt.it

L. Aldrighetti et al. (eds.), *Benign Tumors of the Liver*,
DOI 10.1007/978-3-319-12985-3_9

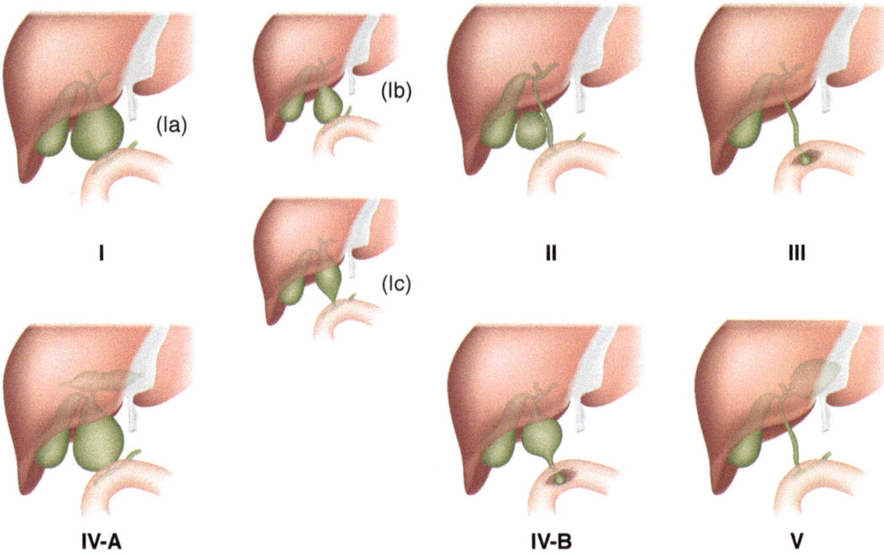

Fig. 9.1 Todani classification of congenital bile duct dilatations (Reprinted from Todani [6] with permission of Springer International Publishing)

Fig. 9.2 MR cholangiography: type IA choledochal cyst (*arrows*). *G* gallbladder

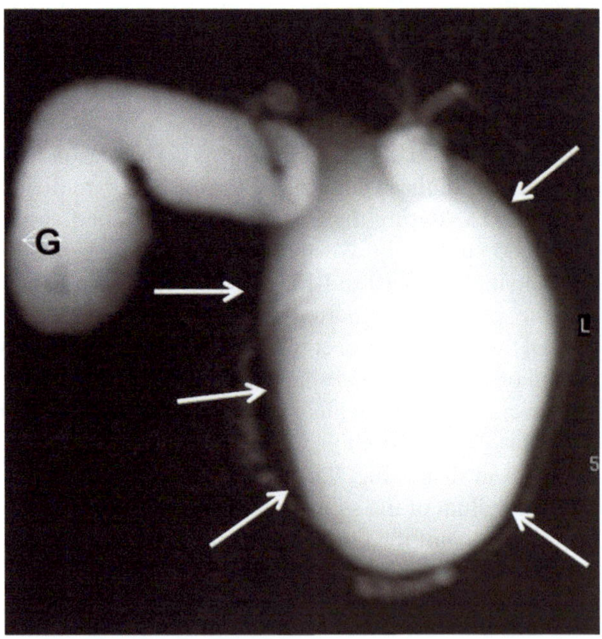

type B diverticular choledochocele, type C duodenal duplication cyst), and identifies two subtypes IV: *type IVA* with both intra- and extrahepatic dilatation of the biliary tree (Fig. 9.5) and *type IVB* with multiple and segmental dilatations of the

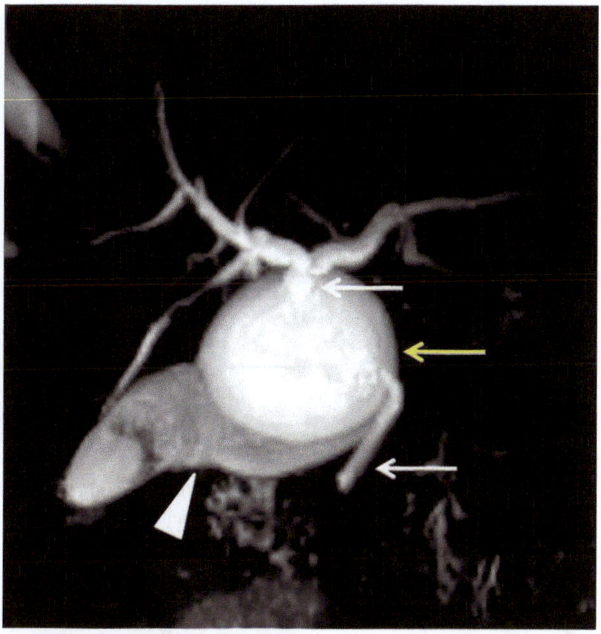

Fig. 9.3 MR cholangiography: type IB choledochal cyst. Segmental cystic dilatation of CBD (*yellow arrow*), with normal proximal and distal CBD (*white arrows*); gallbladder (*head arrow*)

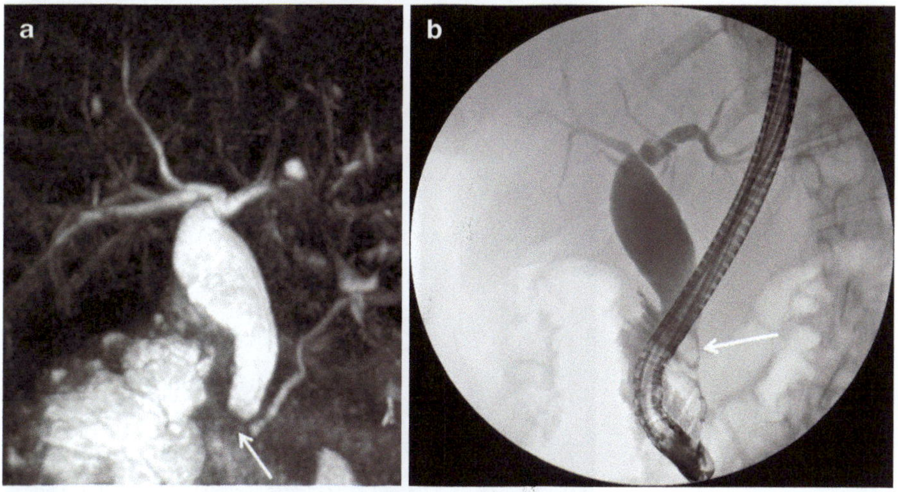

Fig. 9.4 Type IC choledochal cyst; (**a**) MR cholangiography with evidence of distal obstruction (*white arrow*). (**b**) Endoscopic cholangiography: lithiasis of distal CBD (*white arrow*)

extrahepatic biliary tree (Fig. 9.6) [7]; *type V* is characterized by congenital intrahepatic only bile duct dilation (IHBDD), also known as Caroli's disease (Fig. 9.7) [8], and was later classified by Guntz et al. [9] according to shape and extent of intrahepatic bile duct dilatations (type 1 grape-bunch-like saccular of peripheral IHBDD, type 2 fusiform dilatation of large IHBDD, and type 3 saccular dilatation of large

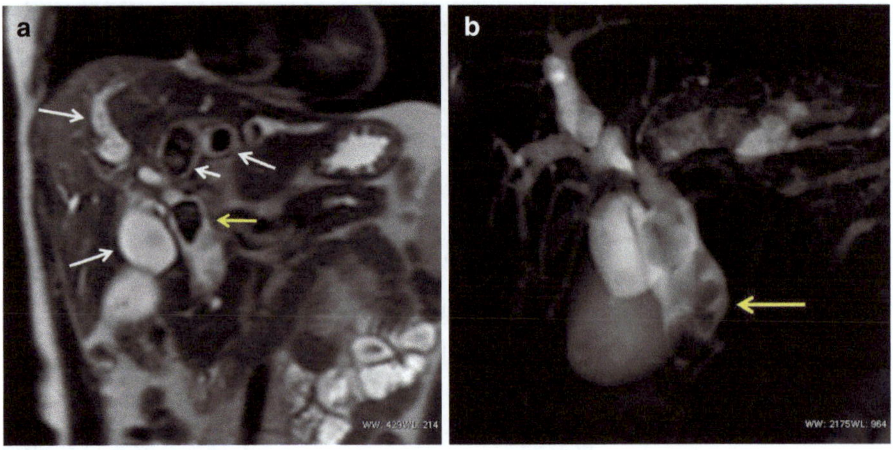

Fig. 9.5 Thirty-six-year-old patient; MR type IVA congenital bile duct dilatation. Choronal view (**a**), MR cholangiography (**b**): bilateral intrahepatic cystic dilatations with lithiasis (*white arrows*) and stones in choledochal cyst (*yellow arrow*)

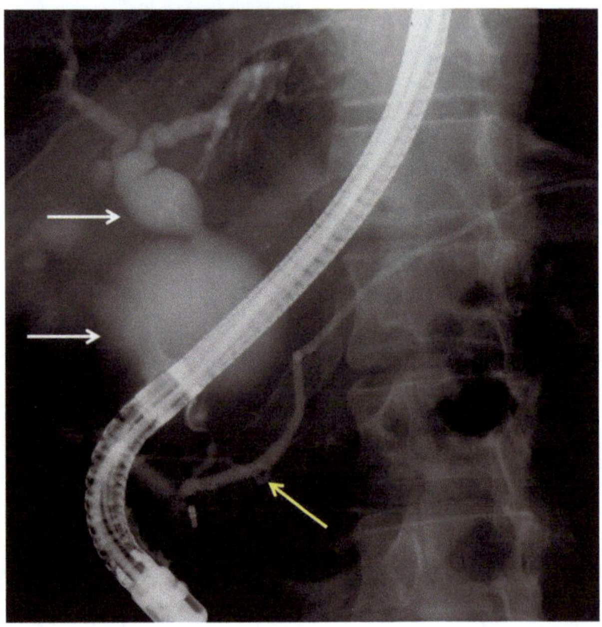

Fig. 9.6 Endoscopic cholangiography: type IVB choledochal cyst. Multiple and segmental dilatations of the extrahepatic biliary tree (*white arrows*). Main pancreatic duct (*yellow arrow*)

IHBDD). Unilobar extension of Caroli's disease is more frequently encountered (80 %) in surgical series [10], especially on the left side of the liver (Fig. 9.8), but the disease may diffusely involve the entire intrahepatic biliary tree. Distribution of the different types of BDD are as follows: 50–80 % are type I, 2 % type II, 1.4–4.5 % type III, 15–35 % type IV, and 20 % type V [5].

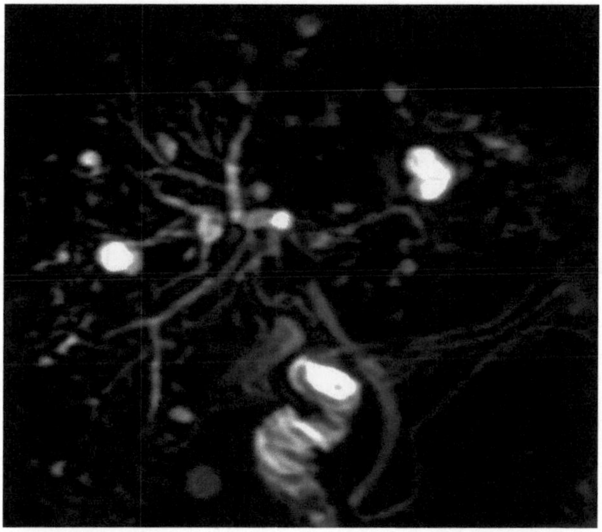

Fig. 9.7 MR cholangiography: type V congenital bile duct dilatation (Caroli's disease)

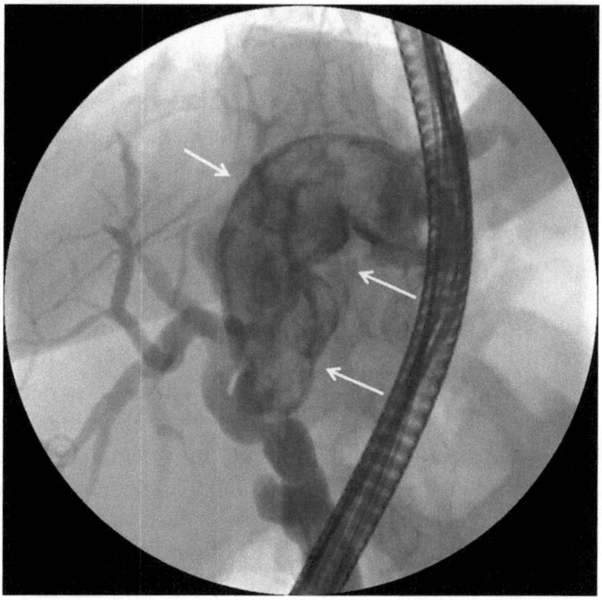

Fig. 9.8 Endoscopic cholangiography; type V congenital bile duct dilatation (type 3 according to Guntz classification): saccular dilatation of left hepatic duct with intrahepatic lithiasis (*white arrows*)

9.2 Etiology

The etiology of congenital bile duct dilatations is not fully understood. As regards Todani's types I–IV BDD, several theories have been proposed, but the most widely accepted hypothesis is the long common channel theory of Babbitt [4, 7, 11]. An anomalous biliopancreatic junction (ABPJ) (Fig. 9.9) with a common channel

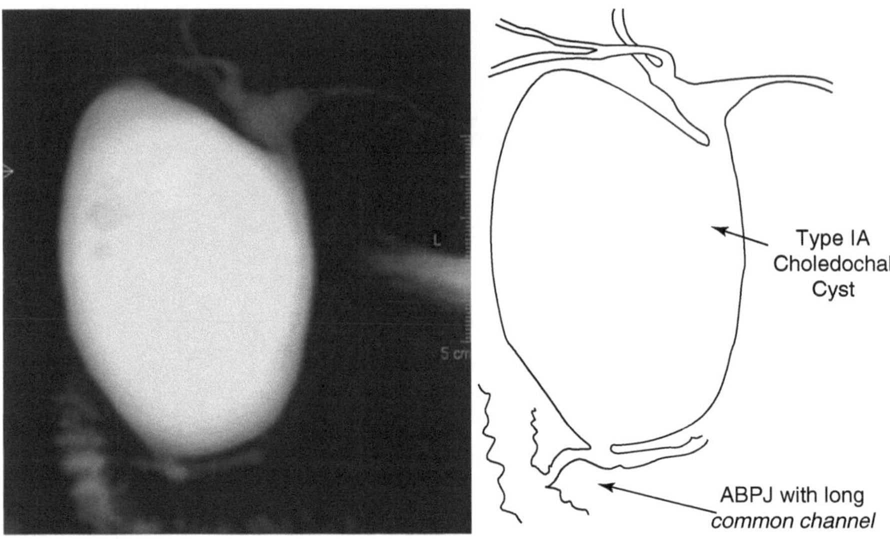

Fig. 9.9 MR cholangiography and sketch: type IA choledochal cyst, with evidence of ABPJ with long common channel

longer than 10–15 mm may allow pancreatic juice to reflux into the biliary tree, with activation of pancreatic enzymes. These active enzymes cause inflammation and deterioration of the biliary duct wall, leading to dilatation [12]. This hypothesis is supported by the detection of high concentrations of amylase in the bile of these patients [7, 13]. Furthermore, greater pressures in the pancreatic duct can further dilate weak-walled cysts [5, 14]. The incidence of ABPJ ranges from 96 to 100 % in pediatric series and from 68 to 94 % in adult series [4, 7, 11]. However, it should be considered that long common channels are arbitrarily defined in terms of length, with wide variation in measured length, from 10 to 45 mm, based on imaging modality and angles [5, 15].

Congenital nature of choledochal cysts has also been reported as a possible etiology of BDD [16]. This theory states that embryologic overproliferation of epithelial cells results in dilatation during the cannulation period of development [5]. Davenport and Basu [17] reported that all neonatal choledochal cysts were cystic in nature and pathologically had fewer neurons and ganglions than those in normal bile ducts. Their theory was that round cysts are congenital in nature, with distal obstruction due to aganglionosis, dysmotility, and functional CBD obstruction (equivalent to achalasia of the esophagus or to Hirschsprung's disease of the colon) [5]. Other authors speculate that all adult cysts are acquired due to distal obstruction, with longer, narrower stenosis leading to round lesions and shorter wider stenosis leading to fusiform lesions [17, 18]. The distal obstruction may be due to sphincter of Oddi dysfunction or scarring and stone formation into an ABPJ [19, 20]. The same authors argue that Todani's type IVA cysts result from combined distal as well as hilar and intrahepatic stenosis [5, 18].

Intrahepatic BDC, corresponding to type V in the Todani classification, results from embryological malformation [11]. Embryology of the intrahepatic biliary tree is as follows: a single layer of cells called ductal plate forms around the portal branches, which then duplicate to form a double layer [5]. Remodeling and selective reabsorption of the ductal plate start in the 12th week and progress to form the large bile ducts at the hilum and proceed toward the small ductules in the periphery. When such ductal plate malformation occurs at the level of the large ducts, Caroli's disease results; malformation that continues during later stages involving the development of the peripheral ductules results in Caroli's syndrome, that is, association of intrahepatic biliary cysts, reflecting large duct arrest, and congenital hepatic fibrosis, reflecting ductile arrest [21, 22]. Caroli's disease can be associated with biliary atresia, which is also thought to be due to ductal plate malformation. Caroli's disease can also be associated with both autosomal recessive and, less commonly, autosomal dominant polycystic kidney disease [23–25].

9.3 Clinical Presentation

BDD may remain asymptomatic for many years and diagnosis may be obtained on imaging studies for unrelated causes [7], but 80 % of patients present symptoms before the age of 10 years [26]. The classic triad of abdominal pain, jaundice, and a palpable abdominal mass occurs in less than 20 % of patients, although almost two-thirds of patients have two of these three symptoms [26].

Neonatal patients generally present with obstructive jaundice (58 %), biliary pain (52.3 %), abdominal masses (17 %), and fever (12.5 %) [1]. The classic triad occurs in 3 % of cases [1]. Complications, as cholecystitis or cholangitis occur in 3–6 % of patients and acute pancreatitis was reported in 21 % of cases [1].

In adult patients the most common symptom is biliary pain. In a recent analysis of literature on 1,639 patients, biliary pain occurs in 71.4 % of cases, jaundice in 26.1 %, and a palpable abdominal mass in 2.5 %; the classic triad occurs in only 1 % of cases [1]. Complications are more commonly observed in adult patients, especially in those with a long history of previous biliary surgical and nonsurgical treatments. According to an analysis of 1,581 patients in literature, pyogenic cholangitis is the most common clinical occurrence, occurring in 23 % of cases (15–41 %), and acute pancreatitis is described in 13.6 % (10–55 %), and it is strictly related to the presence of an ABPJ ($p<0.006$) and to the size of BDD ($p<0.004$) [27]. Acute cholecystitis occurs in 18 % of cases. Associated biliary lithiasis is associated in 38–87 % of patients [1].

In the multicenter study on BDD conducted under the auspices of the French Association of Surgery [1], neonatal patients present more frequently more than one symptom ($p<0.0001$), palpable abdominal mass ($p<0.0001$), jaundice ($p=0.0001$), and acute pancreatitis ($p=0.03$). On the contrary complications ($p=0.0466$) and especially cholangitis ($p=0.0023$) are significantly more common in adult patients.

The mean time elapsed from the appearance of symptoms to diagnosis and treatment is significantly longer in adults than in children and for adult patients was estimated to be up to 6 years [7]. Previous hepato-biliopancreatic treatments including cholecystectomy or other surgical/endoscopic/percutaneous biliary procedures before diagnosis are commonly reported in the adult population (10–50 %) [7]. Moreover, patients might also be referred for recurrent pancreatitis related to incomplete resection of the distal part of the extrahepatic dilatation. Previous biliary surgery is associated with more complex management of the disease in adult patients [7].

9.4 Evolution

Stone formation secondary to bile stasis is the most frequent condition occurring in adults, affecting 37.5–74 % of BDD patients [7]. Half of the cases of Todani's type V BDD are associated with coexistent congenital hepatic fibrosis that corresponds to an inherited congenital malformation transmitted as an autosomal recessive trait [7, 28]. The most important late consequences are cirrhosis and portal hypertension. A significant association between BDD and cholangiocarcinoma (CC) is unanimously reported with a clear increasing age-related incidence. In previous series, the risk of developing a CC is estimated from 20 to 30 times higher than in normal population [4]. Recently two epidemiological studies report that presence of BDD increases 47 times the risk of developing a extrahepatic cholangiocarcinoma [29] and from 10.7 to 36.9 times the risk of developing a intrahepatic cholangiocarcinoma [29, 30]. Moreover CC over BDD occurs at a mean age of 32 years that is about two decades earlier than in the general population [4]. Malignant degeneration can occur in all types of bile duct dilatation. The majority of BDD affected by a cancer are types I and IV according to Todani's classification [2]; a cancer can be observed in all other types of BDD, but analysis of incidence is hindered by their rarity. In an analysis of a series of 63 biliary cancers on BDD, Todani et al. [31] reported a tumor incidence of 68 % in type I, 5 % in type II, 1.6 % in type III, 21 % in type IV, and 6 % in type V. Recently a retrospective Korean multicenter study [32] reports a significantly higher-incidence bile duct cancer in BDD type IVA (13/40, 32.5 %) and of gallbladder cancer in type I (28/35: 80 %). Presence of an ABPJ has a 16–55 % risk of malignancy, with or without congenital bile duct dilation [5]. Cancer usually occurs within the cyst in saccular choledochal cyst (type I A) and in the gallbladder in fusiform choledochal cyst (type I C), leading some authors to postulate that malignancy occurs at the site of bile stasis, irritation, and inflammation (within the dilated cyst in cystic choledochal cyst and within the gallbladder when no dilatation or fusiform choledochal cyst exist) [5]. In patients with type II BDD, the incidence of synchronous cancer was 5.3 % in a recent European Multicenter Study of the French Surgical Association [33].

The incidence of malignancy with choledochocele is perceived to be low but an analysis of the literature is difficult for the confusion concerning the presence of a primary ampullary tumor. In a revision of the literature reported in the Monography of the French Surgical Association [1] on 330 patients with choledochocele, the incidence of cancer is 6.6 % (ranging from 3.5 to 27 %), including ampullary and pancreatic tumors in addition to cancers of the biliary tract.

A previous cystoduodenostomy or cystojejunostomy is a significant risk factor for the development of a tumor that typically occurs earlier than in patients not undergoing cysto-digestive anastomosis [1]. Out of the 241 cases of carcinoma collected by Todani et al. [34], 45 (18.6 %) were encountered following previous cyst-enteric drainage procedures with a mean interval between the biliary bypass procedure and the detection of carcinoma of 10 years. These features support the recommendation that low-risk patients, even asymptomatic, should undergo elective excision of BDD, even if previously treated by cystoenterostomy.

Most importantly, patients with Todani's type V BDD are at high risk to develop intrahepatic cholangiocarcinoma, either synchronously or after incomplete resection. The reported average prevalence is close to 7 %, but higher values of up to 25–30 % have been reported [10]. The prevalence of cholangiocarcinoma in a recent French multicenter study [10] was 5.2 %, but the same authors stated that this prevalence may be underestimated because the series is a retrospective and multicentric study and therefore patients with malignancy who did not require surgery were not included in the study.

Histologically, biliary cancer is predominantly a mass-forming intrahepatic cholangiocarcinoma (Fig. 9.10) and less frequently a papillary CC intraductal type (Fig. 9.11).

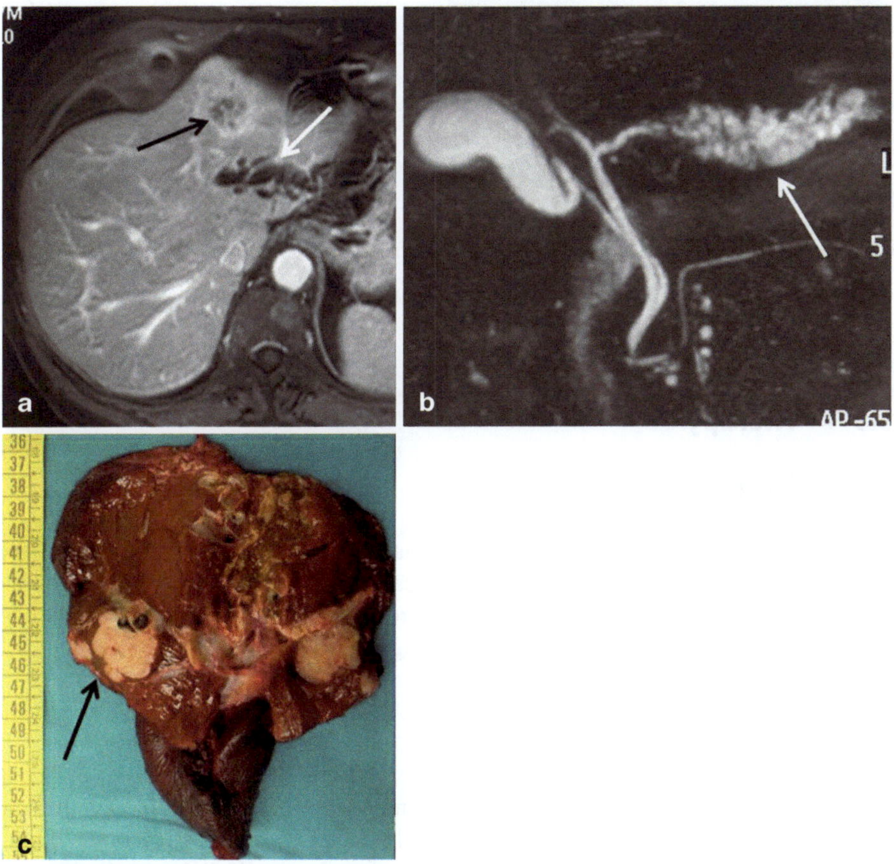

Fig. 9.10 Seventy-five-year-old male patient with left unilateral BDD and intrahepatic cholangiocarcinoma. MRI axial view (**a**) and MR cholangiography (**b**): dilated left biliary tree (white *arrows*) and suspect intrahepatic cholangiocarcinoma (*black arrow*). (**c**) Surgical specimen after left hepatectomy: mass-forming intrahepatic cholangiocarcinoma (*black arrow*) and dilatation with lithiasis of left biliary tree

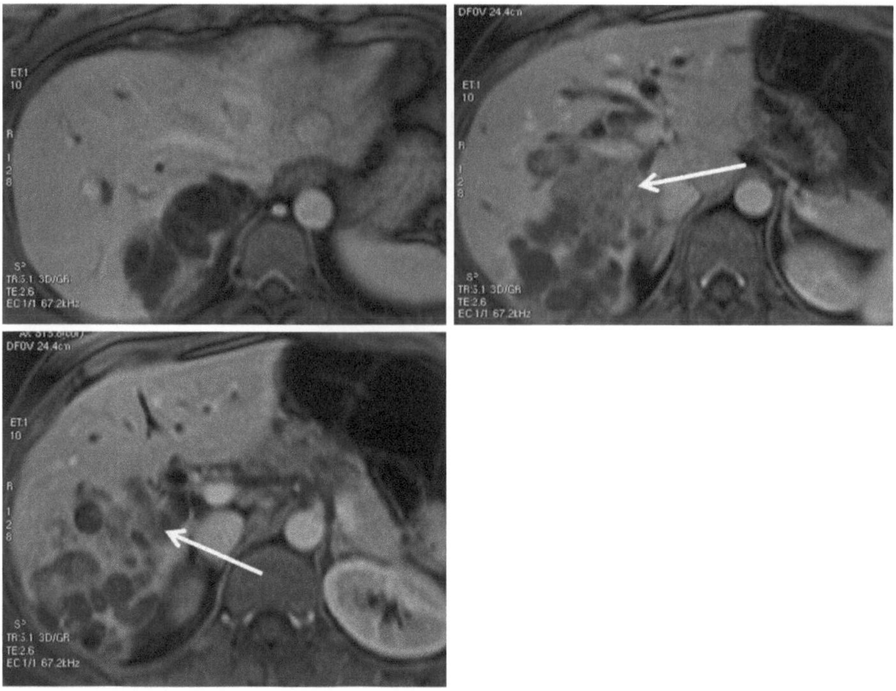

Fig. 9.11 Abdomen MRI: dilated right bile ducts with papillary intraductal-type cholangiocarcinoma (*white arrows*)

9.5 Therapy

9.5.1 Surgical Treatment

Factors to consider during definition of optimal surgical treatment of BDD patients are the following: age, symptoms and complications, coexistent liver or biliopancreatic diseases, previous cyst-related surgical procedures, cyst type on imaging studies, and age-related risk for synchronous malignancy [7].

9.5.2 Type I

Complete cyst excision of the extrahepatic component of BDD combined with cholecystectomy (Figs. 9.12 and 9.13), followed by Roux-en-Y biliary reconstruction, is considered the treatment of choice for type I and type IV BDD [4, 7, 11] . A cholecystectomy is recommended due to the high risk for gallbladder malignancy, especially when ABPJ is present [7]. Treatment of BDD by cystoenterostomy is not recommended [4, 7, 11] because the drainage provided by a cysto-enteric anastomosis is associated with biliary stasis, stone formation, and recurrent cholangitis,

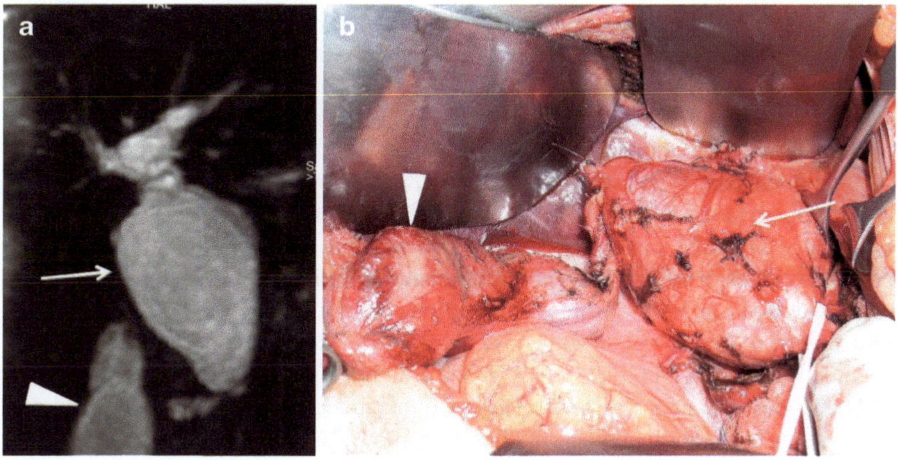

Fig. 9.12 MR cholangiography (**a**) and operative field (**b**): type IA choledochal cyst (*white arrow*). Complete choledochal cyst excision, cholecystectomy, and hepaticojejunostomy at the hilar plate. Gallbladder (*white head arrow*)

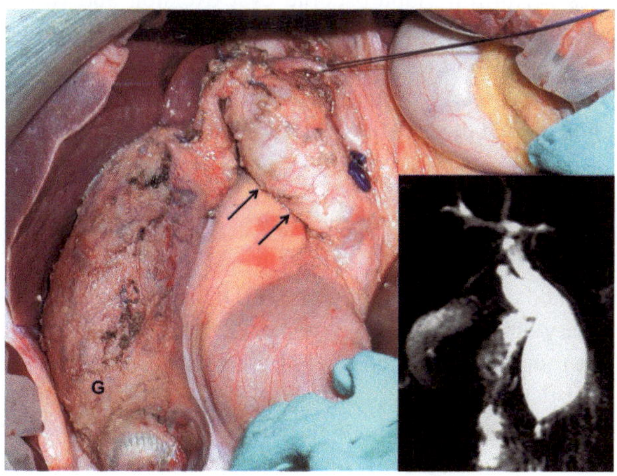

Fig. 9.13 Operative field and MR cholangiography of patient with type IC choledochal cyst (*arrows*). *G* gallbladder

and these lead to malignant transformation [7]. Most importantly, indeed, surgeons found that leaving the cyst intact carried a significant risk of malignant transformation [35]. The overall success rate of internal drainage procedures is 30 %, the risk of postoperative malignancy is 30 %, the mortality rate is 11 %, and more than half who undergo this procedure require reoperation [35]. Therefore, internal drainage is currently thought to be a dangerous and incomplete treatment. In contrast, complete BDD excision appears to be the standard treatment and can be performed safely either as a primary or a secondary procedure (after failure of internal drainage). Complete cyst excision means that the division of the biliary tract should be carried out in healthy biliary tissue, either at the superior and inferior part of the cystic component, with the use of frozen section pathological examination to rule out the presence of cancer [7]. Proximally, the involvement of main biliary convergence and/or of sectorial biliary ducts must be preoperatively or intraoperatively analyzed in order to prevent incomplete resection and reconstruction on non-healthy bile ducts. At their distal part, type I and IV BDD require excision of the intrapancreatic cystic portion down to the healthy distal bile duct [7]. In this setting, precise preoperative knowledge of ABPJ anatomy is a key factor to avoid intraoperative damage of the pancreatic duct or of the long common channel during cyst excision [7]. Biliary reconstruction can be performed using a long 70-cm defunctionalized Roux-en-Y jejunal loop with a wide bilio-digestive anastomosis at the level of the CBD or, more frequently, of the main biliary convergence after having extended the opening on the left hepatic duct (according to the Hepp-Couinaud technique) [7]. The success rate of Roux-en-Y hepaticojejunostomy has been shown to be as high as 92 % [36]. This procedure has a reported complication rate of 7 %, compared with a complication rate of 42 % with hepaticoduodenostomy [37]. Early postoperative complications of cyst excision and hepaticoenterostomy include anastomotic leak and pancreatic fistula with injury to the pancreatic duct. Recently, many authors have reported success performing laparoscopic cyst excision and Roux-en-Y hepaticojejunostomy, with quicker recovery, reduced adhesions, and improved cosmesis and ease of surgery because of magnification of the operative field [35]. With the advent of robot-assisted surgery, which has improved manual dexterity, laparoscopic treatment of choledochal cyst is still evolving and promises further benefits [35].

9.5.3 Type II

Limited cyst excision of type II BDD is recommended. CBD resection may be necessary only in case of a large neck of the cyst at its junction with the CBD and it is not routinely indicated [7, 11]. Surprisingly, despite simple resection of the biliary diverticulum being considered as the standard treatment, associated CBD resection is required in a significant number of patients, 58 % of the cases analyzed in a recent multicenter study [33]. Intimate adhesion of the diverticulum to the extra- or intrahepatic biliary tree according to disease location may explain the technical challenge to dissociate the diverticulum from the bile duct, especially in case of coexistent inflammatory process [33]. Predictive factors of CBD resection are cholangitis, pancreatitis, and jaundice [33]. In case of presence of synchronous cancer, a radical resection with large tumor-free margin is advocated and justifies the need for CBD resection and diverticulum resection, associated with hemihepatectomy or pancreaticoduodenectomy according to cancer location [33]. Despite an increasing use of the laparoscopic approach, very few Todani type II BDD are reported [38], and a laparoscopic approach should be discouraged especially in case of high diverticular location [33]. In the multicenter series reported by Ouaïssi et al. [33] on 19 patients, there was no mortality, the overall complications rate was 15.8 %, and long-term results were excellent for the vast majority of the patients (89 %).

9.5.4 Type III

Transduodenal excision of type III BDD is currently replaced by conservative endoscopic sphincterotomy that is recommended to allow free duodenal drainage of bile and stones [5, 39, 40]. Given the possibility that pancreatic and biliary secretions can mix within the choledochocele and create a precancerous state, some authors recommend sphincterotomy even in asymptomatic patients [40]. In summary most type A choledochoceles should be treated by using either endoscopic sphincterotomy or snare resection, whereas most type B choledochoceles should be completely removed endoscopically by using a polypectomy snare [41]. Although endoscopic intervention may be sufficient in most cases, lesions whose anatomy cannot be defined or varies significantly should be considered for surgery, as well as those that harbor malignancy [41]. Duodenal duplications will more often undergo surgical resection, particularly in young patients [41]. Surveillance for dysplasia should be considered for lesions that are not completely resected. Pancreaticoduodenectomy remains indicated in case of coexistent cancer [7].

9.5.5 Type IV

Treatment of type IV B BDD, as choledochal cyst, is the cyst excision with a wide hilar hepaticojejunostomy; in type IVA patients excision of CBD and Roux-en-Y hepaticojejunostomy is not a complete treatment, and patients often continue to have symptoms because of intrahepatic disease. The management of the intrahepatic component of type IVA BDD remains controversial; if the intrahepatic involvement is localized, a segmental hepatectomy may be performed, especially in case of left unilobar intrahepatic cystic disease (Fig. 9.14), leading thus to complete extra- and intrahepatic disease excision [7]. Furthermore, in type IVA BDC complicated by ductal strictures, intrahepatic stones or abscess, and liver atrophy or malignancy, liver resection is indicated.

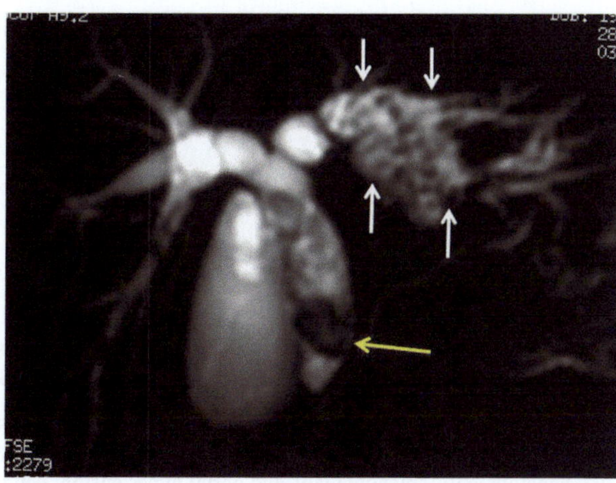

Fig. 9.14 MR cholangiography: type IVA choledochal cyst. Unilateral left intrahepatic cystic dilatations with lithiasis (*white arrows*) and lithiasis in choledochal cyst (*yellow arrow*)

The optimal management of patients with bilateral involvement remains a very complex and challenging task because of the difficulty to obtain a complete cyst excision. Several treatment options have been proposed: bilateral limited liver resections, partial hepatectomy of the most involved side in association with circumferential excision of intraductal stenosis by membranes or septa at the confluence of the major bile ducts by intraoperative cholangioscopy [7], hepaticojejunostomy or hepatico-cutaneo-jejunostomy and placement of large-bored silastic transhepatic stents to facilitate postoperative stone extraction, and orthotopic liver transplantation (OLT). Intrahepatic cystic involvement must be treated as patients with type V BDD.

9.5.6 Type V

The management of Caroli's disease is particularly complex. The extent of the disease (localized or diffuse) into the liver and the presence of concurrent underlying chronic liver (congenital hepatic fibrosis, secondary biliary cirrhosis, CC) or kidney disease are decision-making factors influencing the surgical management. Liver resection (LR) is considered as the treatment of choice for patients with localized forms without underlying chronic liver disease, when the impaired intrahepatic bile ducts can be completely resected [10]. In contrast, a diffuse bilobar disease is more challenging to cure and patients in whom radical resection cannot be performed are candidates for OLT [10] (Fig. 9.15). In the multidisciplinary study conducted under the auspices of the French Association of Surgery [10], collecting the largest series of patients resected for type V BDD, the 5- and 10-year survival rate for the patients who underwent surgery was 88.5 and 81.9 %, respectively, with functional results considered as excellent or good in more than 85 % of the cases whatever the type of the procedure performed (LR or OLT), with an acceptable operative mortality and morbidity, especially taking into consideration the severity of the disease. After LR, biliary reconstruction through a Roux-en-Y hepaticojejunostomy is indicated only

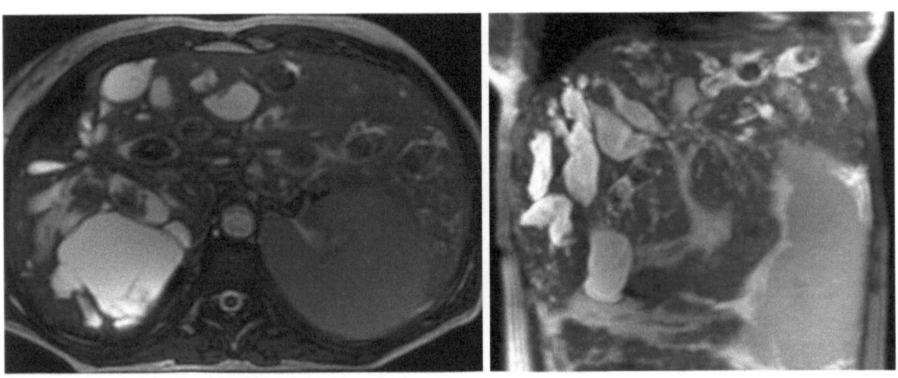

Fig. 9.15 MRI axial and coronal view: Caroli's disease in a 33-year-old female patient with recurrent cholangitis. Bilateral liver involvement (fusiform cystic dilatations and intrahepatic lithiasis), hepatomegaly, splenomegaly, and portal hypertension: candidate for OLT

when the main biliary confluence is involved in the disease. The most common surgical approach for liver resection is open surgery; however, a laparoscopic approach can be attempted when a left hemihepatectomy or a left lateral sectionectomy is indicated. However, the best timing for surgical treatment is of extreme importance, and liver resection has to be avoided in septic conditions. OLT enables a complete resection of diffuse congenital intrahepatic bile ducts whatever the extent, treat underlying liver disease, and to prevent cholangiocarcinoma [10]. OLT is recommend in patients with diffuse bilobar forms of the disease complicated by repeated sepsis or to patients with cirrhosis or portal hypertension [10] and represents less than 0.2 % indications of the whole number of liver transplantations reported in the European Transplant Liver Registry (ETLR) [42, 43]. Some authors [10] have reported some recommendations to limit the risk of postoperative septic complications in patients who underwent transplant under immunosuppressive therapy and propose to perform OLT when biliary sepsis is completely under control. For these reasons (elective basis), living donor OLT has been proposed as an alternative option for Caroli's disease (5.0 % in the American registry [44]). Most importantly, patients with Caroli's disease are at high risk to develop intrahepatic cholangiocarcinoma either synchronously or after incomplete resection. Because of the dismal prognosis of such patients, an early surgical resection is the treatment of choice for invasive lesions diagnosed or suspected preoperatively. Furthermore, because of the high prevalence of septic complications, the risk, and poor prognosis of cholangiocarcinoma, early surgical treatment is recommended, and prophylactic LR should be discussed even in asymptomatic patients with unilobar form of the disease [10]. In patients with diffuse bilobar form of the disease, the sizeable complication rate of OLT must be balanced with the risk of cholangiocarcinoma in asymptomatic patients.

References

1. Mabrut JY, Kianmanesh R, Gigot JF (2012) Dilatations congénitales des voies biliaires, anomalies de la junction biliopancréatique et maladie de Caroli. Rapport présenté au 114ᵉ Congrès Français de Chirurgie 2012. Monographies de l'Association Française de Chirurgie (AFC), Arnette
2. Todani T, Watanabe Y, Narusue M et al (1977) Congenital bile duct cysts: classification, operative procedures, and review of thirty-seven cases including cancer arising from choledochal cyst. Am J Surg 134:263–269
3. Alonso-Lej F, Rever WB, Pessango DJ (1959) Congenital choledochal cyst, with a report of 2, and analysis of 94 cases. Int Abstr Surg 108:1–30
4. Soreide K, Korner H, Havnen J et al (2004) Bile duct cysts in adults. Br J Surg 91:1538–1548
5. Singham J, Yoshida EM, Scudamore CH (2009) Choledochal cysts: part 1 of 3: classification and pathogenesis. Can J Surg 52:434–440
6. Todani T (1997) Congenital choledochal dilatation: classification, clinical features, and long-term results. J Hepatobiliary Pancreat Surg 4:276–282
7. Mabrut JY, Bozio G, Hubert C et al (2010) Management of congenital bile duct cysts. Dig Surg 27:12–18
8. Caroli J, Couinaud C, Soupault R et al (1958) Une affection nouvelle, sans doute congénitale, des voies biliaires: la dilation kystique unilobaire des canaux hépatiques. Sem Hop Paris 34:136–142

9. Guntz P, Coppo B, Lorimier G et al (1991) La maladie de Caroli unilobaire: aspects anatomo-cliniques. Démarche diagnostique et thérapeutique. A propos de 3 observations personnelles et de 101 observations de la littérature. J Chir 128:167–181
10. Mabrut JY, Kianmanesh R, Nuzzo G et al (2013) Surgical management of congenital intrahepatic bile duct dilatation, Caroli's disease and syndrome. Long-term Results of the French Association of Surgery Multicenter Study. Ann Surg 258:713–721
11. Nagorney DM (2000) Bile duct cysts in adults. In: Blumbert LH, Fong Y (eds) Surgery of the liver and biliary tract, vol 2, 3rd edn. Saunders, London, pp 1229–1244
12. Babbitt DP (1969) Congenital choledochal cyst: new etiological concept based on anomalous relationships of the common bile duct and pancreatic bulb. Ann Radiol (Paris) 12:231–240
13. Sugiyama M, Haradome H, Takahara T et al (2004) Biliopancreatic reflux via anomalous pancreaticobiliary junction. Surgery 135:457–459
14. Han SJ, Hwang EH, Chung KS et al (1997) Acquired choledochal cyst from anomalous pancreatobiliary duct union. J Pediatr Surg 32:1735–1738
15. Davenport M, Stringer MD, Howard ER (1995) Biliary amylase and congenital choledochal dilatation. J Pediatr Surg 130:474–477
16. Cheng SP, Yang TL, Jeng KS et al (2004) Choledochal cyst in adults: aetiological considerations to intrahepatic involvement. ANZ J Surg 74:964–967
17. Davenport M, Basu R (2005) Under pressure: choledochal malformation manometry. J Pediatr Surg 40:331–335
18. Todani T, Watanabe Y, Toki A et al (2003) Classification of congenital biliary cystic disease: special reference to type Ic and IVA cysts with primary ductal stricture. J Hepatobiliary Pancreat Surg 10:340–344
19. Elton E, Hanson BL, Biber BP et al (1998) Dilated common channel syndrome: endoscopic diagnosis, treatment, and relationship to choledochocele formation. Gastrointest Endosc 47:471–478
20. Craig AG, Chen LD, Saccone GT et al (2001) Sphincter of Oddi dysfunction associated with choledochal cyst. J Gastroenterol Hepatol 16:230–234
21. Levy AD, Rohrman CA (2003) Biliary cystic disease. Curr Probl Diagn Radiol 32:233–263
22. Fulcher AS, Turner MA, Sanyal AJ (2001) Case 38: Caroli disease and renal tubular ectasia. Radiology 220:720–722
23. Mousson C, Rabec M, Cercueil JP et al (1997) Caroli's disease and autosomal dominant polycystic kidney disease: a rare association? Nephrol Dial Transplant 12:1481–1483
24. Ninan VT, Nampoory MRN, Johny KV et al (2002) Caroli's disease of the liver in a renal transplant patient. Nephrol Dial Transplant 17:1113–1115
25. Sgro M, Rosetti S, Barozzino T et al (2004) Caroli's disease: prenatal diagnosis, postnatal outcome and genetic analysis. Ultrasound Obstet Gynecol 23:73–76
26. Singham J, Yoshida EM, Scudamore CH (2009) Choledochal cysts: part 2 of 3: diagnosis. Can J Surg 52:506–511
27. Swisher SG, Cates JA, Hunt KK et al (1994) Pancreatitis associated with adult choledochal cyst. Pancreas 9:633–637
28. Nagorney DM (2000) Biliary and liver cysts. In: Blumgart LH, Fong Y (eds) Surgery of the liver and biliary tract, vol 2, 3rd edn. Saunders, London, pp 1245–1258
29. Welzel TM, Graubard BI, El-Serag HB et al (2007) Risk factors for intrahepatic and extrahepatic cholangiocarcinoma in the United States: a population-based case–control study. Clin Gastroenterol Hepatol 5:1221–1228
30. Lee TY, Lee SS, Jung SW et al (2008) Hepatitis B virus infection and intrahepatic cholangiocarcinoma in Korea: a case control study. Am J Gastroenterol 103:1716–1720
31. Todani T, Tabuchi K, Watanabe Y et al (1979) Carcinoma arising in the wall of congenital bile duct cysts. Cancer 44:1134–1141
32. Lee SE, Jang JY, Lee YJ et al (2011) Choledochal cyst and associated malignant tumors in adults: a multicenter survey in South Korea. Arch Surg 146:1178–1184

33. Ouaïssi M, Kianmanesh R, Belghiti J et al (2014) Todani type II congenital bile duct cyst: European Multicenter Study of the French Surgical Association and Literature Review. Ann Surg [Epub ahead of print]
34. Todani T, Watanabe Y, Toki A et al (1987) Carcinoma related to choledochal cysts with internal drainage operations. Surg Gynecol Obstet 164:61–64
35. Singham J, Yoshida EM, Scudamore CH (2010) Choledochal cysts: part 3 of 3: management. Can J Surg 53:51–56
36. Tao KS, Lu YG, Wang T et al (2002) Procedure for congenital choledochal cysts and curative effect analysis in adults. Hepatobiliary Pancreat Dis Int 1:442–445
37. Shimotakahara A, Yamataka A, Yanai T (2005) Roux-en-Y hepaticojejunostomy or hepaticoduodenostomy for biliary reconstruction during the surgical treatment of choledochal cyst: which is better? Pediatr Surg Int 21:5–7
38. Liu DC, Rodriguez JA, Meric F et al (2000) Laparoscopic excision of a rare type II choledochal cyst: case report and review of the literature. J Pediatr Surg 35:1117–1119
39. Chatila R, Andersen DK, Topazian M (1999) Endoscopic resection of a choledochocele. Gastrointest Endosc 50:578–581
40. Horaguchi J, Fujita N, Kobayashi G (2005) Clinical study of choledochocele: is it a risk factor for biliary malignancies? J Gastroenterol 40:396–401
41. Law R, Topazian M (2014) Diagnosis and treatment of choledochoceles. Clin Gastroenterol Hepatol 12:196–203
42. De Kerckhove L, De Meyer M, Verbaandert C et al (2006) The place of liver transplantation in Caroli's disease and syndrome. Transpl Int 19:381–388
43. Millwala F, Segev DL, Thuluvath PJ (2008) Caroli's disease and outcomes after liver transplantation. Liver Transpl 14:11–17
44. Harring TR, Nguyen NTT, Liu H et al (2012) Caroli disease patients have excellent survival after liver transplant. J Surg Res 177:365–372

Hepatolithiasis 10

Felice Giuliante, Agostino Maria De Rose,
and Gennaro Nuzzo

10.1 Epidemiology

Hepatolithiasis is endemic in East Asia (including Taiwan, China, Hong Kong, Korea, Malaysia, and Japan) and is less common in Western countries, where, however, it is becoming increasingly recognized. The prevalence of intrahepatic stones in the West is 0.6–1.3 % but in Asian countries ranges from 11.7 % in Malaysia to 47.3 % in Taiwan [1–3].

Differential diagnosis between primary and secondary intrahepatic lithiasis is extremely important in order to correctly approach the patient. Intrahepatic stones secondary to extrahepatic biliary strictures related to previous liver surgery (common bile duct stricture or stricture of hepaticojejunostomy), or secondary to stones migration from gallbladder, can be classified as secondary intrahepatic lithiasis which is the most frequent cause of intrahepatic stones in Western patients (Fig. 10.1). More rarely, stones originate inside the liver within single or multiple dilatations of the intrahepatic biliary tree in association or not with intrahepatic biliary strictures. Such cases can be classified as primary intrahepatic lithiasis (PIL).

10.2 Etiology

The etiology of primary hepatolithiasis remains not fully understood, but genetic, dietary, and environmental factors are thought contributing factors.

In Western countries PIL is strictly related to congenital bile duct dilatation with intrahepatic-only localization corresponding to Todani type V [4]. This entity was first described by Caroli et al. [5] in 1958 and later classified by Guntz et al. [6]

F. Giuliante (✉) • A.M. De Rose • G. Nuzzo
Hepatobiliary Surgery Unit, Catholic University of the Sacred Heart
– A. Gemelli Hospital, Largo A. Gemelli, 8, Rome 00168, Italy
e-mail: fgiuliante@rm.unicatt.it; agostinom.derose@virgilio.it; gennaro.nuzzo@rm.unicatt.it

L. Aldrighetti et al. (eds.), *Benign Tumors of the Liver*,
DOI 10.1007/978-3-319-12985-3_10

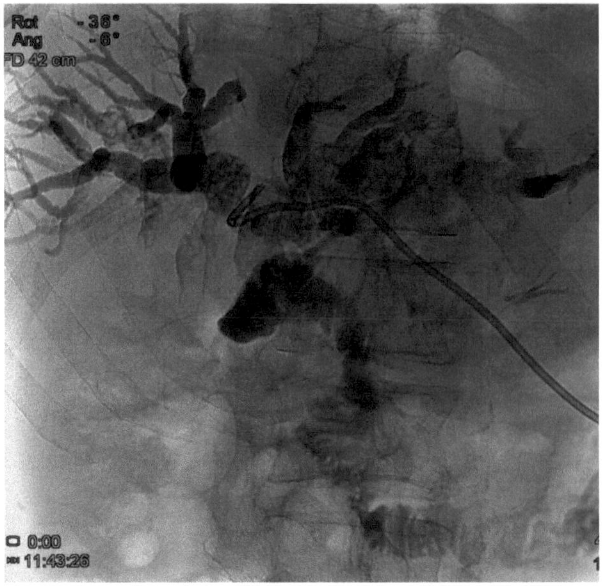

Fig. 10.1 Percutaneous transhepatic cholangiography (PTC): dilated intrahepatic bile ducts with multiple stones over stricture of hepaticojejunostomy (secondary intrahepatic lithiasis)

according to the morphology and the extent of intrahepatic bile duct dilatations. A recent multicenter study conducted by the French Association of Surgery [7] has shown that prevalence of intrahepatic lithiasis in patients with Caroli's disease is above 50 %, whereas in Eastern patients, it seems mainly related to biliary infestations and infections [8].

Typically there are two types of intrahepatic stones: calcium bilirubinate stones (brown pigment stones) and cholesterol stones. Calcium bilirubinate stones, mainly composed of bilirubin, cholesterol, fatty acids, and calcium, represent the majority of intrahepatic stones, whereas cholesterol stones comprise 5.8–13.1 % of all intrahepatic stones [2]. Pathogenesis of intrahepatic stones involves not only the precipitation of calcium bilirubinate, but also an altered cholesterol metabolism.

In addition bile duct stricture, either congenital or acquired, and infection with β-glucuronidase-producing bacteria play a key role in bilirubin precipitation and formation of calcium bilirubinate stones, which are mostly observed in Eastern countries [1, 2, 9]. Lower socioeconomic status and poor hygiene may be involved in the development of intrahepatic stones [10].

Recently, Shoda et al. [11] has shown that pathogenesis of intrahepatic cholesterol stones formation is based upon the dual defects of upregulation of cholesterol synthesis and downregulation of bile-acid synthesis in the liver, possibly in association with defective secretion of phospholipid by its canalicular transporter, multidrug resistance protein (MDR3). Metabolic factors, either acquired or congenital, act synergistically in the development of these intrahepatic stones [1, 12].

Some investigators have reported that anatomic variations of intrahepatic bile ducts can cause hepatolithiasis. Notably, hepatolithiasis is more frequent in the left than in the right lobe, and the acute angle which the left hepatic duct forms at the junction with the common bile duct (CBD), which tends to induce bile stasis when associated

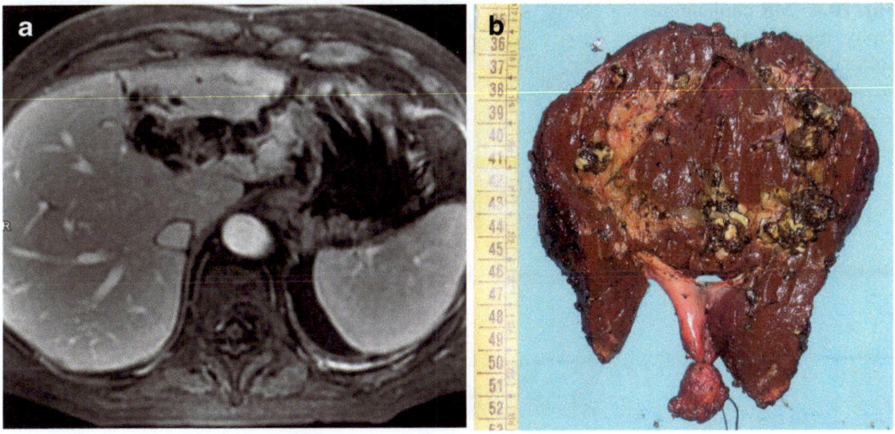

Fig. 10.2 (**a**) Abdominal MRI: intrahepatic lithiasis of the left hemiliver. (**b**) Surgical specimen after left hepatectomy: dilated bile ducts with multiple stones

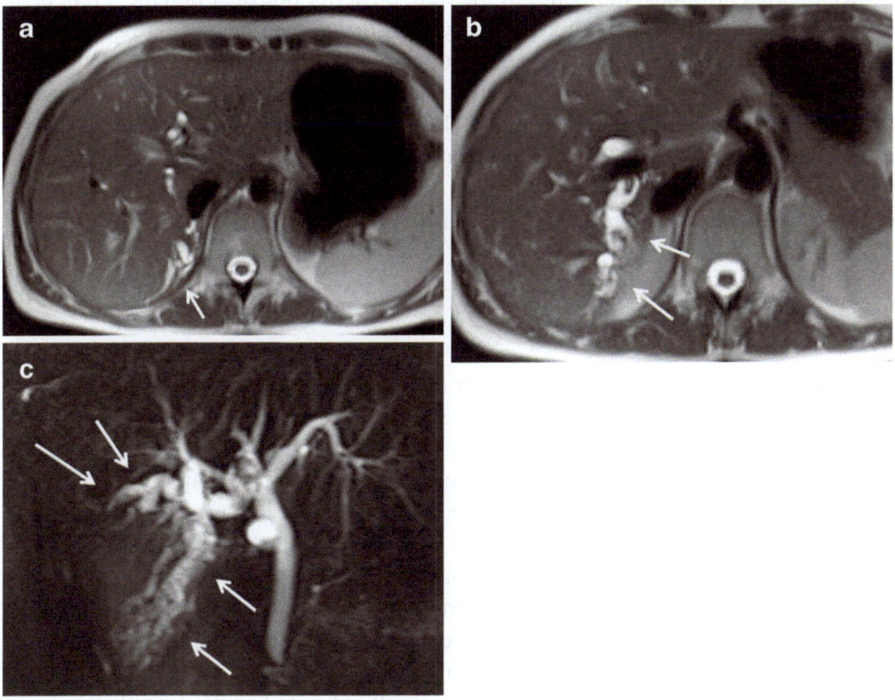

Fig. 10.3 (**a**, **b**) Abdominal MRI, (**c**) MR cholangiography: dilated bile ducts of right posterior sector with stones and parenchymal atrophy of the sector (*arrows*)

with biliary strictures, has been advocated as a key point for this higher rate [1] (Fig. 10.2). In the right lobe the duct of segment 6 alone or of the posterior sector seems the most frequently involved, and also in this case the anatomy of the junction of the ducts of these segment or sector could play a major role (Fig. 10.3). Furthermore,

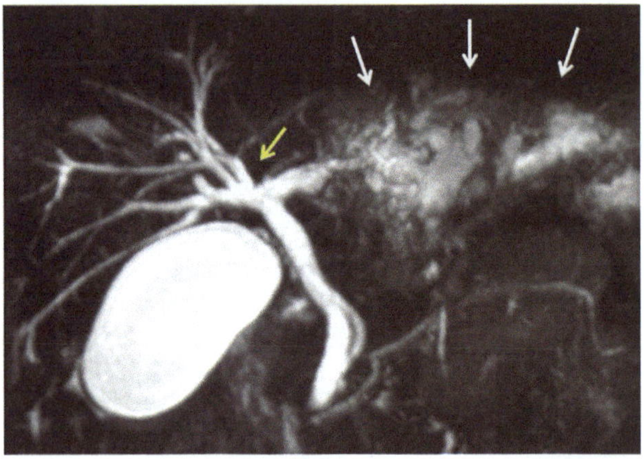

Fig. 10.4 MR cholangiography: dilated left lateral sectorial bile ducts with stones (*white arrows*); anomalous biliary main confluence (*yellow arrow*)

it was reported [13] that confluence of the right posterior bile duct into the left hepatic duct (Norman's anomaly [14]) may also play a role in the development of PIL. However, in a recent comparative study between patients with PIL in Taiwan and Japan, anatomic variations of intrahepatic segmental bile ducts did not seem to play any important role in the pathogenesis of PIL [15]. Therefore, the role of anatomic variations of intrahepatic bile ducts in hepatolithiasis remains unclear, although in clinical practice in Western countries anatomic variations of intrahepatic bile ducts are frequently observed in patients with intrahepatic lithiasis (Fig. 10.4).

10.3 Clinical Presentation

Abdominal pain, either in the right upper quadrant or in the upper abdomen, generally is the most frequent initial symptom. Symptoms of hepatolithiasis include cholangitis, jaundice, and acute pancreatitis. Other abdominal complaints, including abdominal discomfort and vomiting, may be observed. In asymptomatic patients hepatolithiasis may be an incidental finding on abdominal imaging; this occurs with increasing frequency due to the advances in diagnostic imaging modalities and the popularization of routine medical examination.

Most patients have a long history of previous biliary operative and nonoperative treatments and tend to have consequent recurrent pyogenic cholangitis as the most common clinical sign. Pyogenic cholangitis may cause further septic complications such as hepatic abscess and may ultimately result in limited parenchymal atrophy or secondary sclerosing cholangitis. Indeed, the most frequently observed clinical history of patients with PIL includes several endoscopic treatments by endoscopic retrograde cholangiography (ERC) for recurrent stones of CBD. Patients usually first undergo cholecystectomy and then present with recurrent CBD stones misdiagnosed as residual stones that migrated from the gallbladder. For this reason they usually undergo several endoscopic treatments of the CBD stones, frequently without any further complete investigation of all the intrahepatic biliary tree. Patients usually develop recurrent cholangitis which can evolve into intrahepatic abscesses. It is important to consider that after multiple endoscopic or percutaneous treatments and recurrent episodes of cholangitis and medical treatments, it is likely to find multiresistant bacteria into the bile ducts, which strongly influence subsequent clinical history of these patients and the results of treatment. This fact should be strongly emphasized and microbiological cultures of bile should be performed whenever possible from external biliary drainages (percutaneous biliary drainage, naso-biliary drainage).

The Hepatolithiasis Research Group in Japan has proposed a clinical grade classification to quantify the severity of hepatolithiasis [16]: Grade 1, absence of symptoms; Grade 2, abdominal pain; Grade 3, transient jaundice or cholangitis; and Grade 4, persistent jaundice, sepsis, or cholangiocarcinoma.

10.4 Evolution

Late complications of hepatolithiasis include liver abscesses, pyogenic sepsis, parenchymal atrophy, persistent liver dysfunction resulting in secondary biliary cirrhosis, and cholangiocarcinoma. The latter two represent, therefore, the major risks in patients with intrahepatic lithiasis. It is presumed that chronic inflammation of the bile ducts by bile stasis, stones, and infestation with parasites can lead to adenomatous hyperplasia of the epithelium and subsequently to cholangiocarcinoma.

Hepatolithiasis is an established risk factor for intrahepatic cholangiocarcinoma (ICC) in Asian countries, with 2–10 % of patients with hepatolithiasis developing ICC [17]. The Korean, hospital-based, case–control study by Lee et al. found a strong association between hepatolithiasis and ICC, with an OR of 50.0 (95 % CI = 21.2–117.3) [18]. A Chinese, hospital-based, case–control study by Zhou et al. also showed a significant association, with the OR at 5.8 (95 % CI = 1.97–16.9) [19]. There are less data on the relationship between hepatolithiasis and ICC in Western countries, but a recent Italian multicenter study showed that prevalence of ICC in patients who underwent liver resection for intrahepatic lithiasis was 14.3 % [20].

Previous reports showed that bilirubin stones [21], irregular ductal stricture or obstruction, age over 40 years, a long history of hepatolithiasis with weight loss, high level of serum alkaline phosphatase, low level of serum albumin, high level of the serum carcinoembryonic antigen, and/or hepatolithiasis in the right or both lobes [22] were predictive factors for cholangiocarcinoma associated with hepatolithiasis. In a recent Japanese multicenter study, the authors showed that previous choledocoenterostomy and liver atrophy may increase the risk of developing cholangiocarcinoma [23].

Despite the high number of suspected risk factors, preoperative diagnosis of cholangiocarcinoma in these patients is usually difficult because hepatolithiasis and related periductal inflammation hinder clear visualization of bile ducts by imaging techniques; therefore, especially in patients with biliary strictures in whom is very difficult to rule out a malignant stricture with certainty, liver resection should always be considered, and the possibility to find a cholangiocarcinoma should always be kept in mind. Indeed the multicenter Italian study [20] showed that a preoperative suspected diagnosis of ICC was obtained in only 39.1 % of the patients initially evaluated for resection for intrahepatic lithiasis; in the other cases diagnosis of ICC was performed intraoperatively and postoperatively in 26.1 and 34.8 %, respectively. Therefore, the risk of the presence of cholangiocarcinoma in patients with longstanding PIL and of development of cholangiocarcinoma in young patients with PIL, or in patients treated for a long period of time by nonsurgical treatments (Fig. 10.5), should always be considered when choosing the treatment. In case of postoperative diagnosis at pathology of unsuspected cholangiocarcinoma, reoperation to perform more radical procedure (more extended parenchymal resection, resection of main biliary confluence, lymphadenectomy) if necessary should be also considered [24]. Furthermore, development of cholangiocarcinoma has been reported also in patients with previous liver resection for hepatolithiasis; therefore, patients resected for PIL should be carefully followed up for early detection of cholangiocarcinoma [25].

Fig. 10.5 Forty-eight-year-old male patient. Fifteen years previously (33 years old) diagnosis of intrahepatic lithiasis of the right posterior sector (**a**, Abdominal MRI), treated percutaneously: (**b**) PTC, bile ducts of right posterior sector completely filled by stones; (**c**) balloon dilatation of biliary stricture; and (**d**) final cholangiography; clearance of the majority of the stones; residual intrahepatic bile ducts dilation. Five years later cholangitis, with recurrence of intrahepatic lithiasis: (**e**) PTC, stones recurrence (*short arrow*) above sectoral biliary stricture (*thin arrow*); (**f**) percutaneous treatment, double balloon dilatation of biliary stricture; (**g**) final cholangiography after complete removal of lithiasis, residual intrahepatic bile strictures (*arrows*). Nine years later increase of alkaline phosphatases and gamma glutamyl peptidases. (**h**, **i**) Abdominal MRI: atrophy of right posterior sector and hypotrophy of the remnant right hemiliver, with appearance of a dishomogeneous mass in the right posterior sector without portal flow in the relative portal branch. Referral at our unit and indication to surgery. (**j**) Intraoperative field after right hepatectomy, excision of main biliary confluence and CBD, left hepaticojejunostomy, and lymphadenectomy. (**k**) Surgical specimen: intrahepatic cholangiocarcinoma invading the right posterior portal branch

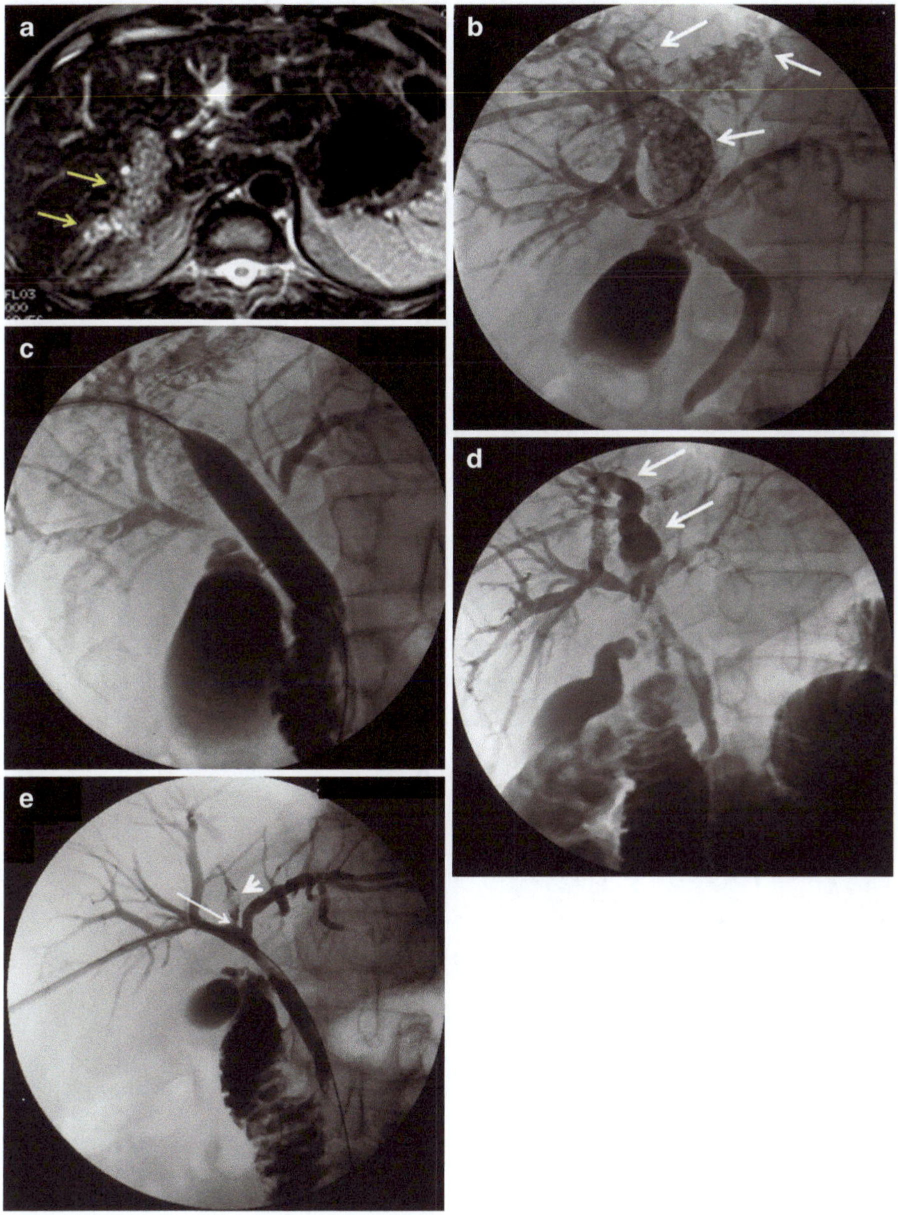
a
b
c
d
e

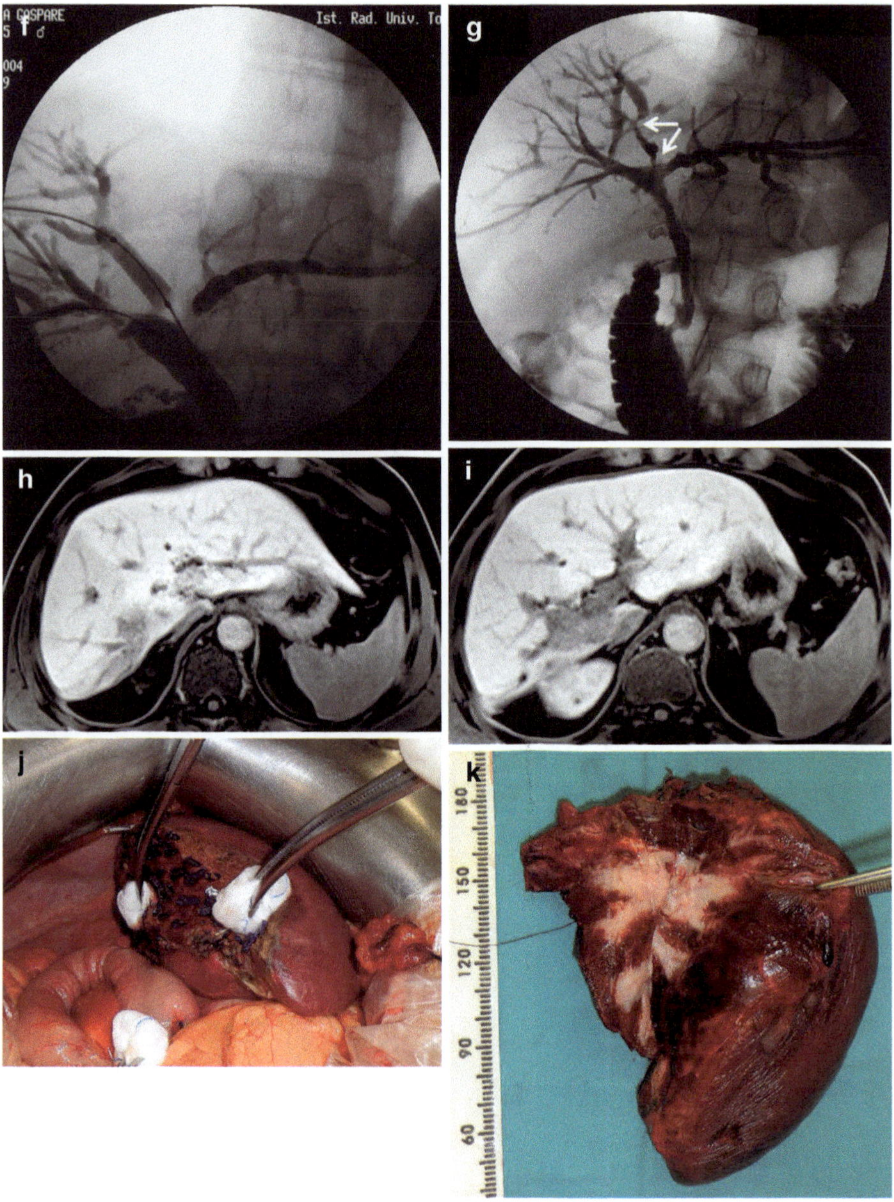

Fig. 10.5 (continued)

10.5 Therapy

Treatment of PIL still remains particularly difficult and controversial. Several surgical, endoscopic, and percutaneous procedures have been reported in the literature, but high recurrence rates are often reported.

10.5.1 Surgical Treatment

Liver resection represents the only treatment which can allow the complete removal of intrahepatic stones together with affected bile ducts. The most frequent indications for liver resection reported in the literature are the following: lithiasis limited to one lobe, sector, or segment; parenchymal hypo-atrophy; liver abscess; failure of previous treatments; and suspected cholangiocarcinoma. Indication in asymptomatic patients is more controversial, but young age of patients, low surgical risk of resection, and risk of early and late complications of other treatments should require liver resection in localized forms of PIL (Fig. 10.6).

Liver resections in patients with PIL have been frequently reported by Eastern centers for the high prevalence of the disease [26–29]. More rarely and with lower number of patients, liver resections are reported by Western centers [7, 30–37]. This is related mainly to the lower incidence of intrahepatic lithiasis in Western countries, but probably also to the relatively unawareness of this disease and of the possible severe late complications, to the wide availability of endoscopic and percutaneous treatments, and to the concern for the operative risk of hepatectomy.

Perioperative mortality of resection of the majority of recent series from all the Western centers was nil [31–37]. Also in Eastern series postoperative mortality was low, ranging from 0 to 3.5 % [26–29, 38] in spite of higher complexity of disease than that reported in Western series (higher rate of bilateral intrahepatic lithiasis and cirrhosis).

Postoperative morbidity rates in Eastern and Western series ranged from 7.4 to 58.8 % [26–38] which mainly include septic complications due to preoperative recurrent cholangitis, frequently related to previous endoscopic or percutaneous treatments. In our experience on 75 patients resected between 1992 and 2012 for PIL, mortality was nil and morbidity rate was 40 % (30 pts); 83 % of complicated patients (29 cases) had septic complications: all these patients had persistent postoperative fever, in 5 cases with subdiaphragmatic abscess and in 12 cases with bile leak. In 79 % of these patients, positive bile cultures were found preoperatively, and the same bacteria were detected from surgical drainages after resection, with positive blood culture in 48 % of these patients. Multivariate analysis identified previous endoscopic or percutaneous treatments and preoperative cholangitis as the only two independent risk factors for septic complications.

Early diagnosis of the disease and surgical treatment at an early stage are key factors for performing liver resections with low operative risk [39]. Noninvasive diagnostic approach by CT and MR for accurate evaluation of the disease and strict avoidance of endoscopic or percutaneous diagnostic approach with consequent

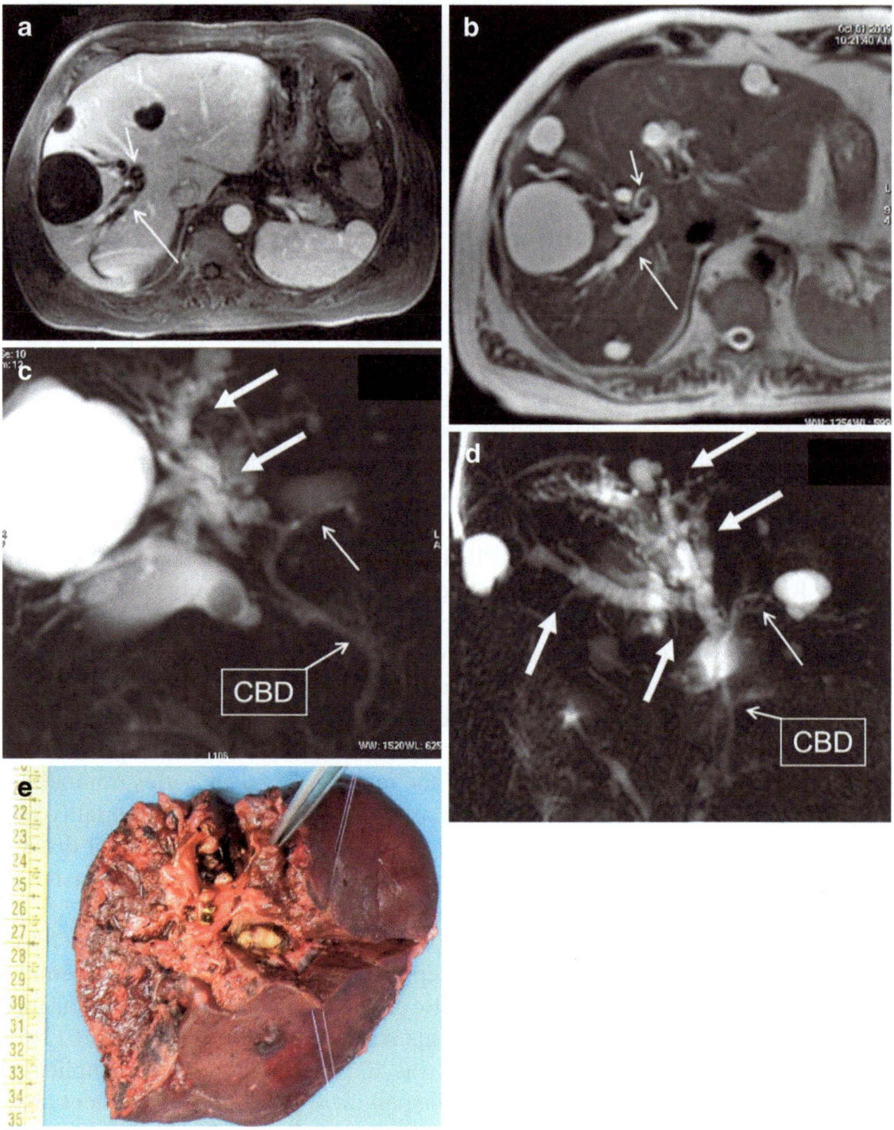

Fig. 10.6 Sixty-seven-year-old male patient, with right intrahepatic lithiasis, simple liver cysts, gallbladder stones; no symptoms. (**a**, **b**) MRI: dilated intrahepatic biliary tree (*arrows*) with stones (*short arrows*). (**c**, **d**) MR cholangiography: diffusely dilation of right intrahepatic bile ducts (*arrows*); CBD and left intrahepatic bile ducts (*thin arrows*) not dilated. (**e**) Surgical specimen after right hepatectomy: dilated bile ducts with multiple stones

biliary infection may prevent postoperative severe septic complications which can explain the high mortality rate of surgery (7.4 %) reported by Kassahun [30]. Actually, effective control of sepsis should be always strongly pursued before liver resection. For patients with acute obstructive suppurative cholangitis with intrahepatic stones, emergency percutaneous transhepatic biliary drainage is indicated and

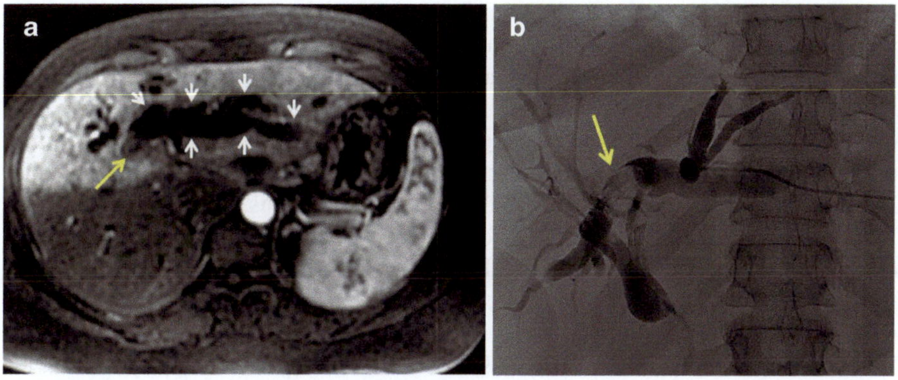

Fig. 10.7 Fifty-six-year-old female with acute cholangitis, already submitted to choledochoduodenostomy for lithiasis. (**a**) Abdominal MRI, dilated left hepatic duct (*short arrows*) above stone (*yellow arrow*); (**b**) PTC: percutaneous treatment of cholangitis; insertion of biliary drainage; stone in the left hepatic duct (*arrow*); subsequent liver resection

Fig. 10.8 Intraoperative field after left hepatectomy with placement of biliary T-tube in the stump of the left hepatic duct

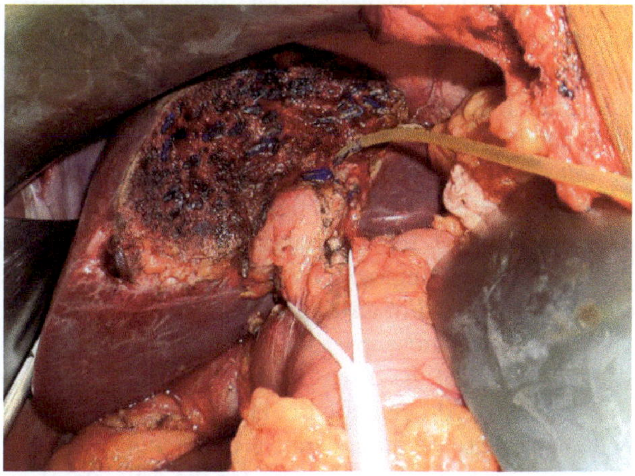

should be preferred to endoscopic transpapillary approaches (Fig. 10.7). Furthermore, in these patients intraoperatively it is mandatory to take samples of bile from intrahepatic bile ducts for microbiological cultures, irrigate all the intrahepatic biliary tree with large amount of saline solution, and leave in place a biliary drainage at the end of resection (Fig. 10.8). In fact the most frequent and severe postoperative complications are sepsis related, and the possibility to get bile samples during the postoperative course is extremely useful. Among septic complications, patients with hepatolithiasis may develop thrombocytopenia and enhanced platelet activation, resulting in coagulation and fibrinolysis disorders, which could be particularly severe after liver resection [40].

When liver resection is considered, operative planning should be decided according to the following issues: location of stones, biliary strictures, and/or dilatations; number of involved liver segments; presence of extrahepatic stones; presence of choledochal cyst; presence of cirrhosis; and suspicion of cholangiocarcinoma. Furthermore, need of other procedures associated with parenchymal resection should be accurately evaluated and planned.

In case of unilateral disease, partial hepatectomy is the treatment of choice which can radically resolve recurrent cholangitis and stone formation and prevent the risk of cholangiocarcinoma [39]. Unilobar extension of the disease, especially left liver location, is more frequently reported than bilateral locations. The incidence of unilobar extent is reported to be 61 % and left involvement ranges from 58 to 86 % of cases [31–33, 39, 41, 42]. Right-side location is less frequently reported; however, these data could be influenced by referral bias in patient's selection to surgical centers.

The exact evaluation of the extension of PIL is of paramount importance for planning the exact extent of liver resection and for reducing the risk of biliary fistula or recurrence of lithiasis. In particular, in left-sided hepatolithiasis, the exact anatomy of the bile duct of segment 4 should be accurately evaluated for the choice between left lateral sectionectomy and left hepatectomy. In our experience left hepatectomy was performed in 67 % (40 out of 60 cases) of left-sided intrahepatic lithiasis, and stone recurrence rate was 2.5 %. Conversely 11 % of patients who underwent left lateral sectionectomy developed stone recurrence.

Also the involvement of the biliary ducts of the caudate lobe should be carefully evaluated. Indeed, biliary ducts of the caudate lobe can be involved, and if this is the case, caudate lobe resection should be associated with left hepatectomy (Fig. 10.9) in order to avoid postoperative biliary fistula and late stone recurrence [36, 37]. In our series caudate lobe resection was associated to left hepatectomy in 9 out of 40 patients (22.5 %). Intraoperative cholangiography should be performed whenever preoperative cholangiography is not complete and the extent of resection is not clearly defined and in any case of unclear intrahepatic biliary anatomy. Also intraoperative cholangioscopy should be always available for further evaluation of the site and extent of the disease (strictures and stones) and for removal of the stones (mechanical, hydroelectrolytic, laser lithotripsy [43]) if needed. Although in these patients the use of intraoperative ultrasonography (IOUS) can be difficult in the study of intrahepatic biliary tree for the artifacts of air in the bile ducts, IOUS is extremely useful to visualize bile ducts filled by stones, not visible to cholangiography, and to guide limited segmental resection (Fig. 10.10).

After surgical treatment, postoperative stone clearance ranged from 95 to 98 %, late stone recurrence from 3.7 to 15.4 %, and recurrent cholangitis from 0 to 24 % [30–39, 41, 43]. The highest rate of stone clearance can be obtained with the addition of intraoperative and postoperative treatments. Immediate and late results depend on extent and severity of disease, presence and site of biliary strictures, time interval from the onset of symptoms and treatment, and duration of preoperative treatments.

Recently laparoscopic liver resection for PIL have been reported with good results, suggesting that laparoscopic hepatectomy could be an effective therapeutic option for these patients in particular in those with left-sided disease, which is the most frequent [44, 45]. It should be emphasized that laparoscopic liver resection for

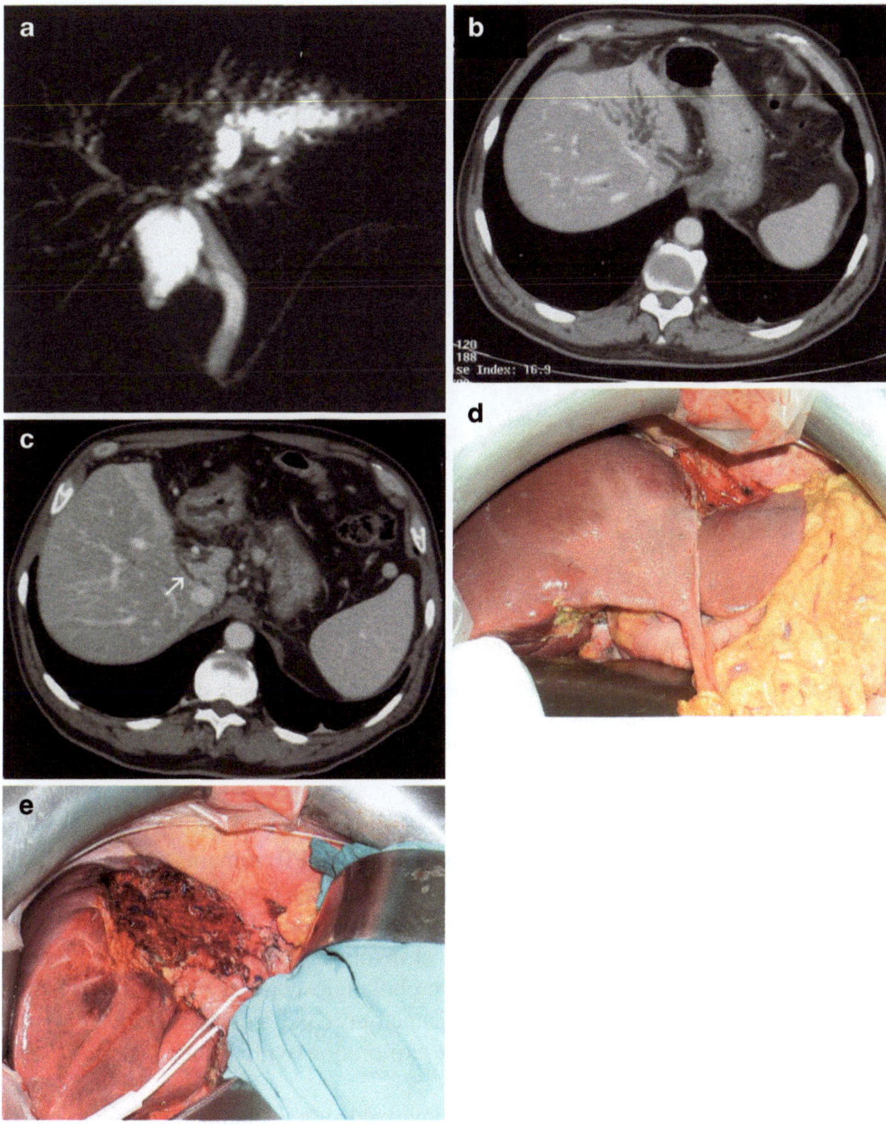

Fig. 10.9 (**a**) MR cholangiography, dilated left bile ducts with lithiasis; (**b**) CT scan, dilation of bile ducts of the entire left hemiliver with parenchymal atrophy; (**c**) CT scan, biliary duct dilation involving also the caudate lobe (*white arrow*); (**d**) operative field, parenchymal atrophy, mainly of segment 4; and (**e**) operative field at the end of left hepatectomy extended to the caudate lobe

PIL should be performed by surgeons with experience in both open hepatobiliary surgery and laparoscopy. In fact liver resections for PIL are frequently more technically demanding than those for tumors for severe perihepatic adhesions, fibrotic parenchyma, deformed intrahepatic biliary anatomy, and atrophic changes.

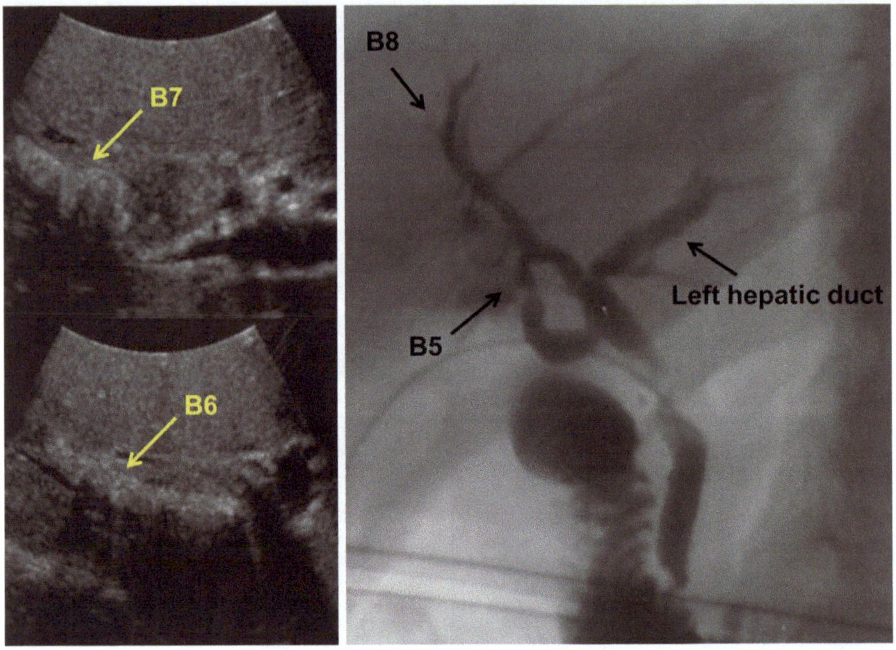

Fig. 10.10 Intraoperative cholangiography from the stump of the cystic duct: left hepatic duct and bile ducts of segment 8 (*B8*) and 5 (*B5*) are visualized; bile ducts of segments 6 and 7 are missing in the cholangiogram. Intraoperative ultrasonography (*left boxes*) shows bile ducts of segments 6 and 7 (*B6*, *B7*) filled by multiple stones

The optimal management of patients with bilateral PIL remains a very complex and challenging task because of the difficulty to obtain a complete stone clearance. Several treatment options have been proposed: bilateral limited liver resections (Fig. 10.11), partial hepatectomy of the most involved side in association with contralateral stone extraction by intraoperative cholangioscopy or by other perioperative nonsurgical procedures, partial hepatectomy and hepaticojejunostomy or hepatico-cutaneous jejunostomy or CBD exploration with T-tube insertion, and liver transplantation (OLT).

When partial hepatectomy of the most involved side is planned, complete clearance of the contralateral bile ducts with removal of the stones from the residual liver should be obtained using all the available tools: intraoperative cholangiography, ultrasonography, and cholangioscopy [46].

In patients with bilateral PIL complicated with liver fibrosis or cirrhosis, OLT may be the treatment of choice [39]. OLT for PIL is rarely reported; in fact indication for OLT represents 0.2 % of the whole number of liver transplants reported in the European Liver Transplant Registry (ELTR) [39].

Historically, biliary-enteric anastomosis (choledochoduodenostomy and Roux-en-Y hepaticojejunostomy) was one of the most common procedures performed for

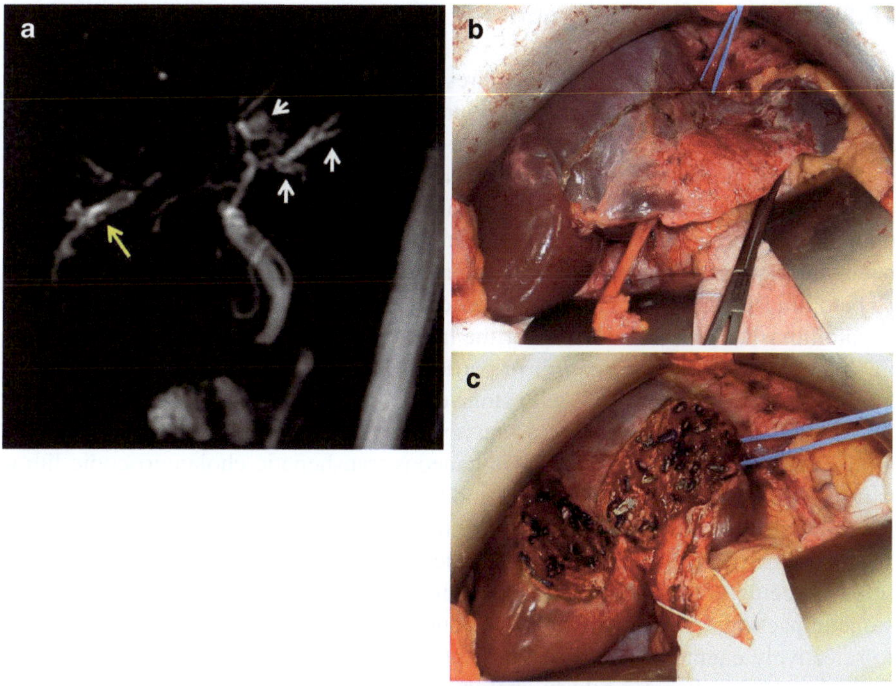

Fig. 10.11 Bilateral lithiasis. (**a**) MR cholangiography, dilated bile ducts of left hemiliver (*short arrows*) and of segment 5 (*yellow arrow*); (**b**) intraoperative field, parenchymal atrophy of left hemiliver and of segment 5 involved by lithiasis; and (**c**) intraoperative field after left hepatectomy and resection of segment 5 (*arrow*)

PIL in order to facilitate postoperative spontaneous discharge of intrahepatic stones into the jejunum. More recently the role of hepaticojejunostomy in the treatment of PIL has been deeply reconsidered. In fact, according to the results reported in recent papers, hepaticojejunostomy is not effective for drainage of residual and recurrent stones and increases the risk of recurrent cholangitis and also of cholangiocarcinoma [23, 47, 48]. Furthermore, hepaticojejunostomy (HJ) eliminates the continuity of CBD and it precludes further endoscopic procedures for removal of recurrent stones. For this last reason, in patients with a high risk of recurrence, that is, patients with complex, bilateral lithiasis, techniques that allow an easy access (percutaneous/endoscopic) to intrahepatic bile ducts have been proposed: hepatico-cutaneous jejunostomy [49–51], hepatoduodenal anastomosis with an interposed jejunal loop [52], and latero-lateral anastomosis between jejunal loop of the H-J and duodenum [53]. For all these reasons hepaticojejunostomy is not recommended as routine treatment for PIL. Indication to perform a hepaticojejunostomy associated to liver resection should be limited to patients with intrahepatic lithiasis and simultaneous presence of cystic dilatation of common bile duct, which is necessary to be also resected.

10.5.2 Nonsurgical Treatment

Percutaneous and endoscopic procedures for treatment of PIL have been widely described in the literature. These procedure are both effective in obtaining bile duct clearance, but the choice between the two techniques depends on location of stones and strictures, presence of associated extrahepatic stones, and local expertise.

Since 1981 Nimura et al. [54] emphasized the role of percutaneous transhepatic drainage and cholangioscopy for treatment of PIL, and percutaneous approach has been reported as the most effective nonsurgical treatment. Recently the Japan Hepatolithiasis Research Group conducted a nationwide survey on patients with hepatolithiasis and showed that over the last 40 years the frequency of nonsurgical treatment significantly increased; in particular the frequency of endoscopic retrograde cholangiography (ERC) with stone extraction changed from 0.2 % in 1998 to 22.7 % in 2011 [55]. Indeed in this survey in 2011 ERC with stone extraction was more frequently performed than percutaneous transhepatic cholangioscopic lithotripsy (PTCSL) (22.7 % vs. 11.7 %), and the authors clarified that the incidence of recurrent stones after ERC was higher than those after PTCSL and surgery (25, 11.4, 0 %, respectively) [55]. However, the role of ERC in the treatment of hepatolithiasis seems to be limited particularly in case of tightened strictures, peripheral stone impaction, or acute angles of bile ducts. The PTCSL provides the possibility to selectively cannulate multiple segmental bile ducts in order to obtain the exact definition of intrahepatic biliary anatomy and the complete removal of the stone especially if associated to electrohydraulic and laser lithotripsy.

As regards indication to nonsurgical treatments of hepatolithiasis, the presence of intrahepatic biliary strictures and dilatation represents the most controversial issues because they are associated with frequent intrahepatic stone recurrence, recurrent cholangitis, and risk of development of cholangiocarcinoma [55].

References

1. Tazuma S (2006) Epidemiology, pathogenesis, and classification of biliary stones (common bile duct and intrahepatic). Best Pract Res Clin Gastroenterol 20:1075–1083
2. Mori T, Sugiyama M, Atomi Y (2006) Management of intrahepatic stones. Best Pract Res Clin Gastroenterol 20:1117–1137
3. Shoda J, Tanaka N, Osuga T (2003) Hepatolithiasis-epidemiology and pathogenesis update. Front Biosci 8:e398–e409
4. Todani T, Watanabe Y, Narusue M et al (1977) Congenital bile duct cyst: classification, operative procedures, and review of 37 cases including cancer arising from choledochal cyst. Am J Surg 134:263–269
5. Caroli J, Couinaud C, Soupault R et al (1958) Une affection nouvelle, sans doute congénitale, des voies biliaires: la dilatation kystique unilobaire des canaux hépatiques. Sem Hop Paris 34:136–142
6. Guntz P, Coppo B, Lorimier G et al (1991) La maladie de Caroli unilobaire: aspects anatomocliniques. Démarche diagnostique et thérapeutique. A propos de 3 observations personnelles et de 101 observations de la littérature. J Chir 128:167–181
7. Mabrut JY, Kianmanesh R, Nuzzo G et al (2013) Surgical management of congenital intrahepatic bile duct dilatation, Caroli's disease and syndrome. Long-term Results of the French Association of Surgery Multicenter Study. Ann Surg 258:713–721

8. Chawla Y, Duseya A (2008) Intrahepatic stones: is it a lifestyle disease? J Gastroenterol Hepatol 23:998–999
9. Nuzzo G, Clemente G, Giovannini I et al (2008) Resection for primary intrahepatic stones: a single-centre experience. Arch Surg 143:570–573
10. Momiyama M, Wakai K, Oda K et al (2008) Lifestyle risk factors for intrahepatic stone: findings from a case–control study in an endemic area, Taiwan. J Gastroenterol Hepatol 23:1075–1081
11. Shoda J, Inada Y, Osuga T (2006) Molecular pathogenesis of hepatolithiasis: a type of low phospholipid-associated cholelithiasis. Front Biosci 11:669–675
12. Kawakami H, Kuwatani M, Onodera M et al (2007) Primary cholesterol hepatolithiasis associated with cholangiocellular carcinoma: a case report and literature review. Intern Med 46:1191–1196
13. Pan S, Liao CH (1951) Intrahepatic stones: probable factors, clinical manifestation and recent advances in diagnosis. J Formos Med Assoc 82:226–238
14. Norman O (1951) Studies on the hepatic ducts in cholangiography. Acta Radiol Suppl 84:1–81
15. Kitagawa Y, Nimura Y, Hayakawa N et al (2003) Intrahepatic segmental bile duct patterns in hepatolithiasis: a comparative cholangiographic study between Taiwan and Japan. J Hepatobiliary Pancreat Surg 10:377–381
16. Nimura Y, Momiyama M, Yamada T et al (2001) The survey of hepatolithiasis. In: Annual reports of the Japanese Ministry of Health and Welfare. Tokyo, Japan: Japanese Government, pp 33–38.
17. Tyson GL, El-Serag HB (2011) Risk factors for cholangiocarcinoma. Hepatology 54:173–184
18. Lee TY, Lee SS, Jung SW et al (2008) Hepatitis B virus infection and intrahepatic cholangiocarcinoma in Korea: a case control study. Am J Gastroenterol 103:1716–1720
19. Zhou YM, Yin ZF, Yang JM et al (2008) Risk factors for intrahepatic cholangiocarcinoma: a case–control study in China. World J Gastroenterol 14:632–635
20. Guglielmi A, Ruzzenente A, Valdegamberi A et al (2014) Hepatolithiasis-associated cholangiocarcinoma: results from a multi-institutional national database on a case series of 23 patients. Eur J Surg Oncol 40:567–575
21. Nakamura Y, Terada T, Tanaka Y, Ohta G (1985) Are hepatolithiasis and cholangiocarcinoma etiologically related? A morphological study of 12 cases of hepatolithiasis associated with cholangiocarcinoma. Virchows Arch A Pathol Anat Histopathol 406:45–58
22. Kim YT, Byun JS, Kim J et al (2003) Factors predicting concurrent cholangiocarcinomas associated with hepatolithiasis. Hepatogastroenterology 50:8–12
23. Suzuki Y, Mori T, Abe N et al (2012) Predictive factors for cholangiocarcinoma associated with hepatolithiasis determined on the basis of Japanese multicenter study. Hepatol Res 42:166–170
24. Lesurtel M, Regimbeau JM, Farges O et al (2002) Intrahepatic cholangiocarcinoma and hepatolithiasis: an unusual association in western countries. Eur J Gastroenterol Hepatol 14:1025–1027
25. Lee JY, Kim JS, Moon JM et al (2013) Incidence of cholangiocarcinoma with or without previous resection of liver for hepatolithiasis. Gut Liver 7:475–479
26. Li SQ, Liang LJ, Peng BG et al (2007) Bile leakage after hepatectomy for hepatolithiasis: risk factors and management. Surgery 141:340–345
27. Chen ZY, Yan LN, Zeng Y et al (2008) Preliminary experience with indications for liver transplantation for hepatolithiasis. Transplant Proc 40:3517–3522
28. Huang ZQ, Huang XQ, Zhang WZ et al (2008) Liver resection in hepatolithiasis: 20-year's evolution. Zhonghua Wai Ke Za Zhi 46:1450–1452
29. Liu ZY, Zhou YM, Shi LH et al (2011) Risk factors of intrahepatic cholangiocarcinoma in patients with hepatolithiasis: a case control study. Hepatobiliary Pancreat Dis Int 10: 626–631
30. Kassahun WT, Kahn T, Wittekind C et al (2005) Caroli's disease: liver resection and liver transplantation. Experience in 33 patients. Surgery 138:888–898
31. Herman P, Perini MV, Machado MA et al (2006) Liver resection as the definitive treatment for unilateral non-oriental primary intrahepatic lithiasis. Am J Surg 191:460–464

32. Catena M, Aldrighetti L, Finazzi R et al (2006) Treatment of non-endemic hepatolithiasis in a western country. The role of hepatic resection. Ann R Coll Surg Engl 88:383–389
33. Bockhorn M, Malagó M, Lang H et al (2006) The role of surgery in Caroli's disease. J Am Coll Surg 202:928–932
34. Vetrone G, Ercolani G, Grazi GL et al (2006) Surgical therapy for hepatolithiasis: a western experience. J Am Coll Surg 202:306–312
35. Ulrich F, Pratschke J, Pascher A et al (2008) Long-term outcome of liver resection and transplantation for Caroli disease and syndrome. Ann Surg 247:357–364
36. Clemente G, Giuliante F, De Rose AM et al (2010) Liver resection for intrahepatic stones in congenital bile duct dilatation. J Visc Surg 147:e175–e180
37. Tabrizian P, Jibara G, Shrager B et al (2012) Hepatic resection for primary hepatolithiasis: a single-center western experience. J Am Coll Surg 215:622–626
38. Uenishi T, Hamba H, Takemura S et al (2009) Outcome of hepatic resection for hepatolithiasis. Am J Surg 198:199–202
39. Mabrut JY, Partensky C, Jaeck D et al (2007) Congenital intrahepatic bile duct dilatation is a potentially curable disease: long-term results of a multi-institutional study. Ann Surg 246:236–245
40. Feng WM, Bao Y, Fei MY et al (2003) Platelet activation and the protective effect of aprotinin in hepatolithiasis patients. Hepatobiliary Pancreat Dis Int 2:602–604
41. Chen DW, Poon RTP, Liu CL et al (2004) Immediate and long-term outcomes of hepatectomy for hepatolithiasis. Surgery 135:386–393
42. Clemente G, De Rose AM, Giordano M et al (2009) Primary intrahepatic lithiasis: indications and results of liver resection. Chir Ital 61:273–280
43. Jiang ZJ, Chen Y, Wang WL et al (2013) Management hepatolithiasis with operative choledochoscopic FREDDY laser lithotripsy combined with or without hepatectomy. Hepatobiliary Pancreat Dis Int 12:160–164
44. Yoon YS, Han HS, Shin SH et al (2009) Laparoscopic treatment for intrahepatic duct stones in the era of laparoscopy: laparoscopic intrahepatic duct exploration and laparoscopic hepatectomy. Ann Surg 249:286–291
45. Dagher I, Diop PS, Lainas P et al (2010) Laparoscopic liver resection for localized primary intrahepatic bile duct dilatation. Am J Surg 199:131–135
46. Yang T, Lau WY, Lai EC et al (2010) Hepatectomy for bilateral primary hepatolithiasis: a cohort study. Ann Surg 251:84–90
47. Li SQ, Liang LJ, Peng BG et al (2006) Hepaticojejunostomy for hepatolithiasis: a critical appraisal. World J Gastroenterol 12:4170–4174
48. Herman P, Perini MV, Pugliese V et al (2010) Does bilioenteric anastomosis impair results of liver resection in primary intrahepatic lithiasis. World J Gastroenterol 16:3423–3426
49. Fang K, Chou TC (1977) Subcutaneous blind loop: a new type of hepaticocholedochojejunostomy for bilateral intrahepatic calculi. Chinese Med J [Engl] 3:413–418
50. Hutson DG, Russell E, Schiff E et al (1984) Balloon dilatation of biliary strictures through a choledochojejuno-cutaneous fistula. Ann Surg 199:637–647
51. Fan ST, Mok F, Zheng SS et al (1993) Appraisal of hepaticocutaneous jejunostomy in the management of hepatolithiasis. Am J Surg 165:332–335
52. Di Carlo I, Sauvanet A, Belghiti J (2000) Intrahepatic lithiasis: a western experience. Surg Today 30:319–322
53. Monteiro Cunha JE, Herman P, Machado MC et al (2002) A new biliary access technique for the long-term endoscopic management of intrahepatic stones. J Hepatobiliary Pancreat Surg 9:261–264
54. Nimura Y, Hayakawa N, Toyada S (1981) Percutaneous transhepatic cholangioscopy. Stomach Intestine 16:681–689
55. Suzuki Y, Mori T, Yokoyama M et al (2014) Hepatolithiasis: analysis of Japanese nationwide surveys over a period of 40 years. J Hepatobiliary Pancreat Sci 21(9):617–622

Hemangioma

11

Alessandro Ferrero, Nadia Russolillo, Serena Langella, and Lorenzo Capussotti†

11.1 Epidemiology

Liver hemangiomas are the most common benign solid liver tumors. The first report of a liver hemangioma was by Frerichs [1] in 1861. Adami [2], in 1910, described 20 cases (1.4 %) of cavernous hemangioma in 1,400 autopsies, while Ochsner and Halperts [3] described a 2.3 % incidence of hepatic hemangioma a half century later. Globally, the incidence reported is between 0.4 and 20 % and prevalence ranging from 1.4 to 7 % in necropsy or surgical series [4]. The highest estimates have been derived from autopsy studies suggesting that these lesions are common in the general population. This observation is confirmed by the increasing recognition of hemangiomas in asymptomatic patients undergoing radiologic imaging of the abdomen for other reasons. In fact, the extensive use of noninvasive abdominal imaging modalities has led to increase the detection of asymptomatic lesions in vivo. In one series of 549 patients who underwent magnetic resonance imaging for evaluation of focal hepatic lesions, 585 of 805 lesions (72 %) were hemangiomas [5].

Hepatic hemangiomas can occur at all ages but the majority are diagnosed between 30 and 50 years. Usually, the average age of patients presenting with symptomatic lesions is approximately 45 years. In general, female patients often present at a younger age and with larger tumors. Rarely, hepatic hemangiomas may be seen in infancy or detected prenatally in a growing fetus [6]. Women, especially with a history of multiparity, are affected more often than men with a female-to-male ratio of 4–6:1 [4].

†Author was deceased at the time of publication.

A. Ferrero (✉) • N. Russolillo • S. Langella • L. Capussotti
Department of General and Oncologic Surgery, Ospedale Mauriziano, Largo Turati 62, Torino 10128, Italy
e-mail: aferrero@mauriziano.it; nrussolillo@mauriziano.it; slangella@mauriziano.it

L. Aldrighetti et al. (eds.), *Benign Tumors of the Liver*,
DOI 10.1007/978-3-319-12985-3_11

It has been observed that in patients with focal nodular hyperplasia [7], the prevalence of hemangioma is higher than that in the general population. Among patients who had primary hepatic masses other than focal nodular hyperplasia, the prevalence of hemangioma is significantly lower. Several authors have speculated that both lesions may have causative factors in common, including focal disturbance of the hepatic blood supply that somehow facilitates the hyperplastic development of these benign lesions.

Although no definite familial or genetic mode of inheritance has been described, Moser et al. first reported a large family of Italian origin in which three female patients in three following generations had large symptomatic hepatic hemangiomas [8]. The authors postulated that restriction of the disease to the female sex could be explained by sex-dependent differences in penetrance, the expression of a presumed liver-hemangioma gene, or the production of proliferative factors, such as female sex hormones.

11.2 Aetiology

The aetiology of hemangiomas of the liver is mainly speculative, and their pathogenesis is still not well understood. The huge differences in clinical course that exist between children and adults and the findings of spontaneous regression, growth, and rupture reflect a wide variability in the natural history of this disease. Several authors suggest that these vascular lesions are benign congenital hamartomas that grow slowly from birth [9]. Moore [10] considers hemangiomas to be acquired tumors resulting from areas of focal hepatic necrosis and subsequent regeneration. Robbins [11] suggests that these lesions may be true neoplasms occurring spontaneously and therefore consist of new blood vessels and tissue rather than dilatations of previous telangiectatic lesions.

More recently, it was assumed that cavernous hemangioma was related to a developmental abnormality in vessel formation [12]. It was also supposed that the response of endothelial cell to angiogenic factors may contribute to the occurrence of cavernous hemangioma. As shown, vascular endothelial cell growth factor and its receptor were upregulated in endothelial cells of cavernous hemangioma. Moreover, it was reported that the liver cavernous hemangioma was significantly decreased in size after treatment with bevacizumab, a recombinant humanized monoclonal antibody directed against vascular endothelial cells growth factor [13].

The role of female hormones in the development and growth of hepatic hemangiomas is still debated. Baum et al. [14] first called attention to the possible relationship between the use of oral contraceptives and the subsequent development of hepatic tumors. Since that time, the literature has reflected numerous reports of the diagnosis of benign tumors in women receiving estrogen replacement therapy. Furthermore, it has been suggested that oral contraceptives may affect normal hepatic tissue by inducing hepatomegaly and periportal congestion. These observations have suggested that oral contraceptives may also play a role in the pathogenesis of vascular tumors of the liver. As reported, some hepatic hemangiomas have estrogen receptors, and an accelerated growth of already existing hemangioma has been observed with high estrogen states such as those associated with puberty, pregnancy, oral contraceptive use, and with androgen treatment [15]. A prospective study [16] evaluated 94 women with hepatic hemangiomas, with a mean follow-up period of 7.3 years (range, 1–17 years). An increase in the size of the hemangiomas was seen in 23 % of women who received hormonal therapy as opposed to 10 % of control group ($p=0.05$). However, sex hormones have not been etiologically linked to the development of hemangioma.

11.3 Clinical Presentation

The clinical presentation and course of hepatic hemangiomas cover a spectrum of disease. The most common clinical presentation of hemangioma is an incidental finding of small capillary hemangiomas lesion (<2 cm). Conversely, cavernous hemangiomas may vary in size from 1 to 40 cm or more (defined "giant hemangiomas" when larger than 5 cm). Multiple hepatic hemangiomas are described up to 40 % of cases. Hepatic hemangiomatosis is a rare condition characterized by diffuse replacement of liver parenchyma with hemangiomatous lesions with histology similar to typical cavernous hemangioma. In same case it could be a manifestation of a systemic disease, such as hereditary hemorrhagic telangiectasia (Rendu-Osler-Disease) or systemic angiomatosis. Hepatic hemangiomas can also occur as part of other clinical syndromes such as Klippel-Trenaunay-Weber syndrome (associated with hemiatrophy and nevus flammeus), Kasabach-Merritt syndrome (characterized by thrombocytopenia and intravascular coagulation), and Von Hippel-Lindau disease (marked by cerebellar and retinal angiomas, with lesions also in the liver and pancreas). Finally, multiple hepatic hemangiomas have been reported in patients with systemic lupus erythematosus. Usually, hepatic hemangiomas are asymptomatic. The true incidence of symptoms is unclear, but it is probably lower than that reported in most surgical series. In fact, the presence of symptoms is a major indication for resection, and that could explain the higher rate of symptomatic patients reported. The size of the lesion appears to correlate with symptoms. Goodman reported that symptoms are experienced by 40 % of patients with 4-cm hemangiomas and by 90 % of patients with 10-cm hemangiomas [4]. The most commonly reported symptoms are right upper quadrant pain and feeling of fullness. Early satiety, nausea, and vomiting may occur when large lesions compress the stomach. The acute nature of some symptoms related to hemangiomas may not be related to increase in size but rather to thrombosis and infarction of part of the tumor. Rarely, hemangiomas may present as a large abdominal mass. In this case, physical examination reveals enlarged liver, a palpable non-tender mass, or the presence of an arterial bruit over the right upper quadrant. Although hemangiomas may grow to huge proportions, they typically do not compromise normal liver function.

11.4 Evolution

Natural history is usually a benign course, and significant growth is rarely observed. Nevertheless, giant hemangiomas may give rise to complications in 4.5–19.7 % of cases, consisting of compressive effect on adjacent structures such as the bowel and torsion if they are pedunculated [17]. Tumors rupture spontaneously or after blunt trauma can occur in 1–4 % [18] of patients mainly with giant hemangioma larger than 10 cm. So far, only 36 spontaneous rupture cases in adults have been reported. The change of rupture seems to be related to the size of the lesions, the location on the surface of the liver, the extrahepatic growth, and the steroid therapy [19].

A malignant transformation has never been described. According to benign course in nearly all cases, observation is the most appropriate treatment. However, the optimal duration of follow-up remains unknown. At present, if imaging in a patient fits definitive criteria for hemangioma, follow-up maybe appropriate at some points to ensure the stability of the findings; however, prolonged follow-up with serial imaging is probably unnecessary. In order to schedule conservative approach, the certainty of the diagnosis is of paramount importance. False diagnosis of hemangioma in the presence of malignancy is not rare nowadays and significantly reduces the chances of cure (Fig. 11.1).

The uncertainty of the diagnosis can be related to atypical imaging findings due to altered morphology or structure or unusual flow patterns [20]. Uncommon enhancement patterns included the so-called flash-filling pattern mostly seen in small hemangioma and marked by intense and uniform enhancement on the arterial phase, hemangioma with perilesional enhancement secondary to arteriovenous shunting, and finally the hyalinized or sclerosed hemangioma with loss of the typical globular enhancement on contrast-enhanced studies related to the replacement of the vascular spaces by hyalinized fibrotic tissue. Sometimes in large hemangiomas, thrombosis of sectorial or lobar portal branch is associated (Fig. 11.2).

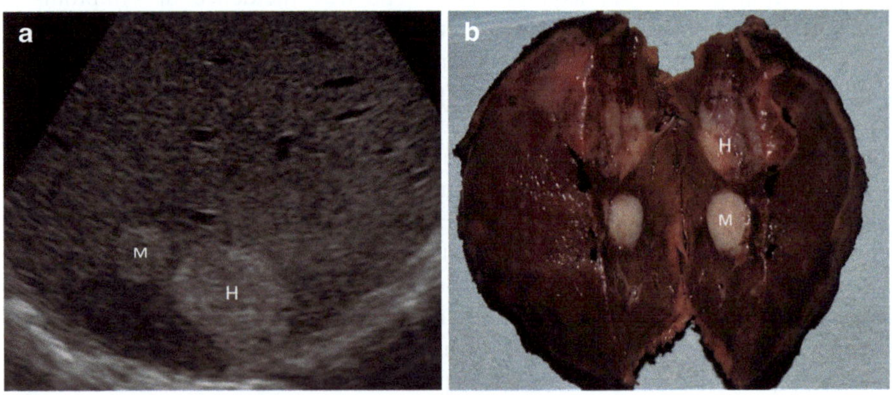

Fig. 11.1 (**a**) Ultrasonography of colorectal liver metastasis and concomitant liver hemangioma, both hyperechoic without peripheral rim. (**b**) Surgical specimen: colorectal metastasis and sclerosed hemangioma. *H* hemangioma, *M* metastasis

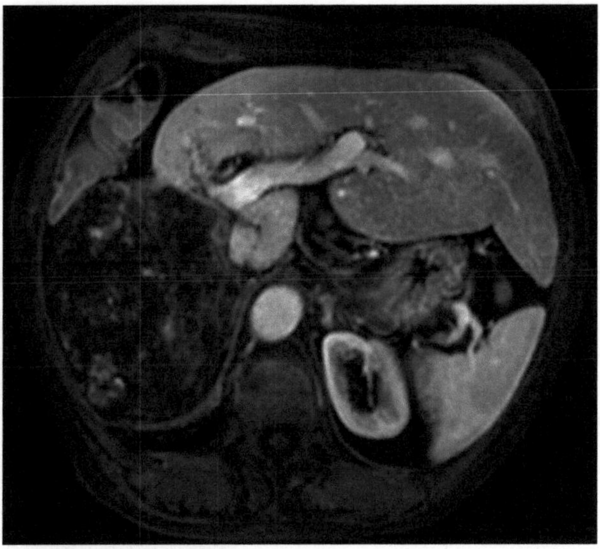

Fig. 11.2 MRI of giant hemangioma of the right liver with thrombosis of the right portal branch and hypertrophy of the left liver

Recently, Portolani et al. [21] analyzed 28 patients with liver cancer who were observed after an initial erroneous diagnosis of hemangioma. The authors reported that the majority of the incorrect diagnoses (75 %) came from low volume center and occurred more frequently with the small nodules in chronic liver disease. For these reasons, as reminded by Duran et al. [22], all cases of hemangioma should be confirmed with at least one MR after 3–6 months, especially in cases of atypical pattern of hemangioma and in chronic liver disease. In situation at risk of having the error (low volume center, poor quality of imaging, etc.), revision of the imaging by an expert radiologist is strongly recommended. On the other hand, it's also possible to perform an overtreatment of a benign lesion because of a false diagnosis of malignancy. Shimizu et al. [23] reported that hemangioma was the most frequent final diagnosis on 32 patients operated because of a false diagnosis of cancer. In a recent study, the authors showed that T2 shine-through effect is approximately observed in half of the lesions (mainly <1 cm) and in two-thirds of a large patient population with hepatic hemangiomas [22]. Radiologists should be aware of this phenomenon considering that T2 shine-through effect is commonly used to distinguish between benign and malignant lesions. Small solid liver tumors, which eluded preoperative radiological examinations, can be a difficult clinical problem for the surgeon. Intraoperative ultrasonography is crucial for accurate diagnosis [24]. At the intraoperative phase, ultrasonography hemangioma typically appears as a well-defined, lobulated, homogenous hyperechoic mass, but it can be also hypoechoic due to hemorrhage or fibrosis. It is known that small hepatocellular carcinomas and some liver metastases (from colorectal, neuroendocrine, and renal cancers) may also appear as hyperechoic lesions. The problem of differentiating benign from malignant lesions on intraoperative ultrasonography exploration becomes crucial. One useful test for diagnosing a hemangioma in cases of not typical ultrasonographic pattern is the finger

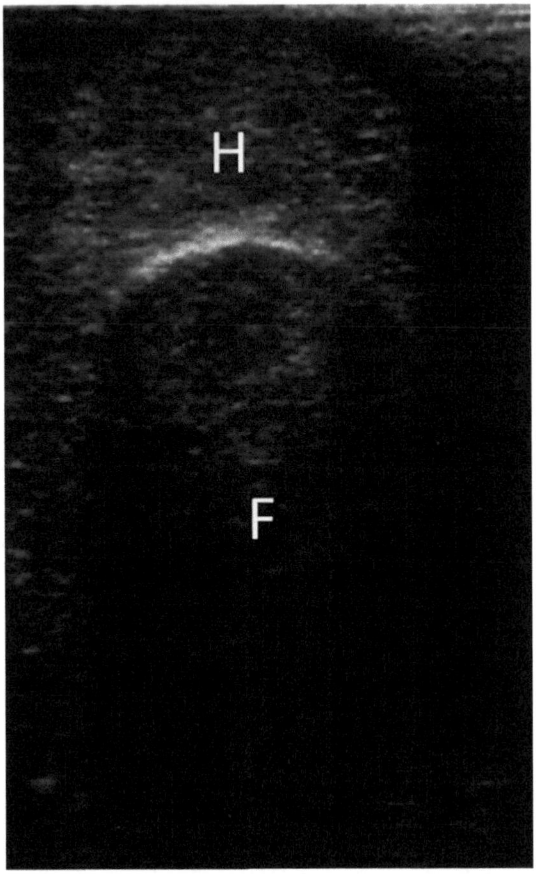

Fig. 11.3 Finger compression maneuver performed to confirm the intraoperative ultrasonography diagnosis of liver hemangioma. *F* finger, *H* hemangioma

compression of suspicious lesions. In fact, when compressed, the hemangioma changes in size and appearance (Fig. 11.3). Nevertheless, in cases of deep lesions or located in the posterior segments, the contrast-enhanced intraoperative ultrasonography provides more useful additional informations. The behavior of lesions during portal and delayed phases has been considered to be helpful in determining the nature of a nodule. The pattern of hypoenhancement in the late phases (washout) is typical of malignancies. In contrast, the benign lesions are isoenhancing or hyperenhancing as hepatic hemangioma [25].

11.5 Therapy

For most patients, the natural history of hepatic hemangiomas remains uneventful, and surgical intervention can be avoided. There is not much controversy over observing small asymptomatic hemangiomas which are discovered incidentally during a surgical procedure or imaging studies for unrelated problems. Nevertheless, in selected cases an intervention could be indicated, mainly on the basis of symptoms.

11.5.1 Indications for Surgery

Since randomized clinical trials assessing the benefits of surgery are lacking, clear indications for surgical resection in the presence of liver hemangiomas are actually missing, and a treatment algorithm remains controversial. The major indication for surgery is commonly a giant hemangioma causing progressive abdominal pain and patient discomfort. Before considering surgical resection, however, it is mandatory to exclude other possible causes of abdominal complaints, such as gallstones, gastroesophageal reflux disease, or peptic ulcer disease. When the abdominal pain is related to the presence of the hemangioma, still a conservative treatment is justified, even in large tumors, when it is possible to control it with analgesics [26]. In surgical series in which patients were carefully evaluated, 82–100 % were relieved of their complaints after surgery [27–29].

A second reason for considering surgery is the rapid enlargement of the hemangioma. Hemangioma size is usually stable. The increasing in size of the tumor can raise the suspicion of malignancy and should carefully be evaluated [28].

The third most common indication for surgery is diagnostic uncertainty. With the combined use of various imaging techniques, nowadays the diagnosis can be established in most patients. However, exceptions to pathognomonic signs do occur, even if rare. Percutaneous biopsy is considered dangerous because of the risk of bleeding and tumor rupture [30]. Patients who undergo surgery to exclude malignancy are more likely to be male, asymptomatic, have a history of cancer, and have smaller lesions [31].

Kasabach-Merritt syndrome requires a surgical intervention, but its incidence is extremely rare. Emergency surgery for complicated liver hemangiomas is seldom necessary, since bleeding, spontaneous rupture, and tumor thrombosis have been exceptionally reported [32].

Some authors support operative treatment for patients with large hemangiomas, mainly in the left liver, whose hobby or occupation carry a risk of hepatic trauma. This prophylactic indication has never been established, but it seems reasonable for the safety of the patient [28]. An interesting study compared resection versus conservative management of liver hemangiomas [33]: the rate of adverse events was similar (14 % of perioperative complications versus 20 % of persistent or new onset of hemangioma-associated symptoms) with an overall low risk for potentially life-threatening complications (7 % versus 2 %). These results could justify surgical indication for patients with giant hemangiomas carrying the risk of trauma.

Patient anxiety and his willingness because of the undesirable feeling of living with a hepatic tumor, even if asymptomatic, should not be considered a good indication for surgery anymore [18]. Even if the patient's wish has to be considered, the surgeon must well explain the risk of liver surgery comparing to the benign natural history of the disease.

During the last 20 years, there has been an increase up to 26 % in laparoscopic procedures for benign tumors of the liver, including hemangiomas [34]. In the present era of spread of mini-invasive liver resections, the above indications should be maintained and cannot be widened by the possible laparoscopic approach.

11.5.2 Surgical Technique

When indicated, liver hemangiomas can be resected with low morbidity and minimal mortality rates (Table 11.1). The first step of the operation should always be an intraoperative ultrasonography in order to assess the tumor relationships with portal pedicles and hepatic veins and to identify small hemangiomas that could be included in the resection plane. Hepatic pedicle clamping can be particularly useful in order to reduce the size of the tumor and to facilitate the manipulation of the tumor and the mobilization of the liver. Selective hepatic vascular exclusion, maintaining the caval flow, has been reported to be safer in patients with giant hemangiomas compressing the major hepatic veins [35].

The most commonly used techniques are resection and enucleation. The use of each method is still an open matter and varies depending on the experience and results of several high volume centers. Some authors prefer enucleation for the following reasons: there is a dissection plane between the hemangioma and the liver

Table 11.1 Surgical series of resected liver hemangiomas

Author	Year	# Observed	# Operation	Median size	Enucleation (%)	Morbidity	Mortality
Schwartz	1987	28	16	10	2 (13)	NR	0
Iwatsuki	1988	411	100	12	0	NR	NR
Baer	1992	NR	10	14.5	10 (100)	1	0
Belli	1992	NR	24	11	0	2	0
Petri	1993	NR	51	5.6	29 (51)	13	0
Brouwers	1997	NR	24	11	0	5	0
Weimann	1997	238	69	8.3	26 (38)	13	0
Ozden	2000	171	39	10	33 (85)	5	1
Reddy	2001	71	34	6.9	0	NR	0
Popescu	2001	NR	57	9	38 (67)	6	0
Yoon	2003	115	52	11	31 (60)	22	0
Lerner	2004	NR	52	10	27 (52)	14	0
Herman	2005	249	8	20	0	0	0
Erdogan	2007	34	14	10	0	3	0
Giuliante	2011	74	40	11.9	12 (30)	4	0
Yuan	2013	NR	589	13.6	0	72	2
Yedibela	2013	307	103	9.1	0	18	0
Miura	2014	NR	241	8.5	NR	14	2

NR not reported

parenchyma, and ligation of the transversing vessels is much simpler, decreasing the risk of blood loss; there are no bile ducts in the enucleation dissection plane so that the risk of postoperative bile leak is minimal; enucleation avoids unnecessary loss of healthy parenchyma for the treatment of a benign lesion [28, 31]. While some authors report fewer intra-abdominal complications after enucleation than after hepatectomy [27], others prefer anatomic liver resections [32]. In the case of enucleation, the centrally located hemangiomas are more likely to be associated to longer operative time and higher blood losses and transfusion rates, compared to peripherally located tumors [36]. Recently, the risk of bleeding and blood transfusions has been reported to be related more to tumor size than to the type of surgical technique [37].

Laparoscopic approach has been dramatically expanded in the recent years even for liver resections [38]. Mini-invasive surgery is particularly indicated for benign lesions because no radical margins are requested, limited resections of the anterior segments of the liver can be easily performed, and normal parenchyma is more manageable than cirrhotic or chemo-treated liver [34]. On the other hand, giant hemangiomas, mainly in the right liver, are usually very close to intrahepatic major vessels and are difficult to be manipulated, leading to increase the risk of the laparoscopic approach.

Liver transplantation has already been employed for the treatment of the extremely rare cases of diffuse hepatic hemangiomatosis and in patients with the Kasabach-Merritt syndrome [39].

11.5.3 Alternative Treatments

Definitive treatment of symptomatic hemangioma remains surgical resection, but other less effective options have been proposed. Hepatic artery ligation was advocated for unresectable lesions. This method has been shown to arrest the growth of some lesions and even effect partial regression of others. However, the experience was limited, the procedure was ineffective in some patients, and in the era of "safe" liver surgery, it should no longer be recommended [28].

Transarterial embolization has been suggested as an alternative treatment for symptomatic hemangiomas [40]. A reduction of symptoms may be possible, but tumor size remains stable after the procedure and recurrence is common. In selected cases, arterial embolization can be performed prior to surgery for very large tumors or in emergency to stabilize a patient with ruptured hemangioma [41].

Local thermal ablation, both with radiofrequency and microwave, is widely used for the management of malignant liver tumors, and an initial experience in the treatment of liver hemangioma has been reported. A recent series of 41 hemangiomas treated with radiofrequency by laparoscopic or tomography-guided percutaneous approach reports low risk of complications and likelihood of complete ablation in tumors between 5 and 10 cm; in contrast, the ablation appears to be an inappropriate method for hepatic hemangiomas larger than 10 cm because of the high occurrence rate of complications [42].

In summary, hepatic hemangiomas are the most common benign tumors of the liver. They are often asymptomatic and are found incidentally on abdominal imaging studies. The natural history is benign, and complications are uncommon. Small hemangiomas and giant asymptomatic or minimally symptomatic hemangiomas can be safely observed. Accepted indications for resection include severe symptoms and the rare complications. When indicated, liver hemangiomas can be resected with low morbidity and minimal mortality rates both with enucleation and liver resection.

References

1. Frerichs FT (1861) A clinical treatise on disease of the liver, vol 2. New Szdenham Society, London
2. Adami GL (1910) Principles of pathology. Lea & Febiger, Philadelphia
3. Ochsner JL, Halpert B (1958) Cavernous hemangioma of the liver. Surgery 43:577–582
4. Ishak KG, Robin L (1975) Benign tumors of the liver. Med Clin North Am 59:995–1013
5. John TG, Greig JD, Krosbie JL et al (1994) Superior staging of liver tumors with laparoscopy and laparoscopic ultrasound. Ann Surg 220:711–719
6. Gandolfi L, Leo P, Solmi L et al (1991) Natural history of hepatic hemangiomas: clinical and ultrasound study. Gut 32:677–680
7. Mathieu D, Zafrani ES, Anglade MC et al (1989) Association of focal nodular hyperplasia and hepatic hemangioma. Gastroenterology 97:154–157
8. Moser C, Hany A, Spiegel R (1994) Familial giant hemangiomas of the liver. Study of a family and review of the literature. Praxis 87:461–468
9. Bockus HL (1965) Gastroenterology: tumors of the liver, vol 3, 2nd edn. WB Saunders, Philadelphia
10. Moore RA (1944) Textbook of pathology. WB Saunders, Philadelphia
11. Robbins SL (1974) Pathologic basis of disease. WB Saunders, Philadelphia
12. Zhang WJ, Wu LQ, Liu HL et al (2009) Abnormal blood vessels formed by human liver cavernous hemangioma endothelial cells in nude mice are suitable for drug evaluation. Microvasc Res 78:379–385
13. Mahajan D, Miller C, Hirose K et al (2008) Incidental reduction in the size of liver hemangioma following use of VEGF inhibitor bevacizumab. J Hepatol 49:867–870
14. Baum JK, Holtz F, Bookstein JJ et al (1973) Possible association between benign hepatomas and oral contraceptives. Lancet 2:926–929
15. van Malenstein H, Maleux G, Monbaliu D et al (2011) Giant liver hemangioma: the role of female sex hormones and treatment. Eur J Gastroenterol Hepatol 23:438–443
16. Glinkova V, Shevah O, Boaz M et al (2004) Hepatic hemangiomas: possible association with female sex hormones. Gut 53:1352–1355
17. Erdogan D, Busch ORC, van Delden OM et al (2007) Management of liver hemangioma according to size and symptoms. J Gastroenterol Hepatol 22:1953–1958
18. D'Angelica M (2013) What's riskier for the patient with an asymptomatic large hepatic hemangioma: observation or the surgeon? World J Surg 37:1313–1314
19. Ribeiro MAF, Papaiordanou F, Gonçalves JM et al (2010) Spontaneous rupture of hepatic hemangiomas: a review of the literature. World J Hepatol 2:428–433
20. Caseiro-Alves F, Brito J, Araujo AE et al (2007) Liver haemangioma: common and uncommon findings and how to improve the differential diagnosis. Eur Radiol 17:1544–1554

21. Portolani N, Baiocchi G, Gheza F et al (2014) Impact on liver cancer treatment of a first erroneous diagnosis of hemangioma. World J Surg. doi:10.1007/s00268-014-2643-7
22. Duran R, Ronot M, Kerbaol A et al (2014) Hepatic hemangiomas: factors associated with T2 shine-through effect on diffusion-weighted MR sequences. Eur J Radiol 83:468–478
23. Shimizu S, Takayama T, Kosuge T et al (1992) Benign tumors of the liver resected because of a diagnosis of malignancy. Surg Gynecol Obstet 174:403–407
24. Ferrero A, Langella S, Giuliante F et al (2013) Intraoperative liver ultrasound still affects surgical strategy for patients with colorectal metastases in the modern era. World J Surg 37:2655–2663
25. Kong W-T, Wang W-P, Huang B-J et al (2014) Value of wash-in and wash-out time in the diagnosis between hepatocellular carcinoma and other hepatic nodules with similar vascular pattern on contrast-enhanced ultrasound. J Gastroenterol Hepatol 29:576–580
26. Farges O, Daradkeh S, Bismuth H (1995) Cavernous hemangiomas of the liver: are there any indications for resection? World J Surg 19:19–24
27. Terkivatan T, Vrijland WW, den Hoed PT et al (2002) Size of lesion is not a criterion for resection during management of giant liver hemangioma. Br J Surg 89:1240–1244
28. Ozden EA, Alper A, Tunaci M et al (2000) Long term result of surgery for liver hemangiomas. Arch Surg 135:978–981
29. Kammula US, Buell JF, Labow DM (2001) Surgical management of benign tumors of liver. Int J Gastrointest Cancer 30:141–146
30. Weimann A, Ringe B, Klempnauer J et al (1997) Benign liver tumors: differential diagnosis and indications for surgery. World J Surg 21:983–990
31. Yoon SS, Charny CK, Fong Y et al (2003) Diagnosis, management and outcome of 155 patients with hepatic hemangioma. J Am Coll Surg 19:392–402
32. Yedibela S, Alibek S, Muller V et al (2013) Management of hemangioma of the liver: surgical therapy or observation? World J Surg 37:1303–1312
33. Schnelldorfer T, Ware AL, Smoot R et al (2010) Management of giant hemangioma of the liver: resection versus observation. J Am Coll Surg 211:724–730
34. Toro A, Mahfouz AE, Ardiri A et al (2014) What is changing in indications and treatment of hepatic hemangiomas. A review. Ann Hepotol 13:327–339
35. Yang Y, Zhao LH, Fu SY et al (2014) Selective hepatic vascular exclusion versus pringle maneuver in partial hepatectomy for liver hemangioma compressing or involving the major hepatic vein. Am Surg 80:236–240
36. Fu XH, Lai EC, Yao XP et al (2009) Enucleation of liver hemangiomas: is there a difference in surgical outcomes for centrally or peripherally located lesions? Am J Surg 198: 184–187
37. Giuliante F, Ardito F, Vellone M et al (2011) Reappraisal of surgical indications and approach for liver hemangioma: single-center experience on 74 patients. Am J Surg 201:741–748
38. Aldrighetti L, Cipriani F, Ratti F et al (2013) The Italian experience in minimally invasive surgery of the liver: a national survey. In: Calise F, Casciola G (eds) Minimally invasive surgery of the liver, Updates in surgery. Springer, Milan
39. Browers MA, Peeters PM, de Jong KP et al (1997) Surgical treatment of giant haemangioma of the liver. Br J Surg 84:314–316
40. Srivastava DN, Gandhi D, Seith A et al (2001) Transcatheter arterial embolization in the treatment of symptomatic cavernous hemangiomas of the liver: a prospective study. Abdom Imaging 26:510–514
41. Seo HI, Jo HJ, Sim MS et al (2009) Right trisegmentectomy with thoracoabdominal approach after transarterial embolization for giant hepatic hemangioma. World J Gastroenterol 15:3437–3439
42. Gao J, Ke S, Ding X et al (2013) Radiofrequency ablation for large hepatic hemangiomas: initial experience and lessons. Surgery 153:78–85

Focal Nodular Hyperplasia

12

Enrico Pinotti, Francesca Ratti, Federica Cipriani, Michele Paganelli, Marco Catena, Renato Finazzi, and Luca Aldrighetti

12.1 Epidemiology

Focal nodular hyperplasia (FNH) is a benign tumorlike condition of the liver with an indolent course and no known potential for malignant transformation. FNH accounts for approximately 8 % of all primary hepatic tumors and is the second most common benign liver tumor after hemangioma; it is reported to occur with a frequency between 0.31 and 3 % in the population [1]. FNH occurs in both sexes and at all ages. It is found most commonly in women (80–95 % of the cases) in their third to fourth decades of life (female to male ratio is between 8:1 and 12:1). Luciani et al. [2] analyzed incidence and characteristic of a large cohort of patients with FNH. In this study, female to male ratio was 12:1 with significantly smaller diameter in men than in women (37.5 mm vs. 63.4 mm; $p < 0.001$). When occurring in men, FNH is diagnosed at an older age compared to women (41.6 vs. 36.2; $p < 0.01$) frequently presenting with atypical features (38.9 % vs. 22.2 % in women) [2].

12.2 Aetiology

Vascular theory, proposed by Wanless et al. [3], postulates that FNH originates from a hyperplastic lesion composed of reactive polyclonal proliferating hepatocytes. The genesis of FNH is probably secondary to a vascular malformation leading to blood

E. Pinotti • F. Cipriani • R. Finazzi, MD • L. Aldrighetti (✉)
Hepatobiliary Surgery Unit, IRCCS San Raffaele Hospital,
Via Olgettina 60, Milan 20132, Italy
e-mail: enricopinotti@hotmail.it; cipriani.federica@hsr.it; finazzi.renato@hsr.it; aldrighetti.luca@hsr.it

F. Ratti • M. Paganelli • M. Catena
Hepatobiliary Surgery, San Raffaele Hospital, Via Olgettina 60, Milan 20132, Italy
e-mail: ratti.francesca@hsr.it; paganelli.michele@hsr.it; catena.marco@hsr.it

L. Aldrighetti et al. (eds.), *Benign Tumors of the Liver*,
DOI 10.1007/978-3-319-12985-3_12

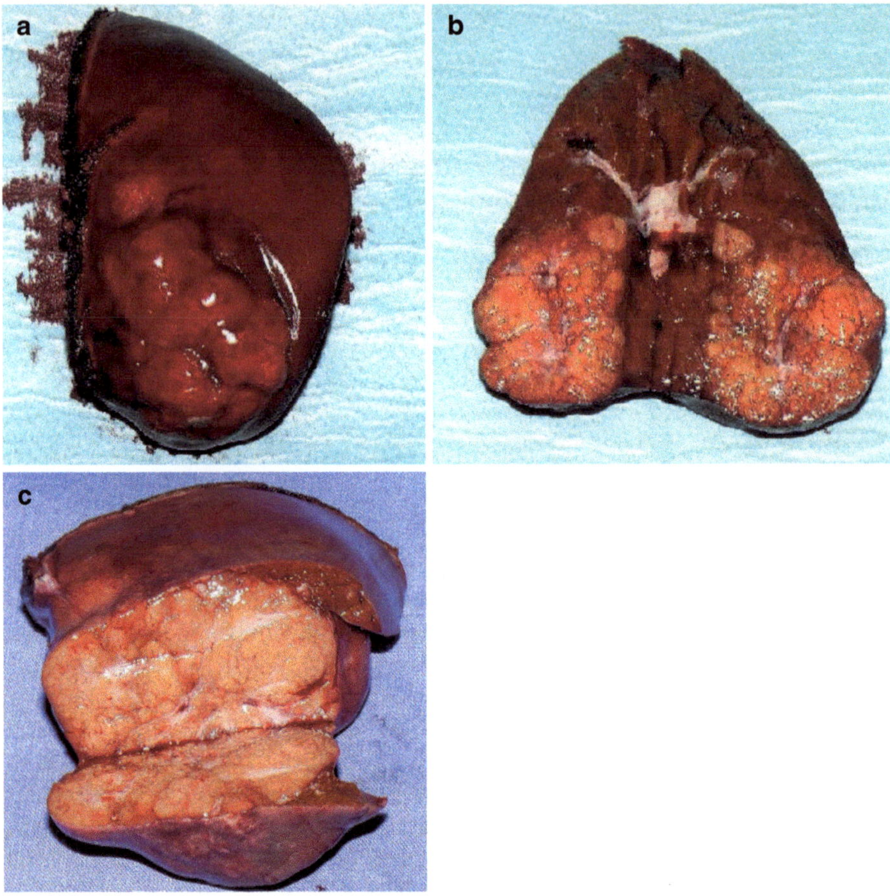

Fig. 12.1 (**a**) Left lateral sectionectomy performed for FNH, surgical specimen. (**b**, **c**) Central fibrous scan with fibrotic arterial vessel in surgical specimen

hyperperfusion in an area of liver parenchyma and resulting in a hyperplastic reaction. FNH is histopathologically defined by normal-like hepatocytes arranged in 1- to 2-cell-thick plates with a plurinodular pattern separated by fibrous bands and surrounding a central fibrous scar with a dystrophic arterial vessel [1]. The lesion is also characterized by absence of portal vein and presence of a ductular reaction at the interface of fibrous band parenchyma (Fig. 12.1). However, FNH appears to better correspond to a hyperplastic lesion than to a neoplastic one. No somatic mutations in genes involved in benign and malignant tumorigenesis have been described in FNH, thereby confirming the polyclonal origin of these tumors [4].

Despite its polyclonal origin, FNH is usually considered a benign hepatocellular tumor due to its mass-forming presentation. Besides this typical form of FNH (80 %), several variants are described and commonly classified as "atypical FNH" (20 %). Abnormal histoarchitecture or vascular malformations may be absent in atypical forms, but bile duct proliferation is always present [5]. Atypical FNH is a heterogeneous group including FNHs without central fibrous scar, FNH with prominent steatosis, or lesions presenting telangiectasia or features of adenoma. Interestingly, molecular studies demonstrated that among "atypical FNHs," lesions displaying telangiectatic changes are clonal processes [6].

Most important risk factors for developing FNH are the following:

- *Gender*. Female to male ratio is between 8:1 and 12:1 [2].
- *Oral contraceptives and estrogens*. Several studies have been conducted to rule out a possible association of focal nodular hyperplasia with oral contraceptives. It was first proposed that oral contraceptives may not promote de novo formation of focal nodular hyperplasia [7] but just increase tumor size. Mathieu et al. showed that neither the size nor the number of focal nodular hyperplasia lesions could be influenced by oral contraceptive use [8]. In a recent study, Rifai et al. [9] followed 20 pregnant women with FNH: during pregnancy, growth of FNH was observed in only 3 patients, while FNH size was stable in 7 patients and even reduced by 11 ± 6 % in 10 patients. So authors concluded that women with FNH are not at risk of significant growth progression or FNH-related complications.
- *Chemotherapy and radiations*. Focal nodular hyperplasia may be a late complication of high doses of alkylating agents and liver radiotherapy, probably as a consequence of vascular endothelium injury and subsequent circulatory disorders. In a recent study, Bouyn et al. [10] showed that incidence of FNH in people who underwent chemotherapy or radiotherapy at a young age is significantly higher compared to the general population (0.45 % vs. 0.02 %; $p < 0.001$).
- *Extrahepatic congenital portosystemic shunt (Abernethy malformation)*. It is a very rare congenital condition: venous flow from splanchnic district bypasses the liver and drains directly into the inferior vena cava, left renal vein, left hepatic vein, iliac veins, or right atrium. This condition is frequently associated to hepatic tumors (40 %) including focal nodular hyperplasia, adenoma and hepatocellular carcinoma. The development of focal nodular hyperplasia may be related to an alteration of liver vascular perfusion [11].
- *Hereditary hemorrhagic telangiectasia (HHT, Rendu–Osler–Weber disease)*. It is a genetic disease characterized by widespread cutaneous, mucosal, and visceral telangiectasias that can involve the lung, brain, and liver. Livers with HHT show hepatocellular regenerative activity, and it is a trigger for development of FNH. Prevalence of FNH in patients with HHT is 100-fold greater than in general population [12]. Association between HHT and focal nodular hyperplasia further reinforces the theory of vascular etiology of FNH.

12.3 Clinical Presentation

The majority of patients with FNH are asymptomatic, and FNH is usually detected incidentally during radiologic examinations, autopsies, or operations performed for other indications. Most FNH are solitary, although 20 % of patients may have multiple FNH nodules at diagnosis. Mean size at diagnosis is 3.3 cm (range 1–9.9 cm) [13] even though in literature cases of FNH larger than 20 cm are reported [1]. In blood tests, liver chemistry is usually unaltered, and the serum tumor markers alpha-fetoprotein (AFP), Ca19.9 (GICA), and carcinoembryonic antigen (CEA) are invariably negative, showing that blood tests are not accurate for FNH diagnosis. If FNH is large, it can lead to compression of intrahepatic bile ducts resulting in mildly elevated serum gamma-glutamyl transferase level. When symptoms occur, they may include palpable mass, hepatomegaly, and loss of appetite. Large subcapsular lesions may cause stretching of Glisson's capsule and therefore produce vague abdominal pain. Large FNH may cause displacement of adjacent organs even though this happens very rarely; indeed, Eris et al. reported a case of gastric obstruction due to focal nodular hyperplasia of the liver [14]. There are several reports describing presentation of FNH with acute abdominal pain due to intratumoral hemorrhage and subsequent hemoperitoneum [15]: this risk, even rare, may occur in the presence of a large exophytic tumor. However, FNH is detected incidentally in most of cases (74 % in the series of Cherqui et al. [16]). Diagnostic confirmation of FNH relies solely on imaging findings if typical features are shown. When clinical, biochemical, or imaging data are not typical of FNH, histological diagnosis is mandatory.

12.3.1 Ultrasound and Contrast Ultrasound

Most of FNH are fortuitously discovered on an ultrasound routine exam. FNH usually appears as a round mass hypoechoic or slightly hyperechoic compared with liver parenchyma. Sometimes it may be detected only because of displacement of the surrounding vessels. The central scar is rarely seen at baseline ultrasound, but it is easily visualized by color Doppler ultrasound [17]. In contrast-enhanced ultrasound (CEUS), FNH presents an early homogeneous filling in the arterial phase and subsequently becomes isoechoic.

12.3.2 Computed Tomography

Computed tomography (CT) can be used to characterize lesions of medium to large size, but it has limitations in the diagnosis of small lesions. On non-contrast examination, FNH is hypodense or isodense and may show occasional mass effect and lobulated contours. After contrast, FNH shows strong homogeneous enhancement during the arterial phase with rapid change to isodensity of the lesion during portal and delayed phases [18]. The central scar on the contrast is typically hypoattenuating during the arterial phase. On CT, the detection rate of the central scar is 35 % for nodes smaller than 3 cm and 65 % for those exceeding 3 cm [19]. An atypical FNH may show less arterial enhancement, absence of a central scar, and the presence of an enhancing pseudocapsule. In these situations, other diagnosis should always be considered, and sometimes biopsy or excision may be indicated.

12.3.3 Magnetic Resonance Imaging (MRI)

Contrast-enhanced MRI is the most accurate imaging method for characterization of FNH. FNH is usually hypo-isointense with respect to normal liver parenchyma on T1-weighted images and slightly hyper-isointense on T2-weighted images. Owing to hypervascularization, the central stellate scar is hypointense on T1-weighted images and hyperintense on T2-weighted images. Because its vascular supply is predominately arterial, following the administration of gadolinium, FNH typically shows intense uniform enhancement during arterial phase sparing the central scar [20]; the lesion usually fades to become isointense to the liver on portal venous and equilibrium phases.

Atypical findings that can be misleading include the following:

- Heterogeneous T1 and T2 signal intensity
- Hyperintense signal on precontrast T1-weighted images
- Hypointense signal relative to the liver during hepatic venous and equilibrium phases suggesting "washout"
- Presence of a pseudocapsule
- Presence of fat accumulation (a finding usually suggestive of hepatic adenoma or hepatocellular carcinoma [21])

Small FNH lesions often lack a visible center. Grazioli et al. showed that the 80 % of FNH lesions smaller than 3 cm lacked a central scar [22]. Conversely, central scars may be seen in other lesions, including fibrolamellar carcinoma and HCC [23].

12.3.4 Biopsy

When conventional imaging does not allow to determine a certain diagnosis, needle biopsy can be considered. If an adequate specimen is obtained, the diagnosis of FNH can usually be established on hematoxylin and eosin sections [24]. Fabre et al. [25] identified four major diagnostic criteria for focal nodular hyperplasia (including fibrous septa without portal tracts, thick-walled blood vessels, ductular proliferation, and hepatocellular nodules) along with two minor criteria (sinusoidal dilatation and perisinusoidal fibrosis). Fabre classified the results of biopsy in the following:

- Definite FNH: 3 or 4 major features
- Possible FNH: 2 major and 2 minor features
- Negative for FNH 2 or fewer major features without minor features

Fibrous septa were recognized in needle biopsies in 78 % of FNH, abnormal vessels in 61 %, ductular proliferation in 67 %, and hepatocellular nodules in 56 % [25]. In the study of Fabre et al., 22 % of biopsies lacked all major criteria for diagnosis, although the lesions later proved to be atypical FNH. Special stains as well as immunostains can be carried out to confirm the diagnosis of FNH. Specific stainings of copper and copper-binding protein in hepatocytes (i.e., rhodanine and Victoria blue stains) have very high specificity [24]. Immunostaining with monoclonal antibodies to biliary type CK (i.e., CK7 and CK19) also supports the diagnosis of FNH because the presence of ductular structures is among atypical features of FNH.

12.4 Evolution

Focal nodular hyperplasia is in most of cases an asymptomatic incidental finding. Once the nature of FNH has been established with imaging technique or biopsy, no specific treatment is required if the patient is asymptomatic, and most authors advocate a "wait and see" approach [16, 26, 27]. Natural history of FNH is to remain asymptomatic in most of cases. A change of size is relatively frequent, while occurrence of complications is rare.

1. *Change in size.* Changes in the size of FNH lesions are common: a study that followed patients with FNH for a mean period of 42 months showed that 71 % of nodules are stable in size, 3 % increase in diameter by more than 30 %, and 27 % even regresses in size over the follow-up period [28]. It has been postulated that lesion regression occurs as a result of thrombosis of the feeding artery, a pathological finding that was confirmed in one large autopsy study [3]. Even though low dose of estrogen is safe to be used in patients with FNH [8], anyway clinicians generally recommend treatment with oral contraceptives discontinuation. Women with FNH are not considered at risk of growth progression during pregnancy [9], but the nodules should be closely monitored during pregnancy.
2. *Transformation in malignant lesion.* In literature, there are no documented cases of transformation of a histologically proven FNH into a malignant lesion. Lesions evolving into malignancies should be considered for an initial different diagnosis.
3. *Hemorrhage.* While hepatic adenoma has a high risk of rupture, patients with focal nodular hyperplasia have a very low bleeding risk, and rupture is reported only in few case reports [29, 30].

12.5 Therapy

12.5.1 Watchful Waiting

The stability in size of most FNH lesions, the lack of potential for malignant transformation, and the extremely low risk of rupture and hemorrhage support a conservative approach for management of most patients with radiologically convincing or histologically proven FNH. Watchful waiting is currently the most diffused approach if the patient is asymptomatic [16, 27]. Ultrasound examination every 6 months for the first 3 years after diagnosis is generally suggested. The frequency can be reduced once the disease has stabilized with no change in nodule size or number.

12.5.2 Surgery

Surgical resection should be considered in the following situations:

- Impossibility to exclude malignancy
- Evidence of progressive growth
- Large lesions (>10 cm in diameter) with increased risk of hemorrhage related to trauma (especially subcapsular lesions)
- Presence of symptoms of compression

Thanks to development of surgical technique, liver resection is presently a procedure with low mortality (0–2 %) and acceptable morbidity (20–30 %) [31]; for these reasons, hepatic resections for benign tumors are frequently reported in the last few years. Poon et al. [32], in an analysis of 1,222 hepatectomies, reported that liver resection was performed for benign liver lesions in 15.4 % of the patients. Similarly, Jarnagin et al. [33], in an analysis of 1,803 hepatectomies, stated that 9 % of these were benign liver lesions.

Recently, laparoscopic approach has become increasingly used in surgical treatment of benign liver tumors [34]. In 1992, Gagner et al. [35] performed the first laparoscopic nonanatomic resection for FNH, and in 1996, Azagra et al. performed the first laparoscopic anatomic liver resection (left lateral sectionectomy) for FNH [36]. Gigot et al. analyzed the outcome of 64 patients who underwent laparoscopic liver surgery for benign hepatic tumors and compare it with the outcome of patients who underwent open surgery for the same disease. The laparoscopic group was associated with a similar complications rate, a decreased blood loss, reduction of postoperative morphine administration, and reduction of hospital stay [37]. Even cosmetic result, a goal that frequently is not specifically addressed in oncological surgery, may be an issue of primary importance in benign disease surgery especially considering the young median age of patients with benign liver tumors. Furthermore, subcostal incision may be responsible for early and late complications following surgery (pain, infection, dehiscence, muscular relaxation, sensitive defect, etc.).

The largest series of laparoscopic liver resections for benign disease performed in a single unit is the series of Ardito et al. [34]. In this study, the authors analyzed the outcome of 50 patients who underwent laparoscopic liver surgery for benign disease; in 22 cases (44 %), the resection was performed in patients with FNH. In 4 patients (8 %), the operation was converted to laparotomy, and the cause of conversion was RA Quality (1 case) and bleeding control in 3 patients. In this study, mortality was nil and postoperative complications occurred in 5 patients (10 %): pulmonary complications occurred in 2 patients, cardiac arrhythmia in 1 patient, and incisional hernias in 2 patients. All symptomatic patients had complete symptom relief after hepatic resection, and most patients were discharged from the hospital in less than 1 week. Laparoscopic liver resections appear safe and feasible, especially for lesions located in left lateral and anterior right segments. Resections in posterior and superior segments of the liver and major liver resections should be reserved for centers with significant experience in laparoscopic liver surgery [38]. Anyway, the use of laparoscopic approach should not modify or widen indications for liver resections. FNH does not require resection except in rare cases of symptomatic or doubtful lesions [34].

12.5.3 Transarterial Embolization (TAE)

A treatment alternative to surgery in patients with symptomatic FNH is transarterial embolization (TAE). TAE can offer to patients the resolution of symptoms. In a recent report, two patients who underwent TAE presented no complications after procedures, and the pain completely disappeared [39]. Anyway the limited data available do not exactly clarify the indications for this procedure in patients with focal nodular hyperplasia. TAE is not free of potential complications, such as post-embolization syndrome (pain, nausea, vomiting, fever, leukocytosis, etc.) or necrosis of the embolized tissue and abscess. Transarterial embolization can be considered an alternative treatment to surgery in the cases of symptomatic focal nodular hyperplasia, but there are few studies in literature about this topic, so indications for this procedure are not still established.

References

1. Nguyen BN, Flejou JF, Terris B, Belghiti J, Degott C (1999) Focal nodular hyperplasia of the liver: a comprehensive pathologic study of 305 lesions and recognition of new histologic forms. Am J Surg Pathol 23(12):1441–1454
2. Luciani A, Kobeiter H, Maison P, Cherqui D, Zafrani ES, Dhumeaux D et al (2002) Focal nodular hyperplasia of the liver in men: is presentation the same in men and women? Gut 50(6):877–880
3. Wanless IR, Mawdsley C, Adams R (1985) On the pathogenesis of focal nodular hyperplasia of the liver. Hepatology 5(6):1194–1200
4. Rebouissou S, Bioulac-Sage P, Zucman-Rossi J (2008) Molecular pathogenesis of focal nodular hyperplasia and hepatocellular adenoma. J Hepatol 48(1):163–170
5. Vilgrain V (2006) Focal nodular hyperplasia. Eur J Radiol 58(2):236–245
6. Bioulac-Sage P, Rebouissou S, Sa Cunha A, Jeannot E, Lepreux S, Blanc JF et al (2005) Clinical, morphologic, and molecular features defining so-called telangiectatic focal nodular hyperplasias of the liver. Gastroenterology 128(5):1211–1218
7. Klatskin G (1977) Hepatic tumors: possible relationship to use of oral contraceptives. Gastroenterology 73(2):386–394
8. Mathieu D, Kobeiter H, Maison P, Rahmouni A, Cherqui D, Zafrani ES et al (2000) Oral contraceptive use and focal nodular hyperplasia of the liver. Gastroenterology 118(3):560–564
9. Rifai K, Mix H, Krusche S, Potthoff A, Manns MP, Gebel MJ (2013) No evidence of substantial growth progression or complications of large focal nodular hyperplasia during pregnancy. Scand J Gastroenterol 48(1):88–92

10. Bouyn CI, Leclere J, Raimondo G, Le Pointe HD, Couanet D, Valteau-Couanet D et al (2003) Hepatic focal nodular hyperplasia in children previously treated for a solid tumor. Incidence, risk factors, and outcome. Cancer 97(12):3107–3113
11. Murray CP, Yoo SJ, Babyn PS (2003) Congenital extrahepatic portosystemic shunts. Pediatr Radiol 33(9):614–620
12. Buscarini E, Danesino C, Plauchu H, de Fazio C, Olivieri C, Brambilla G et al (2004) High prevalence of hepatic focal nodular hyperplasia in subjects with hereditary hemorrhagic telangiectasia. Ultrasound Med Biol 30(9):1089–1097
13. Halankar JA, Kim TK, Jang HJ, Khalili K, Masoom HA (2012) Understanding the natural history of focal nodular hyperplasia in the liver with MRI. Indian J Radiol Imaging 22(2):116–120
14. Eris C, Yildiz MK, Odabasi M, Akbulut S, Abuoglu H, Ozkan E (2013) Gastric outlet obstruction caused by focal nodular hyperplasia of the liver: a case report and literature review. Int J Surg Case Rep 4(8):681–683
15. Demarco MP, Shen P, Bradley RF, Levine EA (2006) Intraperitoneal hemorrhage in a patient with hepatic focal nodular hyperplasia. Am Surg 72(6):555–559
16. Cherqui D, Rahmouni A, Charlotte F, Boulahdour H, Métreau JM, Meignan M et al (1995) Management of focal nodular hyperplasia and hepatocellular adenoma in young women: a series of 41 patients with clinical, radiological, and pathological correlations. Hepatology 22(6):1674–1681
17. Gaiani S, Piscaglia F, Serra C, Bolondi L (1999) Hemodynamics in focal nodular hyperplasia. J Hepatol 31(3):576
18. Carlson SK, Johnson CD, Bender CE, Welch TJ (2000) CT of focal nodular hyperplasia of the liver. AJR Am J Roentgenol 174(3):705–712
19. Brancatelli G, Federle MP, Grazioli L, Blachar A, Peterson MS, Thaete L (2001) Focal nodular hyperplasia: CT findings with emphasis on multiphasic helical CT in 78 patients. Radiology 219(1):61–68
20. Buetow PC, Pantongrag-Brown L, Buck JL, Ros PR, Goodman ZD (1996) Focal nodular hyperplasia of the liver: radiologic-pathologic correlation. Radiographics 16(2):369–388
21. Mortelé KJ, Praet M, Van Vlierberghe H, Kunnen M, Ros PR (2000) CT and MR imaging findings in focal nodular hyperplasia of the liver: radiologic-pathologic correlation. AJR Am J Roentgenol 175(3):687–692
22. Grazioli L, Morana G, Federle MP, Brancatelli G, Testoni M, Kirchin MA et al (2001) Focal nodular hyperplasia: morphologic and functional information from MR imaging with gadobenate dimeglumine. Radiology 221(3):731–739
23. Blachar A, Federle MP, Ferris JV, Lacomis JM, Waltz JS, Armfield DR (2002) Radiologists' performance in the diagnosis of liver tumors with central scars by using specific CT criteria. Radiology 223(2):532–539
24. Makhlouf HR, Abdul-Al HM, Goodman ZD (2005) Diagnosis of focal nodular hyperplasia of the liver by needle biopsy. Hum Pathol 36(11):1210–1216
25. Fabre A, Audet P, Vilgrain V, Nguyen BN, Valla D, Belghiti J et al (2002) Histologic scoring of liver biopsy in focal nodular hyperplasia with atypical presentation. Hepatology 35(2):414–420
26. Vilgrain V, Fléjou JF, Arrivé L, Belghiti J, Najmark D, Menu Y et al (1992) Focal nodular hyperplasia of the liver: MR imaging and pathologic correlation in 37 patients. Radiology 184(3):699–703
27. Herman P, Pugliese V, Machado MA, Montagnini AL, Salem MZ, Bacchella T et al (2000) Hepatic adenoma and focal nodular hyperplasia: differential diagnosis and treatment. World J Surg 24(3):372–376
28. Kuo YH, Wang JH, Lu SN, Hung CH, Wei YC, Hu TH et al (2009) Natural course of hepatic focal nodular hyperplasia: a long-term follow-up study with sonography. J Clin Ultrasound 37(3):132–137
29. Chang SK, Chung YF, Thng CH, Loo HW (2005) Focal nodular hyperplasia presenting as acute abdomen. Singapore Med J 46(2):90–92

30. Bathe OF, Mies C, Franceschi D, Casillas J, Livingstone AS (2003) Massive hemorrhage and infarction complicating focal nodular hyperplasia of the liver. HPB (Oxford) 5(2):123–126
31. Hyder O, Pulitano C, Firoozmand A, Dodson R, Wolfgang CL, Choti MA et al (2013) A risk model to predict 90-day mortality among patients undergoing hepatic resection. J Am Coll Surg 216(6):1049–1056
32. Poon RT, Fan ST, Lo CM, Liu CL, Lam CM, Yuen WK et al (2004) Improving perioperative outcome expands the role of hepatectomy in management of benign and malignant hepatobiliary diseases: analysis of 1222 consecutive patients from a prospective database. Ann Surg 240(4):698–708
33. Jarnagin WR, Gonen M, Fong Y, DeMatteo RP, Ben-Porat L, Little S et al (2002) Improvement in perioperative outcome after hepatic resection: analysis of 1,803 consecutive cases over the past decade. Ann Surg 236(4):397–406
34. Ardito F, Tayar C, Laurent A, Karoui M, Loriau J, Cherqui D (2007) Laparoscopic liver resection for benign disease. Arch Surg 142(12):1188–1193
35. Gagner M, Rheault M, Dubuc J (1992) Laparoscopic partial hepatectomy for liver tumor. Surg Endosc 6:99
36. Azagra JS, Goergen M, Gilbart E, Jacobs D (1996) Laparoscopic anatomical (hepatic) left lateral segmentectomy-technical aspects. Surg Endosc 10(7):758–761
37. Gigot JF, Hubert C, Banice R, Kendrick ML (2004) Laparoscopic management of benign liver diseases: where are we? HPB (Oxford) 6(4):197–212
38. Nguyen KT, Gamblin TC, Geller DA (2009) World review of laparoscopic liver resection-2,804 patients. Ann Surg 250(5):831–841
39. Gómez García MP, Cruz González I, Peña Baranda B, Atín del Campo VM, Méndez Martín JJ (2014) Treatment of symptomatic focal nodular hyperplasia by arterial embolization. Cir Esp 92(2):135–137

Hepatocellular Adenoma 13

Giorgio Ercolani, Chiara Zanfi, Matteo Cescon, and Antonio Daniele Pinna

Hepatic adenoma (HA) is a benign tumor usually occurring in an otherwise normal liver. There are two entities described so far: the first is the solitary adenoma, associated with the use of oral contraceptives or anabolic steroids; the second is hepatic adenomatosis, first described by Flejou and colleagues [1], whereby the patient develops multiple adenomas (usually ten or more).

HA are composed of hepatocytes which are arranged in liver cell plates that are only mildly thickened or irregular; the tumor parenchyma is supplied by numerous arteries which are unaccompanied by bile ducts; tumor hepatocytes are of normal size.

Although they are benign tumors, they present major clinical issues in terms of their identification and distinction from focal nodular hyperplasia (FNH) or other benign liver tumor such as hemangioma, because of the demonstrated link between HA and hepatocellular carcinoma (HCC) and the increased risk of life-threatening hemorrhagic complications [2].

13.1 Epidemiology

HAs are rare tumors which are more common in females, seen predominantly in young women taking oral contraceptives in the third to fifth decades of life with an annual incidence of 3–4 women per 100,000 users of oral contraceptives [3, 4], whose potency in the last years, however, has been reduced and accounts for a reduction in the incidence of HA. Despite this, the detection rate may have increased due to a better and more frequently applied imaging techniques.

G. Ercolani (✉) • C. Zanfi • M. Cescon • A.D. Pinna
Department of Emergency, Surgery and Transplantation,
Sant'Orsola Hospital, University of Bologna, Via Massarenti, 9, Bologna 40138, Italy
e-mail: giorgio.ercolani@aosp.bo.it; nufito@libero.it; matteo.cescon@unibo.it; antoniodaniele.pinna@aosp.bo.it

L. Aldrighetti et al. (eds.), *Benign Tumors of the Liver*,
DOI 10.1007/978-3-319-12985-3_13

Distribution in HA incidence is different in the world: in Europe, North America, and Southeast Asia, a female predominance is observed (91, 78, and 73 %, respectively). In contrast, Chinese literature shows that only 37.7 % of patients with HA is female and only 11 % of them has a history of oral contraceptives/anabolic steroid use, probably because the criterion for the surgical treatment of HA may be more rigorous in China, considering the large prevalence of liver cancer: surgeons should rather advise tumor resection even if the presumptive diagnosis is adenoma, especially in male patients [5].

13.2 Etiology

Female gender (in the period of reproductive years), oral contraceptives, and anabolic steroids are universally considered risk factors for the development of HA; they can also arise in association with the state of abnormal carbohydrate metabolism, such as diabetes mellitus, glycogen storage disease and galactosemia, tyrosinemia, and familial polyposis coli. Interestingly the development of hepatic adenomatosis has little correlation with steroid use and has equal incidence in male and female gender. Further, glycogen storage disease (GSD), especially type I (von Gierke's disease) and type III, is a well-known risk factor for hepatic adenomatosis development [6], such as maturity-onset diabetes of the young (MODY3), a monogenic form of noninsulin-dependent diabetes.

Finally, HA are monoclonal tumors in which several recurrent mutations have been identified (see below).

13.2.1 Association with Estrogen Therapy

Numerous previous reports associated young women on oral contraceptives with a tendency to develop HAs; rarely they can be discovered in prepuberal adolescents (constitutional HA) and in postmenopausal women. Solitary adenoma, in fact, typically occurs in the setting of hepatocellular stimulation, and this is usually in the form of exogenous sex hormones with oral contraceptives or anabolic androgenic steroids. More importantly, withdrawal of estrogen therapy has been associated with regression of HA, even when they are of considerable size [7]. The roles of estrogen in the development of HA were speculated on the basis of several clinical observations: firstly, history of hormone therapy was confirmed between 55 and 77 % of patients with HAs; secondly, there is a relatively rare incidence of HA in male patients. Together, this implicated the potential roles of estrogen and its cognate receptors in stimulating hepatocyte proliferation and HA formation. Further, estrogen and progesterone receptors have been found in HA lesions, with a variable expression (26–73 %) [8].

13.2.2 Association with Glycogen Storage Disease

GSD is an inherited autosomal recessive disorder characterized by intracellular accumulation of glycogen. Type I GSD is the most common form and results from defects in glucose-6-phosfatase system. Type III GDS on the other hand is due to deficiency of glycogen-debranching enzyme. Both diseases result in impaired glycogenolysis and excessive glycogen accumulation in organs, especially in the liver and kidney. Approximately 22–75 % of patients with type I GDS develop hepatic adenomas, usually diagnosed by the second decade of life [6]. In type III GDS, only 4.4–25 % of the patients develop HAs [9]. Further, the estimated risk of malignant transformation of type I GSD-related HAs is as high as 10 % [6]; the same risk is very low in type III GSD (there are only six reported cases) [10]. The biological consequence of excessive glycogen storage seems to induce carcinogenesis in the liver, but the exact mechanism is uncertain [11].

13.2.3 Genetic Mutation

13.2.3.1 HNF1A (Also Called TCF1) Gene

The HNF1α gene is located at chromosome 12q24.2 and encodes the hepatocyte nuclear factor 1 (HNF1) α, a 681 amino-acid homeodomain transcription factor that is involved in hepatocyte differentiation. HNF1α controls the expression of liver-specific gene, such as β-fibrinogen, α1-antitripsin, and albumin. It is also recognized as a human tumor suppressor gene involved in liver tumorigenesis [12]. Biallelic inactivating mutations of this gene are generally observed in 35–40 % of HAs. HNF1α mutations occurring in HAs are somatic in 90 % of cases; heterozygous germline mutations are also the cause of MODY3.

13.2.3.2 β-Catenin Gene

β-Catenin-activating mutations have been identified in a number of HAs: it leads to an activation of the Wnt/β-catenin pathway that plays a key role in liver development and physiology, such as lineage specification, differentiation, stem cell renewal, epithelial–mesenchymal transition, zonation, proliferation, cell adhesion, and liver regeneration. So far, no HA cases with both β-catenin-activating and HNF1α biallelic inactivating mutations have been observed, suggesting that these two tumorigenic pathways are mutually exclusive. β-Catenin mutation is also found in 20–34 % of HCC.

13.2.3.3 gp130 Gene

It has been shown that some HAs are associated with gain-of-function mutations caused by inframe somatic deletions in the IL6 signal transduction gene which encodes for the signaling coreceptor gp130 [13]. The recurrent gain-of-function gp130 mutations fully explain the activation of the acute inflammatory phase observed in tumor hepatocytes. gp130 and β-catenin mutation may coexist in the same HA.

According to genotype and phenotype characteristics, HA can be classified in four groups (Bordeaux classification):

- *HAs with HNF1A gene mutation*: they represent 35–40 % of HA. On the pathological and clinical point of view, they correspond to a histologically homogeneous group of tumors, characterized by marked steatosis, usually sparing the arterialized zones, no cytological abnormalities, and no inflammatory infiltrates. The sharp contrast between tumor and adjacent liver in terms of steatosis enables delineation of tumor borders which are often irregular and lobulated, with often small HA foci in the immediate surrounding parenchyma. Lack of liver fatty acid binding protein (LFABP) on immunohistochemistry readily confirms the diagnosis of HNF1α HA (in the other subtypes, LFABP is normally expressed and is comparable to the corresponding non-tumor tissues, with a specificity and sensibility of 100 %). This kind of HA occurs almost exclusively in women. Germline mutation of HNF1A inactivation has been reported in hepatic adenomatosis, and this seems to be associated with MODY3.
- *HAs with β-catenin gene mutation*: they represent approximately 10–15 % of HA. Correlation with corresponding pathological and clinical data has shown that tumor with β-catenin mutations are usually characterized by the presence of cytological and architectural abnormalities and acinar pattern, whereas they are not steatotic [14]. Due to the cytological and architectural abnormalities, these tumors are often extremely difficult to distinguish from well-differentiated hepatocellular carcinoma (HCC). Moreover, they are more frequently associated with the development of unequivocal HCC than other HA types [15]. Furthermore, this type of HA is overrepresented in male patients and specific risk factors are often found, such as male hormone administration, metabolic syndrome, glycogenosis, and familial polyposis.
- *Inflammatory HAs*: they account for more than 50 % of all HAs, in which activation of the IL6 signaling pathway is observed, and are associated with high body mass index and alcohol consumption [16]. These patients may have signs and symptoms of an inflammatory syndrome, including elevated serum C-reactive protein (CRP) levels. These tumors are morphologically characterized by the presence of inflammatory infiltrates, marked sinusoidal dilatation or congestion, numerous thick-walled arteries, and a more or less obvious ductular reaction, lying inside a small amount of connective tissue, and they are often recognized grossly by their light red color alternating with streaks of dark red areas. Lesions with these features have often been misdiagnosed in the past as "telangiectatic FNH." Immunohistochemical detection of inflammatory proteins (serum amyloid A – SAA – and CRP) in tumoral hepatocytes is a very good argument for the diagnosis because they are strongly and usually diffusely expressed with a sharp demarcation from the surrounding non-tumoral liver. Steatosis may be present in this kind of HA, but is usually not as extensive. The risk of HCC does not exist in these inflammatory HA.
- *HA without markers*: tumors in this group represent only 5–10 % of cases. They neither show HNF1A nor β-catenin gene mutation and do not express inflammatory proteins.

Table 13.1 resumes the genotype and phenotype classification of hepatic adenomas.

Table 13.1 Genotype–phenotype classification of hepatic adenomas (Bordeaux classification)

Subtype	Prevalence	Clinical	Genotype	Histological appearance	Immunohistochemistry	MRI features	Comments
HNF1α-inactivated	15–18		Biallelic inactivation of TCF1	Steatosis	↓LFABP	Homogeneous fat distribution	
β-Catenin activated	35–50		β-Catenin activation		↑Nuclear β-catenin ↓Glutamine synthetase		Increased risk of malignant transformation
Inflammatory	25–35	Predominantly in female patients and frequently associated with alcohol use and obesity	Wild-type TCF1 and β-catenin IL6ST gene mutation	Inflammatory infiltrates, sinusoidal dilatation/ telangiectasia, dystrophic vessels, ductular reactions	↑SAA, ↑CRP	Hyperintense signal on T2W images, strong arterial enhancement, persistent enhancement on delayed phase	1/6 cases also have β-catenin mutation
Unclassified			Wild-type TCF1 and β-catenin				Diagnosis of exclusion

HNF1α hepatocyte nuclear factor 1 alpha, *TCF1* transcription factor 1, *LFABP* liver fatty acid binding protein, *SAA* serum amyloid A protein, *CRP* C-reactive protein, *MRI* magnetic resonance imaging, *T2W* T2-weighted images

13.3 Clinical Presentation

Patients may be completely asymptomatic, and the diagnosis may only be made as an incidental finding by imaging studies, e.g., during the course of investigation of abnormal liver function tests, liver mass on ultrasound, or research for metastasis in patients with a history of cancer.

The clinical presentation is either with a palpable mass lesion or its complications including chronic or acute upper abdominal pain as a result of intratumoral hemorrhage, necrosis, or hepatomegaly and hemorrhagic shock.

The diagnosis may be suspected from MRI characteristics (with typical arterial-type hypervascularized attenuation pattern), but diagnostic biopsy should be considered to confirm the diagnosis of HA.

HA mostly presents as solitary nodule, but two or more tumors may be found; if more than ten nodules are detected, hepatic adenomatosis must be considered. Tumor size is variable with a range of 1–30 cm (usually 8–15 cm). In reports from Southeast Asia and North America, the rate of solitary lesions is 80 and 65.2 %, respectively; in European reports, more than half of patients with HA have multiple lesions: the reason for this difference is unclear [5].

13.4 Evolution

HA is of clinical importance because its tendency is to *bleed* and to *rupture* spontaneously, with catastrophic consequences and intraperitoneal bleeding. There is no conclusive evidence to prove a correlation of the size of HA and rupture; some authors report an increased risk of rupture in tumors more than 6.5 cm in size [17]. A report, analyzing the evolution of HAs and their risk of rupture, found that the mean diameter of the lesions in China, Europe, and North America were 10.8, 12.4, and 14 cm, respectively [5]. There are two types of hemorrhage which are mostly observed in HA: hemorrhage inside the HA nodule, usually admixed with necrotic changes, and spontaneous hemorrhagic rupture which can cause subcapsular hematoma and possible hemoperitoneum. In reported series, the incidence of bleeding is around 20–25 % of cases (see Table 13.2), and it is more frequent in HA with sinusoidal dilatation and congestion.

Further, *malignant transformation* of HAs to HCC has been described by several groups and occurs in 5–9 % of cases ([29, 48], see Table 13.2). The issue of when HA develops into malignancy and which factors influence malignant degeneration are still being investigated. In some reports [5] a total of 5.6 % showed HCC foci within an adenoma upon final pathology; the mean size of the tumor with HCC was larger than the mean tumor diameter in benign HA (11.2 cm vs 7.8 cm). The risk of malignancy is particularly higher for β-catenin mutation HA, which are most frequently associated with glycogenosis type I, androgenic hormone intake, and familial adenomatous polyposis.

World literature actually available suggests that small tumors (<4 cm) are unlikely to become malignant.

Table 13.2 Published series with more than 15 cases and completed data

Study	Year	HA (*n*)	Mean diameter (cm)	HCC transformation (%)	Hemorrhage (%)	Resected
Edmondson et al. [18]	1976	42	–	0	69	41
Kerlin et al. [19]	1983	23	9	8.6	69.5	17
Mathieu et al. [20]	1986	27	7.5	0	40.7	27
Leese et al. [21]	1988	18	13	0	50	17
Iwatsuki et al. [22]	1990	25	12	0	16	25
Arrivé et al. [23]	1994	29	5.4	10.3	51.7	21
Pertschy et al. [24]	1994	30	–	0	0	29
Chung et al. [25]	1995	16	5.4	0	75	15
Nagorney [26]	1995	24	9	4.1	16.6	19
De Carlis et al. [27]	1997	19	7.9	10.5	26.3	19
Ott and Hohenberger [28]	1998	23	–	–	17.4	23
Closset et al. [29]	2000	16	8.1	6.2	43.7	16
Ichikawa et al. [30]	2000	24	–	8.3	41.6	13
Reddy et al. [31]	2001	25	5.9	4	12	25
Terkivatan et al. [32]	2001	33	–	0	36.3	19
Decotte et al. [33]	2003	17	–	0	0	17
Toso et al. [34]	2005	23	–	8.7	43.4	23
Erdogan et al. [35]	2006	22	7.2	0	100	22
Van der Windt et al. [36]	2006	48	–	0	27	16
Chaib et al. [37]	2007	28	8	0	10.7	28
Koffron et al. [38]	2007	47	–	0	–	47
Reddy et al. [39]	2007	25	8.5	0	–	25
Buell et al. [40]	2008	25	–	0	–	25
Cho et al. [41]	2008	41	–	4.8	29.2	41
Petri et al. [42]	2008	22	7.7	0	–	22
Bioulac-Sage et al. [16]	2009	128	7	3.6	17.9	128
Deneve et al. [43]	2009	124	–	4	25	119
Dokmak et al. [44]	2009	91	–	9.8	24.1	91
Mounajjed and Wu [45]	2011	35	–	0	20	35
Bunchorntavakul et al. [46]	2011	60	–	0	11.6	25
De Angelis et al. [47]	2014	62	7.2	–	11.8	62

Among the previously mentioned 5–9 % of HAs with HCC foci, 35 % were female; interestingly, it has been estimated that the risk of malignant transformation of HA in men is 47 %, ten times greater than in women [2].

Therefore, HA size and sex appear as possible risk factors for malignant transformation, but it is not clear whether HA eventually can transform into HCC and at which time point this transformation will occur.

There is no additional risk of bleeding or HCC transformation whether the nodule is solitary or multiple. From a clinical perspective, size, genotype, and underlying disease are far more important than the number of lesions. It has been shown that in patients presenting hepatic adenomatosis, the tumors are often of the same subtype [49].

13.5 Therapy

The management of HA requires a tailored approach, given the lack of robust clinical data. So far, it is defined by clinical parameters: first of all, women with HA should be advised to stop the use of oral contraceptives and other hormone replacement therapy.

The optimal management of HAs remains controversial. Any decision regarding the selection of *conservative* (observation) versus *surgical approach* will depend on the clinical context. However, the molecular analyses of HAs have contributed significantly by providing several molecular characteristics that predict high risk of malignant change.

Giving the difficulty in distinguishing HA from well-differentiated HCC and the risk of spontaneous rupture, large HAs are generally resected [50]. HA can take varying durations of time to progress to malignancy, and in some cases, progression can be very slow or rapid. A decrease in size, documented by radiological imaging, after stopping oral contraceptives, may lead to a discharge or reduction in surveillance, particularly if no β-catenin mutation is detected at biopsy; in case of growth or β-catenin positivity, surgery may be required. Of note, the α-fetoprotein levels are often in the normal range; as such, this is a poor indicator of malignant transformation.

Corroborating the actually known clinical features and the new molecular data, surgical resection of HA is indicated if:

- Large size of HA (>5 cm) with the impending risk of rupture or hemorrhage
- Presence of symptoms
- Evidence of β-catenin activation in any HA
- Any HA in male patients (need to establish a definitive diagnosis)
- Evidence of dysplasia or atypia within an adenoma
- Clinical features of malignant transformation (i.e., increasing size, malignant features on imaging)

Data coming from main reported series are described in Table 13.2.

In case of solitary HA with the above high-risk factors, hepatic resection should be offered as it provides a change of long-term cure. The rationale is that resection prevents future occurrence of malignancy, as there has not been any report of HCC recurrence following resection of HA. After resection a close monitoring is mandatory even if HA are benign tumors, because they have the tendency to recur (8 %). In such situation of recurrent HA, the management is initially nonoperative and based on strict radiological follow-up. Hepatic liver resection is again indicated when HA reaches 5 cm with an increased risk for complications.

From the genetic perspective, it is likely that hepatic adenomatosis have the same genetic mutations as solitary HAs. Therefore, it has been suggested that liver resection should be indicated in the same conditions as solitary HAs (i.e., lesions >5 cm in size or harbors β-catenin activation). Of note there is higher frequency of malignant transformation (and β-catenin activation) in hepatic adenomatosis arising in the context of glycogen storage disease; in this set of patients, liver transplantation is a valid option when the presence of progression to HCC is confirmed, but without evidence of metastatic disease.

Given that biopsy specimen, when performed, can be inconclusive and misleading as some lesions of HCC can be surrounded by HA tissue and the differentiation of HA from well-differentiated HCC remains difficult on histopathological analysis, close follow-up of patients who are treated conservatively should be mandatory.

Although there are limited data on its use in HA cases, it is likely that there is a role for *radiofrequency ablation* in treatment of HA not amenable to resection.

Further, *selective arterial embolization* has been reported to stop bleeding from ruptured adenomas: embolizing them prevents growth of the lesions. The same approach can be adopted also in nonresectable HAs [51].

Also in hepatocellular adenomatosis there are no currently data on the optimal management. Treatment options are therefore dictated by the likelihood of the development of complications. First of all, although there have been conflicting reports on the role of sex hormones, it is prudent to withdraw exogenous steroids as they have been associated with higher rates of bleeding [52]. Antiestrogenic therapy in the form of tamoxifen or surgical oophorectomy has been shown to be ineffective [53]. Surgical removal of large or complicated nodules in symptomatic patients (i.e., ruptured or hemorrhagic HAs) has been shown to significantly improve symptoms. Bleeding seems to be directly related to tumor size: therefore, it has been suggested to remove empirically larger adenomas (>5 cm) as a preventive measure for bleeding [53]. Close follow-up in asymptomatic patients with at least yearly imaging of the liver and measurement of serum α-fetoprotein is crucial to monitor the potential complications.

Rarely, *orthotopic liver transplantation* may be required to treat severe disease with progressive liver failure or malignancy [21].

Actually, hepatic resection for HA should be always attempted when technically feasible, in the cases described above. The postoperative results are excellent even in cases of extended liver resections. Depending on center experience, the morbidity associated to liver resections for benign tumors ranges from 10 to 25 % and mortality from 0 to 3 %. In such situations surgery is often curative, avoids the risk of a liver transplant procedure, and delays the exposition to the immunosuppressor (Fig. 13.1). Moreover, the pathological examination excludes the possibility of malignant transformation that in case of giant adenoma is often not possible through radiology or core needle biopsy.

The indications for liver transplant in patients with HA are very limited to cases of HA (giant, multiple, or recurrent and progressive adenoma) in which hepatic resection is not technically feasible. In PubMed literature only 20 cases of liver

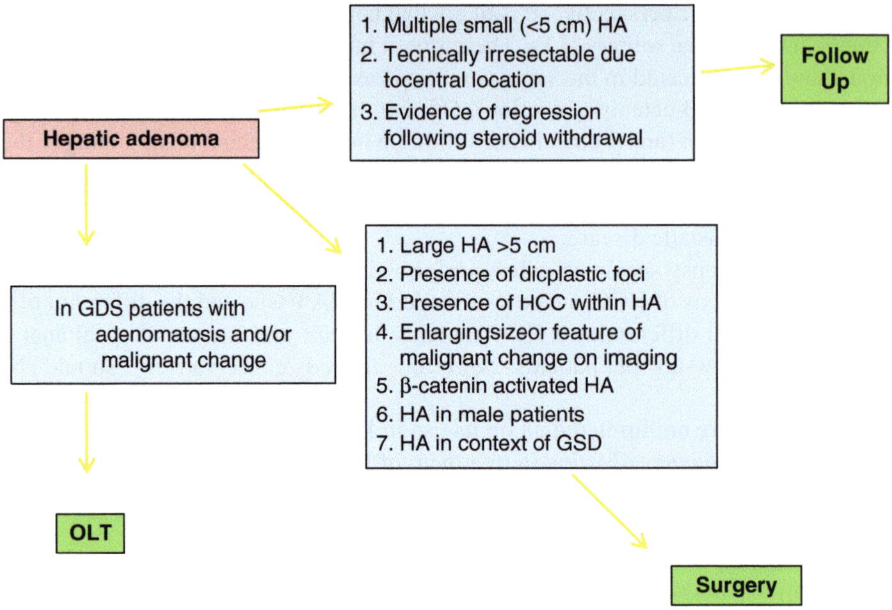

Fig. 13.1 Surgical management of HA

transplantation for HA are reported [54, 55]. However, up to 2008, United Network atransplantation for HA which represent about 6–11 % of all liver transplantation performed for benign liver conditions and 0.085–0.094 % of all indications [56].

Further, liver transplantation for recurrent HA is a technically demanding procedure and shows some different technical aspects if compared to a liver transplantation performed for chronic liver disease. First, surgeons must take into consideration that in such situation a previous hepatectomy is responsible for the presence of adhesions that need to be divided before reaching the liver and the hepatic pedicle. Furthermore, after a previous major hepatic resection, at least one of the major hepatic veins is missing and the hepatic pedicle at bifurcation misses one major branch of portal vein and hepatic artery. These anatomical changes may render the liver implantation more difficult. On the contrary, the absence of portal hypertension could be an advantage when the adhesions are divided since they do not show an intrinsic vascular pattern.

In conclusion, liver resection is considered to be the treatment of choice in case of single HA that can be completely resected. In case of recurrence or in case of complicated liver adenomatosis, liver transplantation represents a definitive and curative treatment, but it should be taken into consideration as the last therapeutic option in patients in whom hepatic resection is indicated but not technically feasible. Moreover, the donor grafts shortage and the high risk of morbidity and mortality related to liver transplantation, let this treatment be not a standard option but an extraordinary choice in a few particular cases.

References

1. Flejou JF, Barge J, Menu Y et al (1985) Liver adenomatosis: an entity distinct from liver adenoma? Gastroenterology 89:1132–1138
2. Farges O, Ferreira N, Dokmak S et al (2011) Changing trends in malignant transformation of hepatocellular adenoma. Gut 60:85–89
3. Jeannot E, Wendum D, Paye F, Mourra N, de Toma C, Flejou JF, Zucman-Rossi J (2006) Hepatocellular adenoma displaying a HNF1alpha inactivation in a patient with familial adenomatous polyposis coli. J Hepatol 45(6):883–886
4. Rooks JB, Ory HW, Ishak KG, Strauss LT, Greenspan JR, Hill AP, Tyler CW (1979) Epidemiology of hepatocellular adenoma. The role of oral contraceptives. JAMA 242(7):644–648
5. Lin H, Van den Esschert J, Liu C, Van Gulik T (2011) Systematic review of hepatocellular adenoma in China and other regions. J Gastroenterol Hepatol 26:28–35
6. Lee PJ (2002) Glycogen storage disease type I: pathophysiology of liver adenomas. Eur J Pediatr 161(Suppl 1):S46–S49
7. Steinbrecher UP, Lisbona R, Huang SN, Mishikin S (1981) Complete regression of hepatocellular adenoma after withdrawal of oral contraceptives. Dig Dis Sci 26(11):1045–1050
8. Torbeson M, Lee JH, Choti M, Gage W, Abraham SC, Montgomery E, Boitnott J, Wu TT (2002) Hepatic adenomas: analysis of sex steroid receptor status and the Wnt signalling pathway. Mod Pathol 15(3):189–196
9. Labrune P, Trioche P, Duvaltier I, Chevalier P, Odievre M (1997) Hepatocellular adenomas in glycogen storage disease type I and III: a series of 43 patients and review of the literature. J Pediatr Gastroenterol Nutr 24(3):276–279
10. Demo E, Frush D, Gottfried M, Koepke J, Boney A, Bali D, Chen YT, Kishnani PS (2007) Glycogen storage disease type III-hepatocellular carcinoma a long term complication? J Hepatol 46(3):492–498
11. Bannasch P, Mayer D, Hacker HJ (1980) Hepatocellular glycogenosis and hepatocarcinogenesis. Biochim Biophys Acta 605(2):217–245
12. Pelletier L, Rebouissou S, Paris A et al (2010) Loss of HNF1αfunction in human hepatocellular adenomas leads to aberrant activation os signaling pathways involved in tumorigenesis. Hepatology 51:557–566
13. Rebouissou S, Amessou M, Couchy G, Poussin K, Imbeaud S, Pilati C et al (2009) Frequent inframe somatic deletion activate gp130 in inflammatory hepatocellular tumors. Nature 57:200–204
14. Zucman-Rossi J, Jeannot E, Nhieu JT, Scoazec JY, Guettier C, Rebouissou S et al (2006) Genotype-phenotype correlation in hepatocellular adenoma: new classification and relationship with HCC. Hepatology 43:515–524
15. Bioulac-Sage P, Rebouissou S, Thomas C, Blanc JF, Saric J et al (2007) Hepatocellular adenoma subtype classification using molecular markers and immunohistochemistry. Hepatology 46:740–748
16. Bioulac-Sage P, Laumonier H, Couchy G, Le Bail B et al (2009) Hepatocellular adenoma management and phenotypic classification: the Bordeaux experience. Hepatology 50:481–489
17. Cobey FC, Salem RR (2004) A review of liver masses in pregnancy and a proposed algorithm for their diagnosis and management. Am J Surg 187:181–191
18. Edmondson HA, Henderson B, Benton B (1976) Liver cell adenomas associated with use of oral contraceptives. N Engl J Med 294:470–472
19. Kerlin P, Davis GL, McGill DB, Weiland LH et al (1983) Hepatic adenoma and focal nodular hyperplasia: clinical, pathologic and radiologic features. Gastroenterology 84:994–1002
20. Mathieu D, Bruneton JN, Drouillard J et al (1986) Hepatic adenomas and focal nodular hyperplasia: dynamic CT study. Radiology 160:53–58
21. Leese T, Farges O, Bismuth H (1988) Liver cell adenomas: a 12-year surgical experience from a specialist hepatobiliary unit. Ann Surg 208:558–564

22. Iwatsuki S, Todo S, Starzl TE (1990) Excisional therapy for benign hepatic lesions. Surg Gynecol Obstet 171:240–246
23. Arrive L, Flejou JF, Vilgrain V et al (1994) Hepatic adenoma: MR findings in 51 pathologically proved lesions. Radiology 193:507–512
24. Pertschy J, Ruckert JC, Manger T (1994) Diagnosis and surgical therapy of benign liver tumors. Zentralbl Chir 119:495–500
25. Chung J, Ferzli G, David A, Kiel T (1995) Laparoscopic resection of a large hepatic tumor. Surg Endosc 9:733–735
26. Nagorney DM (1995) Benign hepatic tumors: focal nodular hyperplasia and hepatocellular adenoma. World J Surg 19:13–18
27. De Carlis L, Pirotta V, Rondinara GF et al (1997) Hepatic adenoma and focal nodular hyperplasia: diagnosis and criteria for treatment. Liver Transpl Surg 3:160–165
28. Ott R, Hohenberger W (1998) Focal nodular hyperplasia and liver cell adenoma: operation or observation? Zentralbl Chir 123:145–153
29. Closset J, Veys I, Peny MO et al (2000) Retrospective analysis of 29 patients surgically treated for hepatocellular adenoma or focal nodular hyperplasia. Hepatogastroenterology 47:1382–1384
30. Ichikawa T, Federle MP, Grazioli L et al (2000) Hepatocellular adenoma: multiphasic CT and histopathologic findings in 25 patients. Radiology 214:861–868
31. Reddy KR, Kligerman S, Levi J et al (2001) Benign and solid tumors of the liver: relationship to sex, age, size of tumors and outcome. Am Surg 67:173–178
32. Terkivatan T, de Witt JH, de Man RA et al (2001) Indications and long term outcome of treatment for benign hepatic tumors: a critical appraisal. Arch Surg 136:1033–1038
33. Descottes B, Glineur D, Lachachi F et al (2003) Laparoscopic liver resection of benign liver tumors. Surg Endosc 17:23–30
34. Toso C, Majno P, Andreas A et al (2005) Management of hepatocellular adenoma: solitary uncomplicated, multiple and ruptured tumors. World J Gastroenterol 11:5691–5695
35. Erdogan D, Busch OR, van Delden OM et al (2006) Management of spontaneous haemorrhage and rupture of hepatocellular adenomas. A single centre experience. Liver Int 26:433–438
36. Van der Windt DJ, Kok NF, Hussain SM et al (2006) Case-oriented approach to the management of hepatocellular adenoma. Br J Surg 93:1495–1502
37. Chaib E, Gama-Rodrigues J, Ribeiro MA et al (2007) Hepatic adenoma. Timing for surgery. Hepatogastroenterology 54:1382–1387
38. Koffron AJ, Auffenberg G, Kung R, Abecassis M (2007) Evaluation of 300 minimally invasive liver resections at a single institution: less is more. Ann Surg 246:385–392; discussion 92–94
39. Reddy SK, Kishnani PS, Sullivan JA et al (2007) Resection of hepatocellular adenoma in patients with glycogen storage disease type Ia. J Hepatol 47:658–663
40. Buell JF, Thomas MT, Rudich S et al (2008) Experience with more than 500 minimally invasive hepatic procedures. Ann Surg 248:475–486
41. Cho SW, Marsh JW, Steel J et al (2008) Surgical management of hepatocellular adenoma: take it or leave it? Ann Surg Oncol 15:2795–2803
42. Petri A, Hohn J, Kokai EL et al (2008) Surgery of benign liver tumors: indications for treatment: twenty years' experience. Hepatogastroenterology 55:592–595
43. Deneve JL, Pawlik TM, Cunningham S et al (2009) Liver cell adenoma management: a multicenter analysis of risk factors for rupture and malignancy. Ann Surg Oncol 16:640–648
44. Dokmak S, Paradis V, Vilgrain V et al (2009) A single center surgical experience of 22 patients with single and multiple hepatocellular adenomas. Gastroenterology 137:1698–1705
45. Mounajjed T, Wu TT (2011) Telangiectatic variant of hepatic adenoma: clinicopathologic features and correlation between liver needle biopsy and resection. Am J Surg Pathol 35:1356–1363
46. Bunchorntavakul C, Bahirwani R, Drazek D et al (2011) Clinical features and natural history of hepatocellular adenomas: the impact of obesity. Aliment Pharmacol Ther 34:664–667

47. De Angelis N, Memeo R, Calderaro J et al (2014) Open and laparoscopic resection of hepatocellular adenoma: trends over 23 years at a specialist hepatobiliary unit. HPB (Oxford) 16(9):783–788
48. Foster JH, Berman NN (1994) The malignant transformation of liver cell adenomas. Arch Surg 129:712–717
49. Lepreux S, Laurent C, Blanc JF, Trillaud H, Le Bail B et al (2003) The identification of small nodules in liver adenomatosis. J Hepatol 39:77–85
50. Flowers BF, McBurney RP, Vera SR (1990) Ruptured hepatic adenoma. A spectrum of presentation and treatment. Am Surg 56:380–383
51. Akovbiantz A, Ackermann D, Buhler H, Schmid M (1980) Management of liver cell adenoma and focal nodular hyperplasia. Helv Chir Acta 47(5):607–609
52. Yoshidome H, McMasters KM, Edwards M (1999) Management issues regarding hepatic adenomatosis. Am Surg 65:1070–1076
53. Ribeiro A, Burgart LJ, Nagorney DM, Gores GJ (1998) Management of liver adenomatosis: results with a conservative surgical approach. Liver Transpl Surg 4:388–398
54. Barthelmes L, Tait IS (2005) Liver cell adenoma and liver cell adenomatosis. HPB (Oxford) 7:186–196
55. Tepetes K, Selby R, Webb M, Madariaga JR, Iwatsuki S, Starzl TE (1995) Orthotopic liver transplantation for benign hepatic neoplasms. Arch Surg 130:153–156
56. Ercolani G, Grazi GL, Pinna AD (2010) Liver transplantation for benign hepatic tumors: a systematic review. Dig Surg 27:68–75

Adenoma and Biliary Cystadenoma 14

Kevin C. Soares, Andrew J. Page, Ihab Kamel, and Timothy M. Pawlik

14.1 Hepatic Adenoma

14.1.1 Epidemiology

The association between hepatic adenomas (HAs) and oral contraceptives pills (OCPs) is well known. The incidence of HA is approximately 0.1 per 100,000 in non-OCP users versus 4 per 100,000 in OCP users [1]. While a precise mechanism underlying OCP use with the pathogenesis of HA is not clear, most studies attribute the exogenous estrogen exposure as a stimulating growth factor for HAs [2]. Furthermore, HAs are more common in women than men, with a female to male ratio of 11:1 [1]. This gender discrepancy is likely secondary to a combination of unregulated estrogen stimulation on hepatocytes, with variable effects of estrogen on hepatic metabolism, immunity, and response to cellular injury [3]. In addition to OCPs, other risk factors associated with HA include hereditary diseases such as galactosemia, glycogenosis, hepatic iron overload related to β-thalassemia, and maturity-onset diabetes of the young type 3 (MODY3) [4–6].

There is increasing evidence that modern formulations of OCPs have less of a pathogenic role in the development of HAs than previously established [7]. Despite this contemporary development, the overall incidence of HA has still increased in the last 30 years in both men and women [7]. The increased widespread use of imaging has detected more incidental HA [7]. Furthermore, there has been a

K.C. Soares • A.J. Page • T.M. Pawlik, MD MPH, PhD (✉)
Division of Surgical Oncology, Department of Surgery, The Johns Hopkins School of Medicine, Blalock 688, 600 N. Wolfe Street, Baltimore, MD 21287, USA
e-mail: tpawlik1@jhmi.edu

I. Kamel
Department of Radiology, The Johns Hopkins School of Medicine, Baltimore, MD USA

L. Aldrighetti et al. (eds.), *Benign Tumors of the Liver*,
DOI 10.1007/978-3-319-12985-3_14

greater relative increase in the incidence of HA in men, and most studies note that this trend may be related to a corresponding increase in metabolic syndrome and obesity [7, 8].

14.1.2 Etiology

The pathomolecular classification for HA distinguishes it from other hepatic lesions. HAs are typically well circumscribed, ranging from microscopic to 30 cm [9]. Patients may present with a solitary HA, multiple HAs, or more than ten adenomas, which is generally termed adenomatosis (Fig. 14.1). Histologically, HAs are defined

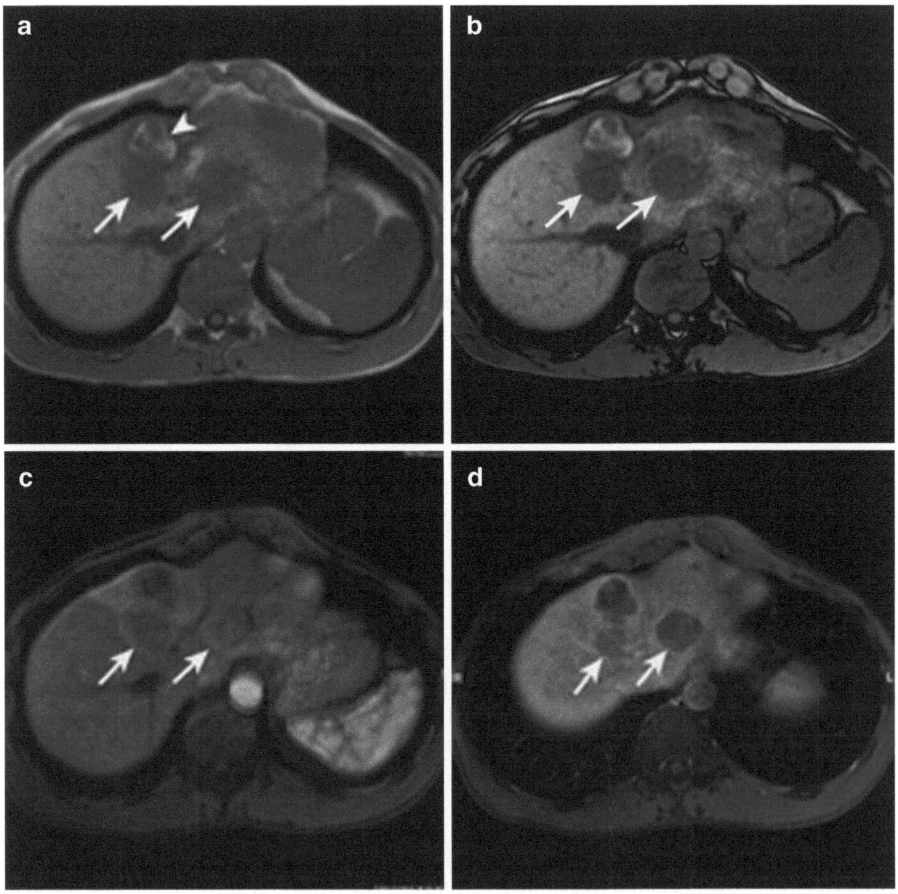

Fig. 14.1 Adenomatosis in a 37-year-old female. Axial non-fat-saturated T1-weighted image (**a**) shows multiple hypointense masses (*arrows*). The presence of bright signal in one of the masses (*arrowhead*) suggests the presence of hemorrhage. Opposed phase image (**b**) shows loss of signal in most of the lesions (*arrows*), suggesting the presence of lipid. These lesions are hypervascular in the arterial phase (*arrows*), post gadolinium injection (**c**), and washout in the portal venous phase (**d**). These MR findings are consistent with adenomatosis

by a proliferation of benign hepatocytes 1 or 2 cell layers thick, with hepatocytes themselves appearing normal, clear, pigmented, or steatotic [8]. Any degree of nuclear irregularity or abnormal nuclear-cytoplasm ratio should raise concern for malignant transformation to hepatocellular cancer (HCC) [10].

In the past decade, improvements in the pathological characterization of HA have led to a more mechanistic understanding of the etiology of HA. There are now recognized distinct HA subtypes described by the World Health Organization [9, 11]. Correspondingly, each subtype demonstrates variable imaging, clinical behavior, and natural history [11].

While different classification schemes have been developed, the most accepted HA subtype designations include: (1) β-catenin-mutated HAs (HA with cellular atypia), (2) hepatocyte nuclear factor-1-α-mutated HAs (steatotic HAs), (3) inflammatory HAs (telangiectatic HA), and (4) unclassified. All of these subtypes may present as solitary lesions to multiple lesions.

β-catenin-mutated HAs represent 10–15 % of all HAs [9, 12]. They are usually solitary and are disproportionately more common in men [8]. With mutation of the β-catenin gene, there is inappropriate upregulation of many of its targets, including glutamine synthetase and the G-protein-coupled receptor 49 [13]. This subsequent aberrant upregulation contributes to the development of cellular atypia and an increased risk of malignant transformation to HCC [11]. Furthermore, the histological distinction between these lesions and HCC can be challenging, and some groups have recently designated some of these lesions as well-differentiated HCC [12].

Hepatocyte nuclear factor-1-α (HNF1α)-mutated HAs are found in 30–50 % of HA patients, with a predisposition in younger women. These often demonstrate evidence of steatosis, and there is an absence of cellular atypia [14]. HNF1α HAs are caused by biallelic mutations in the transcription factor HNF1α [15] resulting in inappropriate hepatocyte differentiation. Adenomatosis in HNF1α-mutated HAs often contain a germline mutation in the HNF1α gene [16]. Emerging evidence also suggests that there is an association with HNF1α adenomatosis and a personal or family history of MODY3 diabetes [5].

The inflammatory HA is the most common, comprising up to 50 % of all HAs, and is also the most directly associated with OCP [13]. Histologically, inflammatory HA has sinusoidal dilation, thickened arteries with absent veins and biliary ducts, and inflammatory infiltrates [17]. Whether an inflammatory event leads to these HAs or whether the HA triggers an inflammatory cascade is unclear. However, in patients with inflammatory HA, activating mutations have been identified in the interleukin-6 receptor gene and Janus kinase-signal transducer and activator of transcription (JAK-STAT) pathway [18]. There is also a characteristic high expression of C-reactive protein and the inflammatory marker serum amyloid-associated (SAA) protein [18]. Furthermore, inflammatory HA is unique in that obesity and alcohol abuse–associated steatohepatitis are associated with the development of this type of HA [19].

The remaining HAs are categorized into the unclassified HA subtype. These unclassified HAs represent up to 10 % of all HAs, and they do not demonstrate any particular histological, morphological, or genetic features [9, 20].

14.1.3 Clinical Presentation

Most HAs are asymptomatic and are discovered incidentally. A subset of patients will present with pain. Another presenting symptom associated with HA includes bleeding – manifesting as acute pain or frank hemorrhage with symptomatic anemia. In general, tumors larger than 5 cm have an increased risk of bleeding and rupture, with up to 11–49 % of all large HAs having bleeding complications [21–23]. Not unexpectedly, the risk of bleeding and malignancy varies based on the subtype. Inflammatory HAs are the most prone to bleeding, with 30 % associated with a bleeding complication. The risk for bleeding is likely a manifestation of sinusoidal dilation and abnormal arterial vasculature [11, 21]. In contrast, HNF1α HAs have a minimal risk of bleeding complications, while the incidence of β-catenin-mutated HA bleeding episodes is unknown [20].

Another possible complication of HA is malignant transformation to HCC. Overall, the risk of HCC is 4–10 %, with risk factors being male sex, anabolic steroid use, and size greater than 5 cm [23–25]. Similar to the risk of bleeding, the risk of malignant transformation varies based on the HA subtype. The subtype most associated with HCC is the β-catenin-mutated HA [10]. This is not surprising as the β-catenin pathway is mutated in approximately 35 % of HCC [26]. While the β-catenin-mutated group has the highest risk of HCC, 10 % of inflammatory HAs also have an increased risk of malignancy, while the risk with HNF1α HA is minimal [11, 20, 21].

14.1.4 Evolution and Therapy

Most patients present with HA detected on imaging performed for other reasons, such as discomfort, stable anemia, or as an incidental finding. The best imaging modality to establish the diagnosis of HA is probably MRI. On MRI most HAs typically have a characteristic isointense or hyperintense appearance on T1- and T2-weighted images. Uniform enhancement on the arterial phase and washout and isointensity with the background liver on the portal phase are also characteristic. Based on the subtype, enhancement patterns vary (Table 14.1). If after MRI the diagnosis is still in question, biopsy may be warranted.

The management of HA is based on the presentation. Resection is offered to patients with symptoms or with risk factors for bleeding or malignant transformation, such as patients with large lesions. Risk factors associated with bleeding and HCC transformation include a history of bleeding, size approaching 5 cm, or concern on imaging or biopsy for HCC [23, 24]. Other relative indications for resection are those patients at risk for malignant transformation – those with glycogen storage diseases, male sex, history of androgen or steroid intake, or concerns by imaging or biopsy of a β-catenin-mutated HA [4, 6, 11]. In women with HA less than 5 cm and taking OCPs, some groups recommend cessation of OCPs and re-imaging at 6–12 months, as regression is possible [27]. However, improvement in symptoms after taking OCPs is unusual and does not eliminate the risk of

Table 14.1 MRI characteristics based on hepatic adenoma subtypes

Subtype	T1-weighted gradient-echo MR images	T2-weighted MR images	Gadolinium-enhanced T1-weighted MR images
Inflammatory HA	Isointense or hyperintense, without signal drop-off with use of chemical shift sequence	Diffusely hyperintense	Intense enhancement during arterial phase that persists in the portal venous and delayed phases
HNF1α-mutated HA	Isointense or hyperintense, with diffuse signal drop-off with the use of chemical shift sequence	Isointense to slight hyperintense	Moderate enhancement in the arterial phase, with no persistent enhancement in the portal venous and delayed phases
β-catenin-mutated HA	No specific MR imaging patterns – strong enhancement during arterial phase, with portal venous washout	No specific MR imaging patterns – strong enhancement during arterial phase, with portal venous washout	No specific MR imaging patterns – strong enhancement during arterial phase, with portal venous washout

Used with permission [20]

malignant transformation or hemorrhage, and careful surveillance is warranted. In the patient with an acutely bleeding HA, interventional radiological (IR) guidance with hepatic artery embolization of the feeding hepatic artery is the treatment of choice, reserving open hepatectomy for a later time when the bleeding has been controlled by IR therapies [28].

14.2 Biliary Cystadenoma

14.2.1 Epidemiology

Biliary cystadenomas (BCAs) are rare epithelial tumors which account for less than 5 % of all cystic liver lesions [29]. BCAs occur predominantly in females and generally present during the fourth or fifth decade of life [30, 31]. Besides female gender, there are no other clearly defined risk factors although the use of OCPs have been postulated in some reports to be associated with BCA [32, 33]. BCA tumors are classified according to the presence of ovarian-like stroma. Unlike BCAs with ovarian stroma, BCAs without ovarian stroma occur equally in both genders. Non-ovarian BCA tumors may, however, occur at a more advanced patient age.

BCAs range from 1 to 30 cm and are slow growing, multiloculated solitary lesions with internal septations, wall nodules, and papillary projections [30]. Although BCA can be seen in both sides of the liver, multiple case series have demonstrated a left hemiliver predominance [30, 34, 35].

14.2.2 Etiology

Nearly 90 % of all BCAs are derived from the intrahepatic biliary tree, while 10 % originate from extrahepatic biliary structures [32, 36]. The etiology of BCA remains unclear, and these tumors have been described as both congenital and acquired lesions [37]. BCAs are believed to derive from ectopic rests of embryonic bile ducts, ovarian cells, or intrahepatic peribiliary glands [32, 38]. BCAs can be premalignant and develop into biliary cystadenocarcinoma (BCAC), which are more likely to occur in older, male patients [31, 32]. In fact, Devaney et al. hypothesized that BCAC originates from either a benign BCA with ovarian stroma or de novo, occurring exclusively in men [32].

Although Hueter first reported BCAs in 1887, Edmonson originally characterized this tumor in 1958 [39]. Wheeler and Edmondson later reclassified BCAs in 1985 according to the following distinct criteria: multilocular cysts, columnar epithelium, and the presence of ovarian stroma [38]. Devaney and colleagues [32] revised this definition in 1994 since 14 % of the cystadenomas in their series of 70 patients did not contain ovarian stroma. Moreover the authors noted that biliary cystic tumors could also be unilocular and therefore suggested that multilocularity not be a qualifying feature of biliary cyst tumor classification [32].

14.2.3 Clinical Presentation

The clinical presentation of BCA is varied. Common patient complaints include nonspecific symptoms such as abdominal pain, abdominal distention, early satiety, and weight loss – although many patients are asymptomatic at the time of diagnosis [30, 35]. Obstructive jaundice and cholangitis are rarely seen and are generally associated with extrahepatic BCA.

More liberal use of cross-sectional imaging as well as the improved sensitivity of imaging techniques has led to increased incidental findings of BCAs. Ultrasound is the most common imaging modality used to characterize these lesions [30]. BCAs typically appear anechoic and internal septations are generally seen [36]. Computed tomography (CT) with intravenous contrast results in nodular enhancement of cystic lesions which are isodense to water. T1- and T2-weighted magnetic resonance imaging often demonstrates a low-intensity T1 signal and high intensity T2 signal [36] (Fig. 14.2).

Although definitive differentiation between BCA and BCAC is not possible with current imaging techniques, certain features are associated with a higher likelihood of malignancy such as the presence of intracystic debris, bile duct dilatation, and mural nodules [34, 36]. CT and MRI demonstrate the anatomic relationships of surrounding structures including hepatic vasculature as well as any biliary dilatation. Cross-sectional imaging is critical for preoperative planning. Magnetic resonance cholangiopancreatography (MRCP) can demonstrate biliary communication and can aid in differentiating BCA from simple cysts through visualization of mural nodules and septations. The role of endoscopic retrograde cholangiopancreatography in BCA is limited and typically only used when tissue diagnosis is needed.

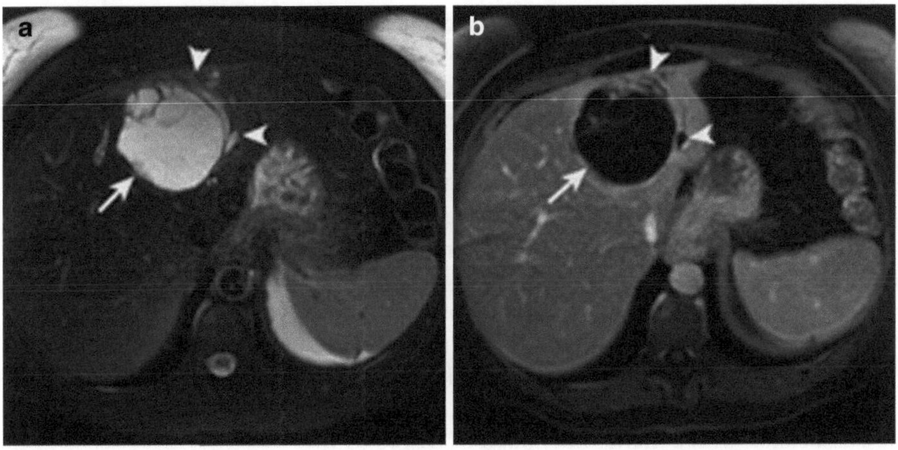

Fig. 14.2 Biliary cystadenoma in a 53-year-old female. Axial T2-weighted image (**a**) and post contrast T1-weighted image in the portal venous phase (**b**) show a large complex mass with thick enhancing septations (*arrow*). There is associated left ductal dilatation (*arrowheads*). These MR findings are consistent with biliary cystadenoma

The differential diagnosis is broad and includes simple cyst, hemangioma, adenoma, hepatic abscess, hemorrhagic cyst, and hydatid cyst. Appropriate therapeutic interventions for each of these entities are varied; therefore, precise preoperative identification of BCA leads to a lower risk of recurrence and malignant transformation. Cysts without internal septations or papillary projections with a well-defined tissue fluid interface are more likely simple hepatic cysts and can be managed conservatively [40, 41]. Daughter cysts are pathognomonic of echinococcal cyst, and fine-needle aspiration in conjunction with serologic analysis is diagnostic [41, 42]. Similarly for liver abscesses, an irregular, contrast-enhanced, thicker cyst wall is common and cyst fluid culture is diagnostic [41].

Measurement of serum tumor markers such as carcinoembryonic antigen (CEA) and carbohydrate antigen 19-9 (CA 19-9) has not proven diagnostic in cases of biliary cystic tumors and is therefore not utilized for clinical differentiation. Core needle biopsy, fine-needle aspiration, and cyst fluid analysis of BCAs remain controversial. CA 19-9 and CEA cyst fluid levels have low sensitivities and specificities and cannot be used to rule out malignancy. Additionally, tissue sampling and cytology are rarely diagnostic, and dissemination of malignant cells with these procedures has been reported [40, 43]. Therefore, the associated low diagnostic yield and potential oncologic ramifications make FNA and core needle biopsy of suspected BCAs relatively contraindicated.

14.2.4 Evolution

BCAs typically appear as endodermal lined cells with cuboidal or columnar epithelium overlying mesenchymal stroma along with an outer layer of collagen connective tissue [36]. This outer fibrous connective tissue layer results in a pseudocapsule separating the cyst from the surrounding hepatic parenchyma. BCA tumors are generally unifocal, fluid filled, and classified according to the presence of "mesenchymal or ovarian stroma" which represents a zone of well-vascularized, spindle cell–rich area expressing estrogen and progesterone receptors [44]. Cytokeratin, CA19-9, and CEA expression is prevalent throughout the epithelium of BCA [36]. Of note, the cellular localization of CEA expression is important. More specifically, luminal CEA expression and cytoplasmic CEA are typical of BCA and BCAC, respectively [45].

The risk of malignant transformation is approximately 20–30 % [32]. The presence of ovarian stroma in BCAC is associated with an improved prognosis, and regression of ovarian stroma during malignant transformation of BCA has been reported [32, 46]. Increased age, male sex, and tumor location in the right hemiliver are associated with a higher likelihood of BCAC [30].

14.2.5 Therapy

Although benign, BCA lesions harbor a risk of malignant degeneration; therefore, appropriate management of BCA requires complete surgical resection with clear margins. In the largest series of BCAs to be reported in the literature, Arnaoutakis et al. [30] reported on 221 cases of BCA. Nearly 85 % of patients underwent formal liver resection, while 15 % of patients underwent unroofing/partial excision, and one patient received a liver transplantation [30]. Techniques such as percutaneous aspiration, marsupialization, and ethanol injection are contraindicated. Approximately 50–90 % of BCA patients who have undergone fenestration or aspiration will eventually recur [30, 47, 48]. Immediate recurrence of a hepatic cyst after aspiration likely indicates misdiagnosed BCA or BCAC. Patients who undergo fenestration or aspiration for a presumed simple cyst which is then diagnosed as a BCA necessitate reoperation and complete cyst excision.

Complete surgical resection consists of hepatic resection or enucleation. The surgical approach is patient dependent, accounting for surgeon experience and anatomic location of the lesion. For example, enucleation of centrally located lesions involving major biliary and vascular structures is acceptable. Formal liver resection is appropriate for peripheral lesions, and biliary resection with restoration of bilioenteric continuity is indicated in extrahepatic BCAs. Appropriate management of these lesions necessitates an R0 resection in order to reduce recurrence rates and avoid the incomplete resection of an unidentified BCAC which is associated with a particularly poor prognosis [43]. Frozen section analysis has a low likelihood of identifying a small focus of malignant cells and is therefore not indicated [36].

Complete resection of BCA with negative margins leads to extremely low recurrence rates (5–10 %), and the overall survival of patients is over 80 % after 5 years [30, 35, 38]. Although most commonly approached via open techniques, minimally invasive approaches have been described with comparable morbidity, R0 resection rates, and long-term outcomes [47]. Few case reports of orthotopic liver transplantation (OLT) have been reported with acceptable outcomes. However, this technique is more applicable in BCAC, and utilization of OLT for both BCA and BCAC necessitates a multidisciplinary team approach with a panel of experts.

References

1. Reddy KR et al (2001) Benign and solid tumors of the liver: relationship to sex, age, size of tumors, and outcome. Am Surg 67(2):173–178
2. Balabaud C et al (2013) Focal nodular hyperplasia and hepatocellular adenoma around the world viewed through the scope of the immunopathological classification. Int J Hepatol 2013:268625. doi:10.1155/2013/268625
3. Guy J, Peters MG (2013) Liver disease in women: the influence of gender on epidemiology, natural history, and patient outcomes. Gastroenterol Hepatol 9(10):633–639
4. Barthelmes L, Tait IS (2005) Liver cell adenoma and liver cell adenomatosis. HPB (Oxford) 7(3):186–196. doi:10.1080/13651820510028954
5. Reznik Y et al (2004) Hepatocyte nuclear factor-1 alpha gene inactivation: cosegregation between liver adenomatosis and diabetes phenotypes in two maturity-onset diabetes of the young (MODY)3 families. J Clin Endocrinol Metab 89(3):1476–1480. doi:10.1210/jc.2003-031552
6. Labrune P et al (1997) Hepatocellular adenomas in glycogen storage disease type I and III: a series of 43 patients and review of the literature. J Pediatr Gastroenterol Nutr 24(3):276–279
7. Chang CY et al (2013) Changing epidemiology of hepatocellular adenoma in the United States: review of the literature. Int J Hepatol 2013:604860. doi:10.1155/2013/604860
8. Bioulac-Sage P et al (2012) Hepatocellular adenoma subtypes: the impact of overweight and obesity. Liver Int 32(8):1217–1221. doi:10.1111/j.1478-3231.2012.02786.x
9. Paradis V (2013) Hepatocellular adenomas: WHO classification and immunohistochemical workup. Surg Pathol Clin 6(2):311–331
10. Farges O et al (2011) Changing trends in malignant transformation of hepatocellular adenoma. Gut 60(1):85–89. doi:10.1136/gut.2010.222109
11. Zucman-Rossi J et al (2006) Genotype-phenotype correlation in hepatocellular adenoma: new classification and relationship with HCC. Hepatology 43(3):515–524. doi:10.1002/hep.21068
12. Evason KJ et al (2013) Atypical hepatocellular adenoma-like neoplasms with beta-catenin activation show cytogenetic alterations similar to well-differentiated hepatocellular carcinomas. Hum Pathol 44(5):750–758. doi:10.1016/j.humpath.2012.07.019
13. Bioulac-Sage P et al (2007) Hepatocellular adenoma subtype classification using molecular markers and immunohistochemistry. Hepatology 46(3):740–748. doi:10.1002/hep.21743
14. Shafizadeh N et al (2014) Hepatocellular adenomas in a large community population, 2000 to 2010: reclassification per current World Health Organization classification and results of long-term follow-up. Hum Pathol 45(5):976–983. doi:10.1016/j.humpath.2013.12.011
15. Bluteau O et al (2002) Bi-allelic inactivation of TCF1 in hepatic adenomas. Nat Genet 32(2):312–315. doi:10.1038/ng1001
16. Bacq Y et al (2003) Familial liver adenomatosis associated with hepatocyte nuclear factor 1alpha inactivation. Gastroenterology 125(5):1470–1475
17. Bioulac-Sage P et al (2011) Pathological diagnosis of hepatocellular adenoma in clinical practice. Diagn Histopathol 17(12):521–529
18. Rebouissou S et al (2009) Frequent in-frame somatic deletions activate gp130 in inflammatory hepatocellular tumours. Nature 457(7226):200–204. doi:10.1038/nature07475
19. Paradis V et al (2007) Telangiectatic adenoma: an entity associated with increased body mass index and inflammation. Hepatology 46(1):140–146. doi:10.1002/hep.21684

20. Katabathina VS et al (2011) Genetics and imaging of hepatocellular adenomas: 2011 update. Radiographics 31(6):1529–1543. doi:10.1148/rg.316115527
21. Bioulac-Sage P et al (2010) Subtype classification of hepatocellular adenoma. Dig Surg 27(1):39–45. doi:10.1159/000268406
22. Dokmak S et al (2009) A single-center surgical experience of 122 patients with single and multiple hepatocellular adenomas. Gastroenterology 137(5):1698–1705. doi:10.1053/j.gastro.2009.07.061
23. van Aalten SM et al (2012) Systematic review of haemorrhage and rupture of hepatocellular adenomas. Br J Surg 99(7):911–916. doi:10.1002/bjs.8762
24. Farges O, Dokmak S (2010) Malignant transformation of liver adenoma: an analysis of the literature. Dig Surg 27(1):32–38. doi:10.1159/000268405
25. Bioulac-Sage P et al (2009) Hepatocellular adenoma management and phenotypic classification: the Bordeaux experience. Hepatology 50(2):481–489. doi:10.1002/hep.22995
26. Takigawa Y, Brown AM (2008) Wnt signaling in liver cancer. Curr Drug Targets 9(11):1013–1024
27. van der Windt DJ et al (2006) Case-orientated approach to the management of hepatocellular adenoma. Br J Surg 93(12):1495–1502. doi:10.1002/bjs.5511
28. Stoot JH et al (2007) Life-saving therapy for haemorrhaging liver adenomas using selective arterial embolization. Br J Surg 94(10):1249–1253. doi:10.1002/bjs.5779
29. Walt AJ (1977) Cysts and benign tumors of the liver. Surg Clin North Am 57(2):449–464
30. Arnaoutakis DJ et al (2014) Management of biliary cystic tumors: a multi-institutional analysis of a rare liver tumor. Ann Surg. doi:10.1097/SLA.0000000000000543
31. Sang X et al (2011) Hepatobiliary cystadenomas and cystadenocarcinomas: a report of 33 cases. Liver Int 31(9):1337–1344. doi:10.1111/j.1478-3231.2011.02560.x
32. Devaney K et al (1994) Hepatobiliary cystadenoma and cystadenocarcinoma. A light microscopic and immunohistochemical study of 70 patients. Am J Surg Pathol 18(11):1078–1091
33. Dixon E et al (2001) Cystadenoma of the liver without mesenchymal stroma in a female following hormonal therapy for acne. HPB (Oxford) 3(2):183–186. doi:10.1080/136518201317077224
34. Seo JK et al (2010) Appropriate diagnosis of biliary cystic tumors: comparison with atypical hepatic simple cysts. Eur J Gastroenterol Hepatol 22(8):989–996. doi:10.1097/MEG.0b013e328337c971
35. Vogt DP et al (2005) Cystadenoma and cystadenocarcinoma of the liver: a single center experience. J Am Coll Surg 200(5):727–733. doi:10.1016/j.jamcollsurg.2005.01.005
36. Soares KC et al (2014) Cystic neoplasms of the liver: biliary cystadenoma and cystadenocarcinoma. J Am Coll Surg 218(1):119–128. doi:10.1016/j.jamcollsurg.2013.08.014
37. Emre A et al (2011) Intrahepatic biliary cystic neoplasms: surgical results of 9 patients and literature review. World J Gastroenterol 17(3):361–365. doi:10.3748/wjg.v17.i3.361
38. Wheeler DA, Edmondson HA (1985) Cystadenoma with mesenchymal stroma (CMS) in the liver and bile ducts. A clinicopathologic study of 17 cases, 4 with malignant change. Cancer 56(6):1434–1445
39. Edmondson HA, Atlas of tumor pathology (1958) Tumors of the liver and intrahepatic bile ducts. Armed Forces Institute of Pathology, Washington, DC
40. Hai S et al (2003) Surgical management of cystic hepatic neoplasms. J Gastroenterol 38(8):759–764. doi:10.1007/s00535-003-1142-7
41. Garcea G et al (2013) Surgical management of cystic lesions in the liver. ANZ J Surg 83(7–8):E3–E20. doi:10.1111/j.1445-2197.2012.06096.x
42. Grisolia A et al (2009) A simple sonographic scoring system combined with routine serology is useful in differentiating parasitic from non-parasitic cysts of the liver(). J Ultrasound 12(2):75–79. doi:10.1016/j.jus.2009.02.004
43. Lauffer JM et al (1998) Biliary cystadenocarcinoma of the liver: the need for complete resection. Eur J Cancer 34(12):1845–1851

44. Zen Y et al (2006) Biliary cystic tumors with bile duct communication: a cystic variant of intraductal papillary neoplasm of the bile duct. Mod Pathol 19(9):1243–1254. doi:10.1038/modpathol.3800643
45. Tomioka T et al (1986) Cystadenoma and cystadenocarcinoma of the liver: localization of carcinoembryonic antigen. Jpn J Surg 16(1):62–67
46. Ishibashi Y et al (2007) Invasive biliary cystic tumor without ovarian-like stroma. Pathol Int 57(12):794–798. doi:10.1111/j.1440-1827.2007.02176.x
47. Koffron A et al (2004) Intrahepatic biliary cystadenoma: role of cyst fluid analysis and surgical management in the laparoscopic era. Surgery 136(4):926–936. doi:10.1016/j.surg.2004.06.031
48. Manouras A et al (2008) Laparoscopic fenestration of multiple giant biliary mucinous cystadenomas of the liver. World J Gastroenterol 14(26):4257–4259

Benign Tumors of Bile Ducts and Gallbladder

15

Marco Massani, Nicolò Bassi, C. Nistri, and B. Pauletti

15.1 Introduction

Benign tumors of the bile ducts are uncommon clinical entities, and therefore, most published papers only describe case reports. Nevertheless, these entities, together with pseudotumors, should be considered in the differential diagnosis of painless jaundice patients.

The accepted classification of these tumors divides benign biliary lesions according to the histological differentiation pattern: epithelial tumors, non-epithelial tumors, and neural tumors and pseudotumors [1]. Benign tumors of the gallbladder are more frequent if compared with biliary ones; in fact, polyps of the gallbladder are detected in 4–6 % of patients studied with abdominal ultrasound (US) [2].

The biliary tract is generally divided into intrahepatic, extrahepatic, and the gallbladder.

The extrahepatic part consists of the choledochus, the proper main biliary tract, the cystic duct, the main right and left branches, and the gallbladder. The term "intrahepatic" refers to all the bile ducts inside the liver, starting from the second-order branches [3, 4].

The anatomy of the bile ducts is very complex and several variations are described: all surgeons should consider them when approaching liver resection.

M. Massani (✉) • N. Bassi • C. Nistri • B. Pauletti
IV Divisone Chirurgica, II Dipartimento Chirurgico,
Centro Regionale di Riferimento per la Chirurgia epatobiliopancreatica
Ospedale Regionale, Piazza Ospedale 1, 31100 Treviso, Italy
e-mail: mmassani@ulss.tv.it

L. Aldrighetti et al. (eds.), *Benign Tumors of the Liver*,
DOI 10.1007/978-3-319-12985-3_15

Table 15.1 Anatomic variations of bile ducts, personal experience

	2008	2009	2010	Total	%
Normal anatomy	122	110	81	313	67.3
Seg 6–7° from main left duct	24	21	19	64	13.8
Trifurcation	9	14	7	30	6.5
Seg 6–7° insertion in the main hepatic duct	8	8	11	27	5.8
Seg 6–7° aberrant duct	3	0	3	6	1.3
Seg 5–8° from left main duct	1	3	1	5	1.1
Seg 2° insertion in the main hepatic duct	0	3	0	3	0.6
Seg 5–8° insertion in the main hepatic duct	0	3	0	3	0.6
Cystic duct insertion in the right main duct	2	1	0	3	0.6
Seg 2° insertion in the right main duct	0	1	0	1	0.2
Seg 6° insertion in the left main duct	0	0	1	1	0.2
Seg 6° aberrant duct	1	0	0	1	0.2
Combinations	4	1	2	7	1.5
Number of patients	169	159	118	465	100.00

Table 15.1 shows our personal experience in the intraoperative study of biliary anatomy: the so-called normal anatomy was found in 67.3 % of patients treated, and the most frequent variation was the abnormal origin of the posterior right branch from the main left duct (13.8 % of cases).

15.2 Embryology

The biliary tract originates from embryonic foregut, simultaneously with liver, at fourth week. The initial phase starts from a diverticulum, arisen from the ventral surface of the foregut, that later will become the duodenum. The liver develops from mesenchymal cells of septum transversum and from the endodermal evagination of the foregut. After the development of liver parenchyma, the cells located between the liver and the foregut generate the bile ducts precursors. The extrahepatic biliary tract and the gallbladder originate from the caudal portion of the liver diverticulum, while the intrahepatic biliary system, together with the hilum, originates from the upper portion of the diverticulum. The well-known similarity between the intrahepatic pattern of portal vein branches and ductal biliary system is given by the growth of ductal cells, which follows the connective tissue of the portal veins system. The formation of the main duct completes later, when the cells of the initial occluding epithelium begin to vacuolate and a continuous epithelial-lined lumen is formed; the same process occurs for the cystic duct and the gallbladder. The main duct originates from the dorsal mesentery of the second portion of the duodenum, as pancreatic duct, thus explaining the fact that some biliary and pancreatic lesions have the same pathological behavior. The development of the sphincter of Oddi and of the papilla of Vater is the last phase of biliary tract growth [4, 5].

Table 15.2 WHO 2010 classification of biliary benign tumors

Benign	Premalignant lesions
Epithelial	Epithelial
Adenoma (peribiliary gland hamartoma and others) Microcystic adenoma Biliary adenofibroma	Biliary intraepithelial neoplasia, grade III (BilIN-3) Intraductal papillary neoplasm with low- or moderate-grade intraepithelial neoplasia Intraductal papillary neoplasm with high-grade intraepithelial neoplasia Mucinous cystic neoplasm with low- or intermediate-grade intraepithelial neoplasia Mucinous cystic neoplasm with high-grade intraepithelial neoplasia Miscellaneous

Modified by the authors [6]

15.3 Clinical Presentations and Diagnosis

Jaundice is the most frequent manifestation of benign biliary neoplasms, and the onset of symptoms may be acute or chronic. Pain, when noticed, has the typical characteristics of hepatic and biliary area: it focalizes in epigastrium and in upper right quadrant with diffusion to the right shoulder and to the back. Weight loss is not as frequent as for pancreatic and biliary tract cancers but can be important in clinical setting, especially because there are not specific typical signs of benign biliary and gallbladder lesions. It is important to remark that sometimes these tumors are slow-growing neoplasms, and therefore symptoms may be intermittent.

Other physical findings are not typical such as gallbladder distension and liver enlargement.

The first diagnosis of a biliary or gallbladder lesion is usually given by the use of US, which has high variability on specificity and sensibility due to tumor size and to the presence of biliary dilatation.

The progress of modern radiology has allowed to avoid an extensive use of invasive exams (that are used mostly to relieve symptoms and rarely to clarify the site and extension of the stenosis), such as endoscopic retrograde cholangiopancreatography (ERCP) and percutaneous transhepatic cholangiography (PTC) which were extensively used in the past. The introduction of modern high-quality computed tomography (CT) and magnetic resonance cholangiopancreatography (MRCP) resulted in a significant improvement in the diagnosis of these lesions, although the differential diagnosis with malignant lesions remains difficult (this is clearly confirmed by the high incidence of intraoperative or postmortem findings). The role of modern radiology in the diagnosis of liver lesions is treated in part II of this book. The use of biliary brushing during ERCP or PTC has high positive-predictive value but only very low negative-predictive value, and this is its great limit for clinical usefulness.

The 2010 WHO classification of digestive system tumors divides epithelial biliary tumors in benign or premalignant lesions (Table 15.2) [7].

Bile duct adenoma is treated in part III, Chap. 13, of this book. Here we examine specifically the intraductal and the mucinous cystic neoplasia that only in recent years have been considered as autonomous entities.

15.4 Intraductal Papillary Neoplasm of the Bile Duct (IPNB)

Intraductal papillary neoplasm of the bile duct (IPNB) is a special form of biliary neoplasm [8] that is associated with better outcome compared with conventional bile duct carcinoma and may represent an alternative carcinogenesis pathway in the biliary tract (flat biliary dysplasia vs. exophytic proliferation of biliary epithelium) [9].

Only recently WHO recognized IPNB as a distinct pathologic entity [6], and therefore IPNB can now be defined as "tumor showing papillary proliferation of neoplastic biliary epithelial cells with delicate fibrovascular stalks within the bile ducts, microscopic or macroscopic presence of mucin, and variable dilatation or multilocular cystic changes in the affected bile ducts" [8].

IPNBs can be separated from mucinous cystic neoplasms of the liver by their origin, their luminal communication with the bile duct, and the absence of ovarian-like stroma in the cyst wall; some authors affirm that they may be a biliary counterpart to IPMN.

Hepatolithiasis, liver flukes, and alcohol intake have been associated with these tumors, while smoking has been not [8, 9].

The most common presenting symptoms are those related to cholangitis such as abdominal pain, jaundice, fever, and mucobilia, but some patients may remain asymptomatic [8, 9]. Symptoms and abnormal laboratory findings (elevation in liver function test, e.g., AST, γGT, and CRP) may be caused by bile duct obstruction due to the tumor itself or to mucin production [8], and they are not significantly different between invasive and noninvasive lesions [8, 9].

These tumors can be histologically classified as low-, intermediate- or high-grade intraepithelial neoplasia (carcinoma in situ) and can have an associated invasive carcinoma [6, 8–10].

Also the neoplastic cells are classifiable cytologically into four phenotypes (pancreatobiliary (PT), intestinal (IT), gastric (GT), and oncocytic type (OT)) that are closely associated with the grade of malignancy (PT and IT with adenocarcinoma, while GT with adenoma or borderline tumor) and with the prognosis (a better outcome after resection for OT and GT and a poorer outcome for PT and IT) [8, 9].

The degree of invasion is highly correlated with outcome, and the tumors showing mucin secretion are associated with decreased invasion and better survival. Instead, the primary site of the lesion does not affect the course of the disease, its prognosis, and the survival [9].

Complete resection of IPNBs contributes to good prognosis, even in patients with an invasive carcinoma [8], and all these lesions should be resected with negative margins in order to achieve long-term survival [9].

15.5 Mucinous Cystic Neoplasm (MCN)

Mucinous cystic neoplasms (MCNs) are well-known lesions of the bile ducts that differ from IPNBs substantially for the presence of an ovarian-like stroma. In the past, these lesions were classed as biliary cystadenoma or cystadenocarcinoma, and only recently they have been considered as a specific entity. The 2010 WHO classification defines these lesions as "cystic forming epithelial neoplasm, usually with no communication with the biliary ducts, composed of cuboidal to columnar, variably mucin-producing epithelium, associated with ovarian-type sub-epithelial stroma" [6]. According to their behavior, MCNs are considered as noninvasive (characterized by low-, intermediate-, and high-grade dysplasia) or invasive tumors [6]. The incidence of MCNs is estimated in less than 5 % of all liver cystic lesions; it is important to notice that there is a prevalence in female, usually around the fifth decade [11]. Symptoms are aspecific and include upper right pain, jaundice, cholangitis, fever, and weight loss; liver function tests are usually abnormal. In literature are reported some cases of major symptoms due to portal or caval compression. It has to be considered that, in 30–56 % of cases, these patients are asymptomatic, and the diagnosis is done incidentally [11].

The differential diagnosis can be difficult and should be considered: hepatic abscess, echinococcal cyst, simple cyst, polycystic disease, hemangioma, hamartoma, Caroli's disease, and a huge variety of liver malignant neoplasms [12]. MCNs are slow-growing tumors and the possible evolution into aggressive diseases suggests surgical resection as the treatment of choice.

Diagnosis of IPNBs and MCNs: US is usually the first exam for patients with cholestasis or other symptoms related to liver diseases. Usually the finding is a dilatation of intrahepatic bile ducts that can be limited and/or diffused with variable enlargement. However, the accuracy is extremely variable, and all patients with the description of biliary dilatation, with or without a mass, should be studied with a second level exam. Contrast-enhanced CT and magnetic resonance imaging (MRI) with gadolinium or hepatocyte-specific contrast agent are the gold standard techniques for definition of biliary neoplasms, although the size of the lesion is still a limit (decreasing accuracy with size smaller than 0.5 cm). ERCP can be useful in the detection of mucin inside the biliary duct. Some authors suggest the use of FDG-PET and PET-CT in the diagnostic workup of these lesions, but these exams may be useful only when malignancy is suspected. Age can be helpful in the differential diagnosis: MCNs are more frequent in younger patients, while IPNBs typically arise most between 50 and 70 years [11–13]. The use of CA 19–9 does not seem to be useful in the differential diagnosis between benign or malignant lesions [13].

15.6 Bile Duct Hamartoma

Hamartoma are very common benign liver lesions; otherwise called Von Meyenburg complex, they represent a ductal plate malformation. Usually asymptomatic and mostly diagnosed intraoperatively, these lesions are typically located in the periphery or in the portal tract. They consist of cuboidal or flattened cells with round nuclei.

There is no description of malignant evolution and no specific treatment is necessary [7].

15.7 Granular Cell Tumors

This tumor is usually located in the oral pharynx and in the skin and is also known as Abrikossoff's tumor. It accounts for less than 1 % of bile duct tumors and is typically located in the common bile duct. It is a soft mass, usually single, that can cause jaundice and/or abdominal pain. Sometimes jaundice can be complicated by a secondary liver cirrhosis due to the slow growth of the tumor. The prevalence is higher in female and diagnosis is difficult. CT and MRI show a lesion that enhances contrast with morphological appearance of regular segmental endoluminal or extrinsic compression. The differential diagnosis with cholangiocarcinoma should be considered in young patients presenting history of initial floating jaundice that slowly worsens. The diagnosis is usually performed with histo-/immune-histochemistry: the lesion originates in the Schwann cells and is therefore positive for S100 protein labeling. Preoperative diagnosis can be useful for avoiding unnecessary major resections, but it is extremely difficult considering the fact that the lesion appearance mimics cholangiocarcinoma. This tumor can be located also in the cystic duct and in the gallbladder, with similar behavior [14].

15.8 Rare Benign Biliary Tumors

Some extremely rare benign neoplasms may involve the biliary system. Among these we mention:

- Serous cystadenoma that is very similar to the form usually located in the pancreas. It consists of small and numerous microcysts formed by lined cuboidal epithelium PAS positive.
- Biliary adenofibroma: this lesion, only recently described, consists of stromal and ductular elements with solid microcysts. As for serous cystadenoma, the epithelium is cuboidal, sometimes low columnar.

Both serous cystadenoma and biliary adenofibroma are benign neoplasms that do not require surgical resection; nevertheless, preoperative diagnosis is extremely difficult and this explains the high incidence of post-resection diagnosis.

15.9 Gallbladder Benign Lesions

Gallbladder (GB) tumors are a rare pathology that occur in 3–7 % of the adult population, but with the frequent use of abdominal US, detection of small polypoid lesion of the gallbladder has been increasing considerably in the last years [15–18].

Table 15.3 Benign lesions of the gallbladder

Neoplastic lesions	Nonneoplastic lesions
Epithelial Adenoma Heterotopic tissues Papillomatosis Adenomyomatosis	Cholesterol polyps Inflammatory polyps Xanthogranulomatous cholecystitis Porcelain gallbladder
Non-epithelial Lipoma Leiomyoma Neural tumors	
Miscellaneous	

Most lesions of the GB are benign and are divided into polypoid lesions and atypical thickening of the gallbladder wall with an uncertain diagnosis, which can mimic malignant lesions.

Polyps of the GB include neoplastic and non-neoplastic lesions, and the majority of them is represented by cholesterol polyps (CPs) that have a prevalence of 60–90 % [15, 17, 18] (Table 15.3). CPs are composed by accumulation of triglycerides and cholesterol esters within macrophages in the GB wall (without a real cellular proliferation) forming a polypoid proliferation usually very small (1–2 mm) and that however do not exceed 10 mm. Clinically asymptomatic in most of cases, this lesion is usually an occasional detection at US analysis. The US aspect is a characteristic hyperechoic intraluminal polyp, without posterior shadowing, fixed on the GB wall (Fig. 15.1); if CPs are correctly recognized, no further investigation with other imaging technique, surveillance, or treatment is necessary, unless it become symptomatic [15, 19].

Inflammatory polyps represent 10 % of GB lesions; they are the result of chronic inflammation and are composed of granulation, fibrous tissue, and lymphocytes. Even if usually they are very small, lesions >10 mm are described; they can mimic GB cancer, so the diagnosis is based on histologic examination [15].

The most common benign tumor of the GB is adenoma, which derives from epithelial cells as pseudoglandular proliferation surrounded by fibrous stroma; it can develop in a sessile polypoid or in a pedunculated aspect with a fibrovascular axis (papillary form). The US aspect is an iso-echoic intraluminal lesion fixed on the GB wall without posterior shadowing; color-doppler imaging can evidence the presence of a vascular axis. The potential malignant degeneration of these lesions is linked to the size: it is widely demonstrated that for polyps <10 mm, malignancy rate varies from 0 to 5 %, while for polyps >15 mm, it increases over than 80 % [15–18]. Contrast-enhanced US has high accuracy on characterizing a malignant lesion and should be performed in patients with diagnostic doubts or in the presence of other risk factors [15, 17, 19] (Figs. 15.2 and 15.3).

Papillomatosis is a rare condition characterized by the diffuse presence of papillary adenomas in the biliary tract, intra- and extrahepatic, including the gallbladder [15, 20, 21]. Pathogenesis is still not clear, but it seems to be associated to chronic inflammatory stimulation due to recurrent infective cholangitis or to bile duct stones [20]. Multiple polyps can be found within the cystic lumen, and they are better recognized at endoscopic US rather than classic US. In CT scan and

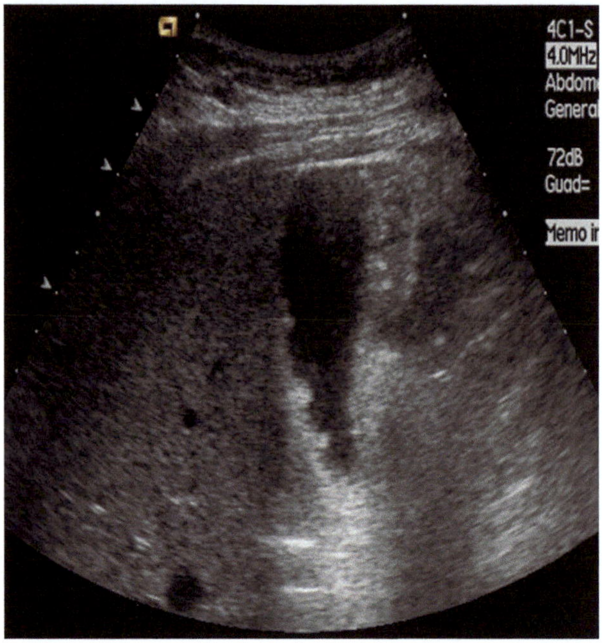

Fig. 15.1 Gallbladder cholesterol polyps at US: *characteristic hyperechoic intraluminal lesion fixed on the gallbladder wall, with no posterior shadowing*

MRI images, the detection of bile duct dilatation is very common, due to obstruction of the lumen by the polyps (Fig. 15.4). This condition has a high potential of cancerous degeneration, and surgical treatment is suggested, adapting surgical technique to the extension of the pathology; liver transplantation should be considered in case of bi-lobar diffusion of papillomatosis or in case of recurrence [15, 20, 21].

Other rare benign lesions of the gallbladder include heterotopic polyps (formed by ectopic tissue as hepatic, gastric, pancreatic, and thyroidal that have no potential for malignant degeneration) and mesenchymal lesions such as leiomyomas, lipomas, and neural tumors (Schwannoma) that do not require surgical treatment unless there are diagnostic doubts [15].

A particular condition of the GB wall thickening is adenomyomatosis; it is localized usually in the cystic fundus and consists in the hyperplasia of smooth muscle layers with invagination of normal epithelial layer (pseudodiverticula) and the formation of cystic structure called Rokitansky-Aschoff sinus. The gold standard imaging technique is MRI with a diagnostic accuracy of 93 %. Malignant degeneration risk of these lesions is still uncertain, but surgical treatment is suggested in the presence of other risk factors for malignancy [15, 22].

Another thickening of GB wall that has a significant relevance is porcelain gallbladder. It is a calcification in the wall that can have a complete intramural diffusion (type 1) or that can involve only mucosal layer completely (type 2) or incompletely (type 3). This condition is associated with GB cancer in 12–60 % of cases and represents an important risk factor. In these patients, preventive laparoscopic cholecystectomy is mandatory [15].

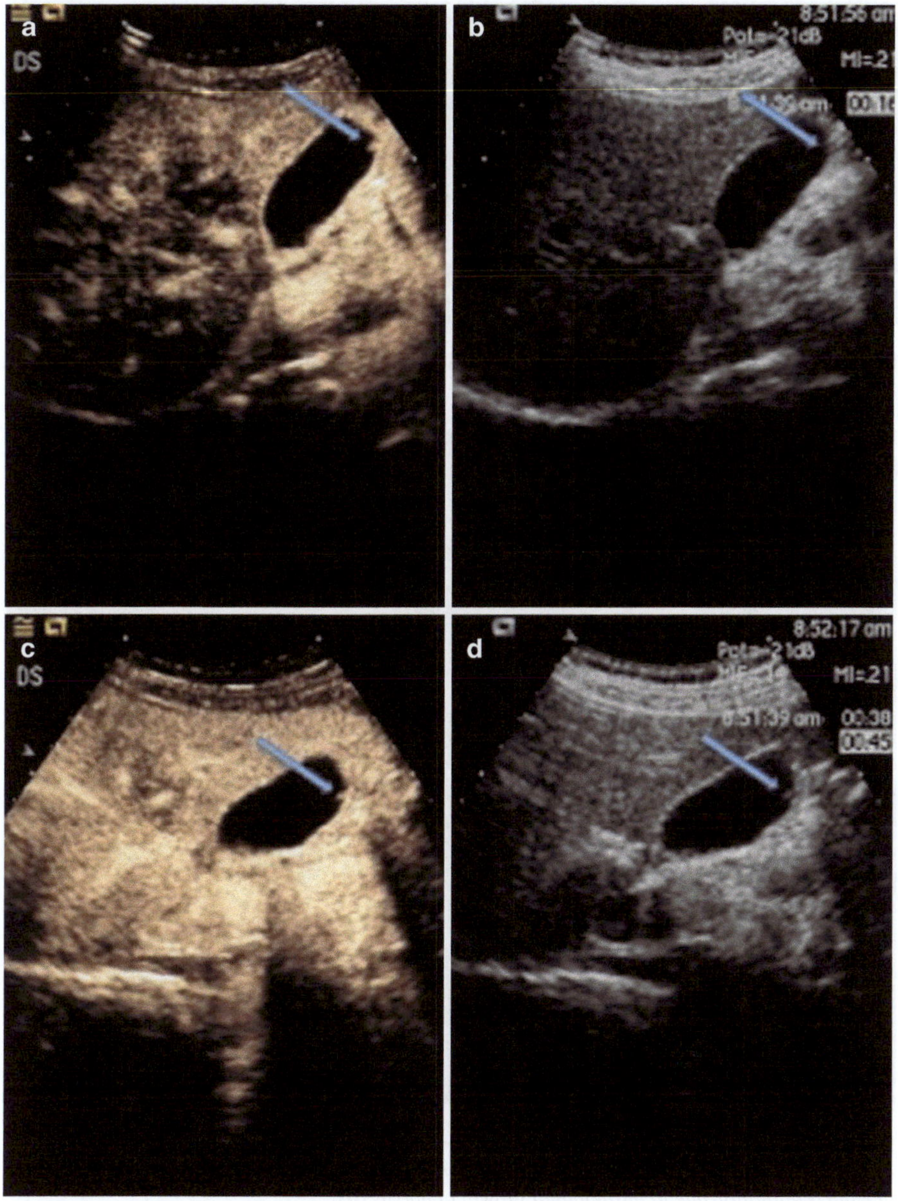

Fig. 15.2 (**a–d**) Gallbladder polyps: *iso-echoic intraluminal lesion fixed on the GB wall, with no posterior shadowing at US* (*blue arrows* **b, d**)*; the same lesions showing contrast enhancement at CEUS* (*blue arrow* **a, c**)

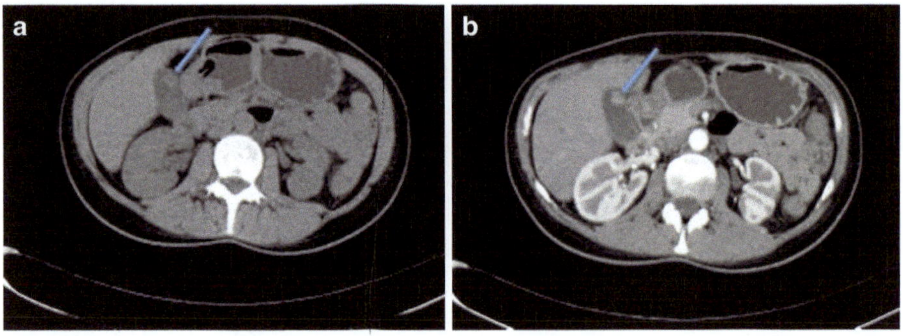

Fig. 15.3 *Blue arrows* shows a gallbladder polyp at CT scan*: direct scan* (**a**), *after contrast enhancing* (**b**)

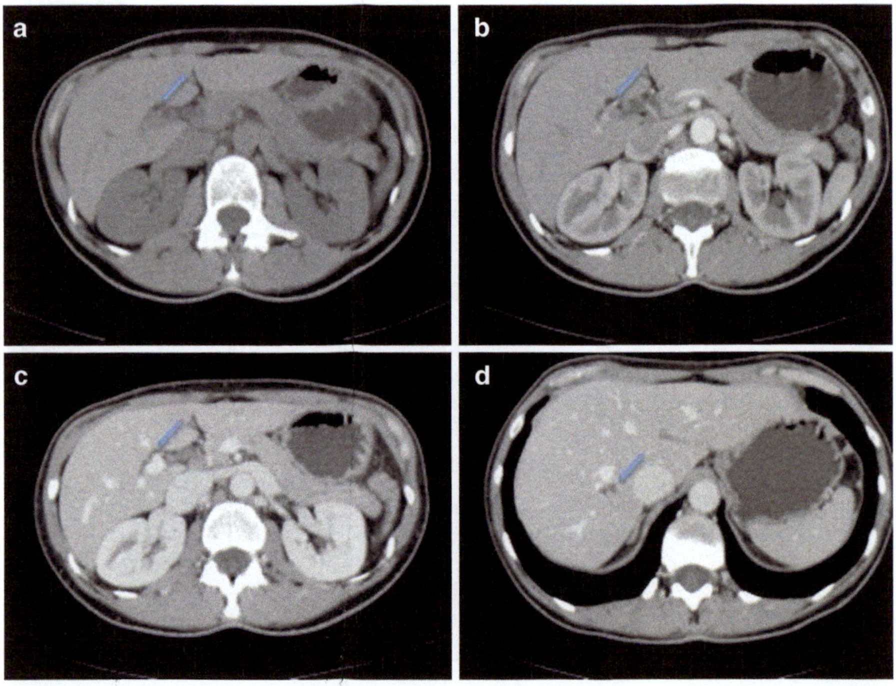

Fig. 15.4 Intrahepatic biliary papillomatosis: *arrow* shows *bile duct dilatation with no presence of gallstones* (**a**) *and with mild contrast enhancing of bile duct wall* (**b**, **c**)*; arrow* shows *sectorial bile ducts dilatation due to intraluminal growth of polyps* (**d**)

15.10 Management

It is widely accepted that polyps greater than 10 mm in size need surgical excision due to the high risk of cancerous degeneration evidenced by numerous studies. Laparoscopic cholecystectomy remains the technique of choice avoiding cystic wall injuries, with eventual frozen section examination to guide extension of resection. However, for polyps >2 cm or with clear signs of malignancy assessed preoperatively, open surgery is suggested by many authors to reduce the risk of tumor seeding [15–19].

Laparoscopic cholecystectomy is also recommended for symptomatic polyps smaller than 10 mm, but what is still debated is the management of small lesions detected occasionally during US examination. It has been reported in various studies that 6–33 % of small polyps disappear at histologic examination [16]. Considering the low risk of cancerous degeneration, a US follow-up every 6 months is suggested; furthermore, it has been demonstrated that small benign lesions with no possibilities of malignancy changes have no growth during follow-up, while malignant lesions have a rapid growth up to fourfold in size within 12 months. So it seems reasonable that a short-term US follow-up may detect eventual cancerous degeneration initially missed [15–18].

Some authors identified risk factor for malignant degeneration in addition to polyp size: age >50 years, primary sclerosing cholangitis, porcelain gallbladder, gallstones, a past history of cancer, and ethnic origins (in some regions such as Chile, Israel, Poland, Mexico, Bolivia, etc., incidence of gallbladder cancer is higher) [15, 17]. In the presence of risk factors, laparoscopic cholecystectomy (considering the reasonable safety of this procedure) is suggested even for small polyps to reduce risk of GB cancer development.

References

1. Levy AD (2002) Benign tumors and tumorlike gallbladder and extrahepatic bile duct: radiologic-pathologic correlation. Radiographics 22:387–413
2. Zileinski MD, Atwell TD, Davis PW et al (2009) Comparison of surgically resected polypoid lesions of the gallbladder to their pre-operative ultrasound characteristics. J Gastrointest Surg 13(1):19–25
3. Vakili K, Pomfret EA (2008) Biliary anatomy and embryology. Surg Clin North Am 88:1159–1174
4. Keplinger KM, Bloomston M (2014) Anatomy and embryology of the biliary tract. Surg Clin North Am 94:203–217
5. Adkins RB, Chapman WC, Reddy VS (2000) Embryology, anatomy and surgical applications of the extrahepatic biliary system. Surg Clin North Am 80(1):363–379
6. Bosman FT, Carneiro F, Hruban RH (eds) (2010) WHO classification of tumours of the digestive system, World Health Organization classification of tumours. IARC, Lyon
7. Odze RD, Goldblum JR (2009) Surgical pathology of the GI, liver, biliary tract and pancreas. Part III, 2nd edn. Saunders/Elsevier, Philadelphia
8. Kubota K, Nakanuma Y, Kondo F et al (2014) Clinicopathological features and prognosis of mucin-producing bile duct tumor and mucinous cystic tumor of the liver: a multi-institutional study by the Japan Biliary Association. J Hepatobiliary Pancreat Sci 21:176–185
9. Rocha FC, Lee H, Katabi N, De Matteo RP et al (2012) Intraductal papillary neoplasm of the bile duct: a biliary equivalent to intraductal papillary mucinous neoplasm of the pancreas? Hepatology 56:1352–1360
10. Nakanuma Y, Curado M-P, Franceschi S et al (2010) WHO classification of tumours of the digestive system, 4th edn. WHO, Lyon, pp 217–224
11. Simo KA, Mckillop IH, Ahrens WA et al (2012) Invasive biliary mucinous cystic neoplasm: a review. HPB (Oxford) 14:725–740

12. Wu JM, Wu YM, Hu RH et al (2008) Surgical treatment of biliary cystadenomas. Int Surg 93:373–376
13. Li T, Ji Y, Zhi X et al (2009) A comparison of hepatic Mucinous Cystic Neoplasms with biliary intraductal papillary neoplasms. Clin Gastroenterol Hepatol 7:586–593
14. Kamaoui I, Pilleul F (2013) Granular cell tumor of the common bile duct: a condition to be aware of. Diagn Interv Imaging 94:324–326
15. Zemour J, Marty M, Lapuyade B et al (2014) Gallbladder tumor and pseudotumor: Diagnosis and management. J Visc Surg 151:289–300
16. Ito H, Hann LE, D'Angelica M et al (2009) Polypoid lesions of the gallbladder: diagnosis and followup. J Am Coll Surg 208(4):570–575
17. Lee KF, Wong J, Li JC et al (2004) Polypoid lesions of the gallbladder. Am J Surg 188(2):186–190, Review
18. Wiles R, Varadpande M, Muly S et al (2014) Growth rate and malignant potential of small gallbladder polyps – Systematic review of evidence. Surgeon 12:221–226
19. Sun XJ, Shi JS, Han Y et al (2004) Diagnosis and treatment of polypoid lesions of the gallbladder: report of 194 cases. Hepatobiliary Pancreat Dis Int 3(4):591–594
20. Yeung YP, AhChong K, Chung CK et al (2003) Biliary papillomatosis: report of seven cases and review of English literature. J Hepatobiliary Pancreat Surg 10(5):390–395
21. Kosemehmetoglu K, Akpinar E, Sokmensuer C et al (2011) Papillary carcinoma with diffuse papillomatosis of gallbladder and cystic duct. Ann Diagn Pathol 15(2):140–144
22. Kim JH, Jeong IH, Han JH et al (2010) Clinical/pathological analysis of gallbladder adenomyomatosis; type and pathogenesis. Hepatogastroenterology 57(99–100):420–425

Liver Focal Localizations of Systemic Diseases

16

Massimo Memoli

Focal liver lesion is defined as solid- or liquid-containing mass foreign to the normal anatomy of the liver that may be detected using imaging techniques.

The hepatic localization of focal lesion in systemic nontumoral nor infectious disease is really uncommon.

It may rarely occur in the course of sarcoidosis, and there are only anecdotal reports for liver involvement in course of other diseases such as extrapelvic endometrioma and cystic lymphangioma of the liver.

16.1 Sarcoidosis

16.1.1 Epidemiology

The disease has a worldwide distribution, with higher rates of prevalence in Scandinavia, Japan, and the United States. The annual incidence is 55–64/10^5 inhabitants in Scandinavia and 11/10^5 in whites and 35/10^5 in Afro-Americans in the United States. Men and women are equally affected, and 99 % of all cases of sarcoidosis occur between 20 and 60 years of age. Hepatic granulomas may be demonstrated in more than 70 % of the cases of pulmonary sarcoidosis. Liver involvement without lung disease occurs in approximately 13 % of cases [1, 2].

M. Memoli, MD
General Medicine and Clinical Immunology,
San Raffaele Hospital, Via Olgettina, 60, Milan 20100, Italy
e-mail: Memoli.massimo@hsr.it

L. Aldrighetti et al. (eds.), *Benign Tumors of the Liver*,
DOI 10.1007/978-3-319-12985-3_16

16.1.2 Etiology

Sarcoidosis is a chronic multisystemic disease characterized by the accumulation of T lymphocytes and macrophages leading to noncaseating granuloma formation in affected organs.

The etiology is unknown, but the disease process is driven by an exaggerated T-helper lymphocyte immune process.

Organ dysfunction occurs from distortion of the normal architecture by the inflammatory infiltrate or by development of fibrosis associated with chronic inflammation.

16.1.3 Clinical Manifestation

The clinical spectrum of hepatic sarcoidosis encompasses asymptomatic patients with mild elevations of alkaline phosphatase and γGT serum levels, a chronic cholestatic liver disease, hepatic vein thrombosis, and nodular transformation of the liver with portal hypertension.

Splenomegaly is most commonly secondary to granulomatous infiltration rather than portal hypertension; ascites formation can be secondary to right heart failure because of pulmonary hypertension, to hypoalbuminemia because of hepatic dysfunction, or rarely to peritoneal sarcoid granulomas [3, 4].

Although sarcoid granulomas are usually 100–200 μm in size, bulky mass-like granulomatous tissue ("sarcoidoma") can mimic malignancy [6].

In a study assessing clinicopathological features in 100 patients with clinical evidence of liver disease and histological evidence of sarcoidosis at liver biopsy, 6 % had dominant mass ("sarcoidoma") which had been biopsied to rule out tumor [5].

16.1.4 Diagnosis

Sonography usually cannot show hepatic or splenic focal sarcoid lesions, although heterogeneous and/or increased echogenicity with organ enlargement has been reported. In sarcoidosis patients hypoechoic, less than 1 cm in diameter nodules in the liver and spleen can occasionally be detected by ultrasound (Figs. 16.1 and 16.2), but diffuse increased homogeneous or heterogeneous echogenicity is more common [6].

Confluent granulomas forming tumorlike nodules ("sarcoidoma") appear as space-occupying lesions and must be further differentiated by biopsy. Enlarged abdominal lymph nodes occur in up to 30 % of cases with abdominal sarcoidosis [6, 7].

MRI appears to demonstrate hepatic nonspecific abnormalities in sarcoid patients more sensitively than ultrasound [6].

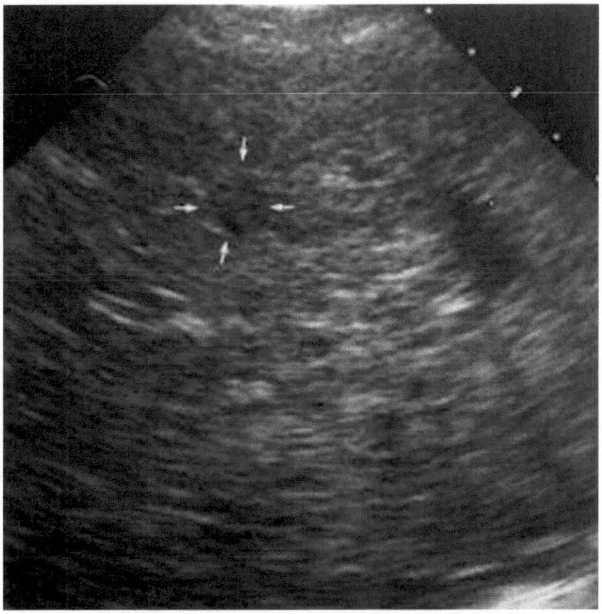

Fig. 16.1 Transverse sonogram of the liver, the *arrows* indicate a hypoechoic nodule due to sarcoidosis (Reprinted with permission from Kessler et al. [6])

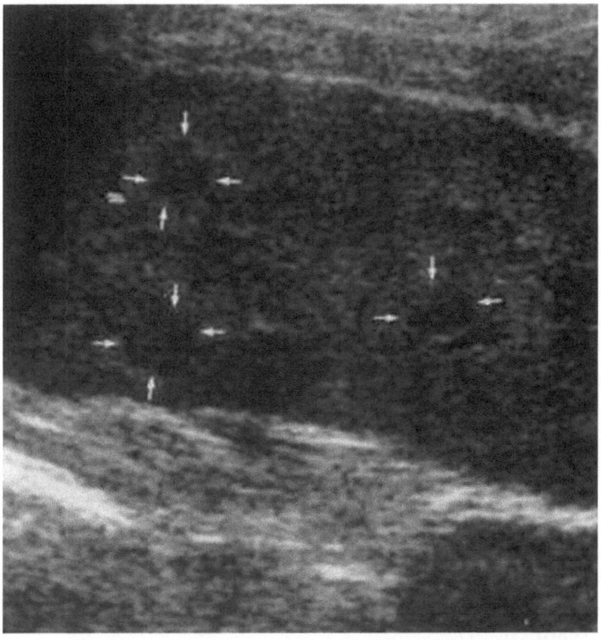

Fig. 16.2 Splenic US, multiple hypoechoic focal lesion, each less than 1 cm in diameter are shown by the *arrows* (Reprinted with permission from Kessler et al. [6])

CT scan can show diffuse hepatosplenomegaly and has detected focal hepatic lesions in 38 % of patients with proved hepatic involvement [6, 8].

In uncomplicated hepatic sarcoidosis, CT and MRI do not add significant diagnostic information to ultrasound findings.

Liver biopsy is the method of choice to demonstrate hepatic granulomas. If granulomas are present on the liver surface, they appear laparoscopically as small (≤2 mm) and well-delineated whitish nodules. Even if no granulomas are seen laparoscopically, liver biopsy usually will yield positive results. Although hepatic nodules are not specific for sarcoidosis, it should be considered among the possible etiologies in appropriate patients.

Histology: Sarcoid granulomas are epithelioid and noncaseating. Occasionally some granulomas may show a central fibrinoid necrosis which must not be mistaken for caseation. Granulomas are spread diffusely throughout the liver and preferentially located in the portal/periportal areas. Usually all granulomas are approximately the same developmental stage. Early acinar granulomas are composed of relatively few loosely assembled epithelioid cells, while mature cells, while mature lesions are sharply rounded and may also coalesce to form granulomatous aggregates.

Large confluent granulomas may form pseudotumors. Involvement of central veins or portal venous branches may cause granulomatous phlebitis. Nodular regenerative hyperplasia, probably due to the disturbance of microcirculation, develops in 6 % of cases. Healing of large granulomas by fibrosis may lead to nodular transformation of the liver with consequent portal hypertension [9–11].

16.1.5 Therapy

The presence alone of granulomas in an organ in sarcoidosis does not dictate treatment.

The decision to treat should be based on symptoms and severity of disease.

Although hepatic involvement usually is asymptomatic, a minority of patients progress to chronic cholestatic disease, portal hypertension, and cirrhosis that may require liver transplantation. Treatment of hepatic sarcoidosis should be reserved for patients who manifest this spectrum of disease.

Glucocorticoid treatment is the first-line therapy for hepatic sarcoidosis, improving symptoms and abnormal laboratory values but generally having no effect on the progression of disease.

In addition to glucocorticoids, immunosuppressive agents such as azathioprine, methotrexate, hydroxychloroquine, and infliximab have been used with some positive effects on symptoms, liver enzyme abnormalities, and hepatomegaly, but none has been shown to prevent progression of disease (Table 16.1).

Ultimately, in case of overt liver failure, liver transplantation is the definitive treatment [4].

Table 16.1 Drugs used in the treatment of severe hepatic sarcoidosis

Prednisone	40 mg/day
Methotrexate	15 mg qw
Azathioprine	20–200 mg/day
Chloroquine phosphate	200–400 mg/day
Ursodeoxycholic acid	10–15 mg/kg body weight/day

Reprinted with permission from Dancygier H [3]

16.2 Hepatic Endometrioma

Endometriosis is a condition characterized by the presence and proliferation of endometrial tissue outside the uterus. Ectopic endometrium has been described in almost every location of the female and even in the male body. The only organ in the abdominal cavity that is apparently refractory to the disease is the spleen [12, 13].

Hepatic endometriosis has an extremely rare occurrence characterized by the presence of ectopic endometrium in the liver. At present only 15 cases of hepatic endometriosis have been previously reported in literature [14].

16.2.1 Clinical Presentation

Abdominal pain is the main symptom, even not related to menses. The physical exam can reveal no palpable mass.

The *gross and microscopic pathological appearances* of endometriosis vary widely depending on the location, extent, age, and endocrine response of lesion. The appearance of endometriotic tissue depends on the degree of its response to the normal hormonal fluctuation of the menstrual cycle. Endometriotic foci may enlarge to produce nodules, cysts, or both.

Because of a wide range of morphological features of endometriomas, there are no characteristic findings with which to distinguish either pelvic or extrapelvic endometriosis from other processes; therefore, clinical history is important for proper diagnosis [15].

Endometriomas typically have a fibrotic wall of variable thickness and are more commonly covered by dense fibrous adhesions that may result in fixation to adjacent structures. The wall structure has been described as smooth, membranous, ragged, or undulating at imaging or morphological examination; the content may be cystic (mostly) or heterogeneous, frequently including septation and/or punctate calcification of the wall. The location of the hepatic lesion has been described as completely intrahepatic and intraparenchymal as well as peripheral and not completely intraparenchymal at surgery [16].

Computed tomography scan can show a well-limited hypovascularized cystic mass with hemorrhagic contents in the lumen, with or without septation [14] (Fig. 16.3).

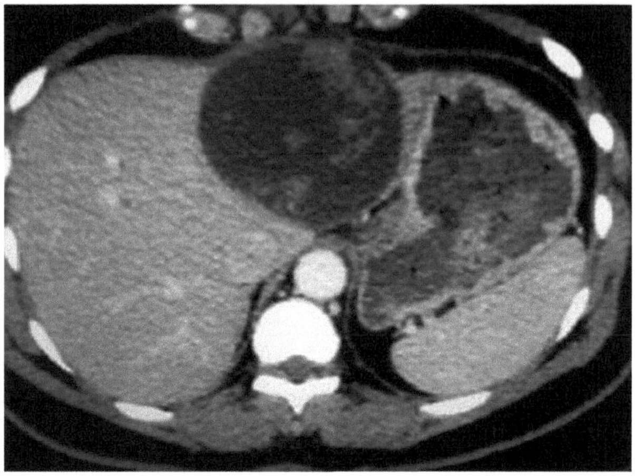

Fig. 16.3 Hepatic CT scan showing a cystic endometriotic mass in the left lobe of the liver (Reprinted with permission from Rivkine et al. [14])

At MRI, endometrial implants usually demonstrate signal intensity similar to that of normal endometrium on T1- ant T2-weighted images. However, because endometrial implants can exhibit various degrees of hemorrhage due to hormonal stimulation, implants may demonstrate a spectrum of appearances depending on the age of hemorrhage [17].

Hepatic endometriosis can be added to the differential diagnosis list of peripherally located cystic or heterogeneous liver mass with septations and wall structure in women, with or without pelvic endometriosis. The radiologist must be aware that the appearance of endometriotic tissue can vary depending on hormonal response, especially on MR.

A diagnosis of hepatic endometriosis is established after *surgery*. The diagnosis is made according to a histological examination of the whole surgical sample.

16.2.2 Therapy

Some authors propose the systematic use of intraoperative frozen sections to avoid radical hepatectomy in order to decrease morbidity and mortality.

A diagnosis of endometriosis must be considered in the differential diagnosis of cystic liver masses, particularly in patients with known endometriosis.

16.3 Cystic Lymphangioma of the Liver

Lymphangiomas are congenital malformations of the lymphatic system.

A hepatic lymphangioma is a rare benign neoplasm that is usually associated with lymphangiomas of other viscera.

It can be solitary or associated with multiple liver lesions and is characterized by cystic dilatation of lymphatic vessels in the hepatic parenchyma. A solitary lymphangioma is unusual.

16.3.1 Clinical Presentation

Lymphangiomas are the results of congenital malformations of the lymphatic system.

The condition is due to the obstruction of lymphatic fluid drainage between the cystic lymphatics and the central veins, or abnormal development of the lymphatic branches, or formation of separated lymphatics and cysts which result in lymphangiomas [18, 19].

Lymphangiomas have been classified into three types: simple lymphangioma, cavernous lymphangioma, and cystic lymphangioma [20]. Other authors have divided lymphangiomas into five types: simple lymphangioma, cavernous lymphangioma, cystic lymphangioma, lymphangio-hemangioma, and lymphangio-sarcoma [21]. Among these five types, cystic lymphangiomas are the most common.

The fluid component of a lymphangioma can be serous or chylaceous, depending on the location of the lymphangioma. In the presence of hemorrhage or infection, a lymphangioma can be bloody or purulent.

Abdominal lymphangiomas are rare (less than 1 %) and usually occur in the mesentery and retroperitoneum.

Although hepatic lymphangiomas are considered as a subset of multiple abdominal lymphangiomas, they rarely occur in the liver alone [21, 23].

Hepatic lymphangiomas are single or multiple occurrences of lymphangiectasia, containing blood in the lumen and lined with endothelial cells which have inconspicuous nuclei on the inner walls (Fig. 16.4) [21, 23, 29].

Normally, most hepatic lymphangiomas are found by routine physical examination or from other complaints and have no specific clinical presentation.

Occasionally, abdominal pain is due to the compression of surrounding tissues or organs [18].

Ultrasonography or CT imaging may lead to a misdiagnosis of hepatic hemangioma or hepatic cystadenocarcinoma. Thickness of the cyst wall, number of cystic

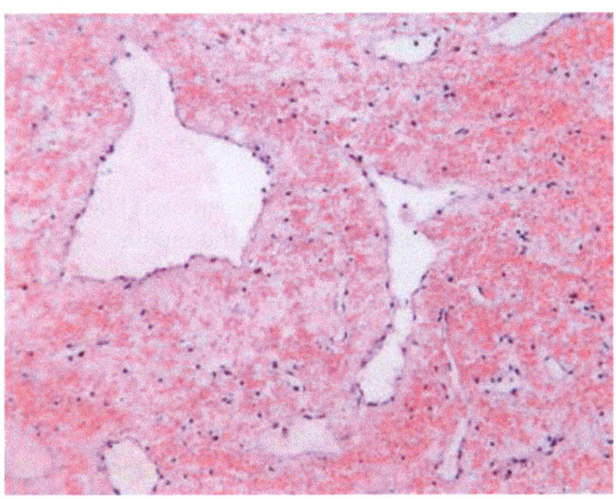

Fig. 16.4 Microscopically the lesion consisting of multiple cystic spaces lined by a layer of cells, morphologically consistent with mature differentiation endothelium (Reprinted with permission from Huang et al. [29])

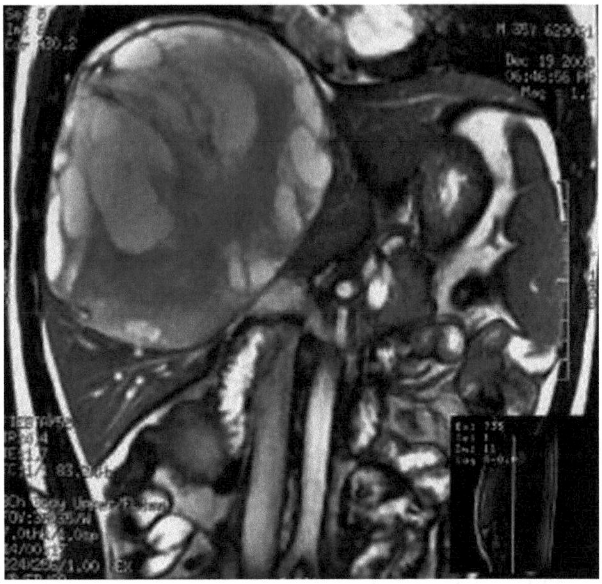

Fig. 16.5 Coronal cover of T2-weighted MRI showing a giant cystic mass involving segment IV, V, VI, VII, and VIII of the liver (Reprinted with permission from Huang et al. [29])

septations, and internal echoes may be helpful to differentiate lymphangioma from other mesenteric cysts [24].

CT imaging can reveal the cystic characteristics. When containing chylous fluid, the cysts may manifest as a negative CT value. CT imaging features of a lymphangioma are a cystic or multicystic lesion with no enhancement in the central region and enhancement in the septa.

Magnetic resonance imaging (MRI) of a lymphangioma usually shows a multiloculated heterogeneous mass with low signal intensity on T1-weighted images and high signal intensity on T2-weighted images because of the content of the lymphangioma [23]. MRI is very helpful for determining such characteristic features of a lesion because T2-weighted and heavily T2-weighted imaging are sensitive to the presence of water (Fig. 16.5) [18, 19, 22, 29].

However, when hemorrhage or infection occurs, the CT value of the cystic region will rise and may lead to misdiagnosis [25]. The image as seen on MRI corresponds to dilated lymphatic spaces and is useful in differentiating a lymphangioma from a true solid neoplasm.

Lymphangiomas are benign hamartomas but have a risk of cancerization.

Continuing enlargement can cause rupture.

Surgical resection of lymphangiomas has been considered standard treatment.

Histopathological examination from frozen section is helpful for intraoperative diagnosis if it is difficult to make a clear diagnosis during the operation.

For huge or multiple lymphangiomas, liver transplantation is also considered [26].

The prognosis of hepatic lymphangiomas is good, and patients have no need for further treatment after resection.

It has been found that a lymphangioma rarely recurs or progresses [27, 28].

References

1. Kennedy PT, Zakaria N, Modawi SB et al (2006) Natural history of hepatic sarcoidosis and its response to treatment. Eur J Gastroenterol Hepatol 18:721–726
2. Newman LS, Rose CS, Maier LA (1997) Sarcoidosis. N Engl J Med 336:1224–1234
3. Dancygier H. Sarcoidosis of the liver. Clinical hepatology. Springer-Verlag Berlin Heidelber 2010, pp 1239–1242
4. Ayyala US, Padilla ML (2006) Diagnosis and treatment of hepatic sarcoidosis. Curr Treat Options Gastroenterol 9(6):475–483
5. Devaney K, Goodman ZD, Epstein MS, Zimmerman HJ, Ishak KG (1993) Hepatic sarcoidosis: clinicopathologic features in 100 patients. Am J Surg Pathol 17(12):1272–1280
6. Kessler A, Mitchell DG, Israel HL, Goldberg BB (1993) Hepatic and splenic sarcoidosis: ultrasound and MR imaging. Abdom Imaging 18(2):159–163
7. Deutch SJ, Sandler MA, Tankanow LB (1987) Abdominal lymphadenopathy in sarcoidosis. J Ultrasound Med 6:237–242
8. Britt AR, Francis IR, Glazer GM et al (1991) Sarcoidosis: abdominal manifestation at CT. Radiology 178:91–94
9. Gitlin N (1997) Sarcoidosis and the liver. In: Gitlin N (ed) The liver in systemic disease. Churchill Livingstone, New York, pp 137–146
10. Ishak KG (1998) Sarcoidosis of the liver and bile ducts. Mayo Clin Proc 73:467–472
11. Tekeste H, Latour F, Levitt RE (1984) Portal hypertension complicating sarcoid liver disease: case report and review of the literature. Am J Gastroenterol 79:389–396
12. Giudice LC, Kao LC (2004) Endometriosis. Lancet 364:1789–1799
13. Bergquist A (1992) Extragenital endometriosis, a review. Eur J Surg 158:7–12
14. Rivkine E, Jakubowicz D, Marciano L, Polliand C, Poncelet C, Ziol M, Barrat C (2013) Hepatic endometrioma: a case report and review of the literature: report of a case. Surg Today 43:1188–1193
15. Inal M, Biçakçi K, Soyupak S, Oguz M, Özer C, Demirbas Ö, Akgül E (2000) Hepatic endometrioma: a case report and review of the literature. Eur Radiol 10:431–434
16. Finkel L, Marchevsky A, Cohen B (1986) Endometrial cyst of the liver. Am J Gastroenterol 81:576–578
17. Stevens SK (1992) The adnexa. In: Higgins CB, Hricak H, Helms CA (eds) Magnetic resonance imaging of the body. Raven, New York, pp 865–889
18. Matsumoto T, Ojima H, Akishima-Fukasawa Y, Hiraoka N, Onaya H, Shimada K, Mizuguchi Y, Sakurai S, Ishii T, Kosuge T, Kanai Y (2010) Solitary hepatic lymphangioma: report of a case. Surg Today 40:883–889
19. Kochin IN, Miloh TA, Arnon R, Iyer KR, Suchy FJ, Kerkar N (2011) Benign liver masses and lesions in children: 53 cases over 12 years. Isr Med Assoc J 13:542–547
20. Alqahtani A, Nguyen LT, Flageole H, Shaw K, Laberge JM (1999) 25 years' experience with lymphangiomas in children. J Pediatr Surg 34:1164–1168
21. Chen CQ, Zhan WH, Wang JP, Chen ZX, Dong WG, Lan P, Peng JS (2000) The clinical characteristics, diagnosis and treatment of abdominal lymphangioma. Chin J Pract Surg 20:421–422
22. Adachi S, Maruyama T, Suetomi T, Morishita Y, Otsuka M, Todoroki T, Fukao K (2001) Retroperitoneal multiple lymphangioma with differential cyst contents causing hydronephrosis and biliary dilatation. Hepatogastroenterology 48:397–400
23. Abe H, Kubota K, Noie T, Bandai Y, Makuuchi M (1997) Cystic lymphangioma of the pancreas: a case report with special reference to embryological development. Am J Gastroenterol 92:1566–1567
24. de Perrot M, Rostan O, Morel P, Le Coultre C (1998) Abdominal lymphangioma in adults and children. Br J Surg 85:395–397
25. Choi WJ, Jeong WK, Kim Y, Kim J, Pyo JY, Oh YH (2012) MR imaging of hepatic lymphangioma. Korean J Hepatol 18:101–104
26. Qin Y, Ni Y, Wang CY, Wang CL (2009) Diagnosis and treatment of the rare tumor-like lesions of liver. Anhui Med J 30:157–159

27. Datz C, Graziadei IW, Dietze O, Jaschke W, Königsrainer A, Sandhofer F, Margreiter R (2001) Massive progression of diffuse hepatic lymphangiomatosis after liver resection and rapid deterioration after liver transplantation. Am J Gastroenterol 96:1278–1281
28. Zhang YZ, Ye YS, Tian L, Li W (2013) Rare case of a solitary huge hepatic cystic lymphangioma. World J Clin Cases 1(4):152–154
29. Huang L, Li J, Zhou F, Yan J, Liu C, Zhou AY, Tang A, Yan Y (2010) Giant cystic lymphangioma of the liver. Hepatol Int 4:784–787

Focal Infectious Diseases 17

Renato Finazzi

17.1 Pyogenic Abscess

17.1.1 Epidemiology

The incidence of pyogenic liver abscess is about 10 cases per million persons per year, or 15 cases per 100,000 hospital admissions, with a lethality rate of 6–14 %, even if treated [1, 2]. The patient usually is middle aged, and the incidence is higher between the fifth and sixth decade (the period in which the incidence of biliary disease is higher as well). No difference can be observed as regards sex and ethnic or geographical origin.

17.1.2 Etiology

Pyogenic liver abscess can recognize several pathogenic mechanisms:

1. *Bacteremia from the portal vein* from an intra-abdominal infection such as appendicitis, diverticulitis, peritonitis, pancreatitis, intestinal obstruction/perforation, and chronic inflammatory bowel diseases, as well as after abdominal or bariatric surgery [3].
2. *Bacteremia from hepatic artery;* this hematogenous route accounts for the localization in the liver of septic processes from systemic bacteremia as seen during sepsis, infective endocarditis, or i.v. line infections; this septic embolization may produce multiple abscesses or microabscesses.

R. Finazzi, MD
Hepatobiliary Surgery Unit, IRCCS San Raffaele Hospital,
Via Olgettina 60, Milan, MI 20132, Italy
e-mail: finazzi.renato@hsr.it

L. Aldrighetti et al. (eds.), *Benign Tumors of the Liver*,
DOI 10.1007/978-3-319-12985-3_17

3. *Spreading from biliary tree.* This pathogenic mechanism accounts for the majority of hepatic abscesses, which are usually multiple, and is the result of ascending cholangitis as seen in partial or complete biliary tree obstruction due to gallstones, extrinsic stenosis, neoplasia, or, more rarely, infestation by *Ascaris lumbricoides*; the presence of biliary-intestinal anastomosis also constitutes a risk factor for hepatic abscesses.
4. *Extension from contiguous infectious sites* as seen sometimes in subphrenic or perinephric abscesses or cholecystitis.
5. *Trauma;* both penetrating (in which the microorganisms are delivered directly in the liver) or blunt trauma (by means of superinfection of resulting hematoma or ischemic zone) may cause liver abscesses, as well as tumor angiographic embolization (e.g., TAE, TACE, DEB-TACE).

The abovementioned mechanisms can explain the majority of hepatic abscesses, but in few cases, none of these can be advocated and the abscess is thus defined *cryptogenic* [4].

The causes and microbiological agents of pyogenic liver abscesses differ between the East and West [2]. In the East, liver abscesses are mainly categorized as cryptogenic, while in the West, it predominates the biliary origin. Usual etiologies include *Enterobacteriaceae*, *Bacteroides*, and enterococci. Among *Enterobacteriaceae*, *Klebsiella pneumoniae* is being reported more and more frequently (especially in Asia), and this has been correlated to the emergence of more virulent strains which have been demonstrated also to be more invasive [5, 6]. In patients who suffer from hemochromatosis, *Yersinia enterocolitica* may also be a pathogen involved.

17.1.3 Clinical Presentation

Symptoms may be very variable and consist mainly of fever, jaundice, and right upper quadrant tenderness. The full classical triad is present in less than 10 % of cases, while fever is frequent, even without localization symptoms and often accompanied by nonspecific symptoms like malaise, nausea, fatigue, anorexia, and weight loss [7].

The duration of symptoms may also be variable, ranging from an acute (few days) to a chronic (weeks to months) pattern. This diversity can be well understood given the wide range of possible etiologies, the clinical picture often being closely correlated to.

Usually hepatic abscesses are single and present with a subacute onset and a protracted course with low-grade, remittent fever as the prominent feature. The nonspecific systemic symptoms abovementioned are usually present; tenderness or swelling in the upper right abdominal quadrant is seen in half of the cases.

Leukocytosis and elevation of alkaline phosphatase, together with CRP, are the main abnormalities of blood tests. Anemia and mild elevation of transaminases and bilirubin may be present. More pronounced elevation of cholestatic indexes may be found in biliary diseases. US and CT scan constitute the main step for diagnosis as well as for therapy (Fig. 17.1).

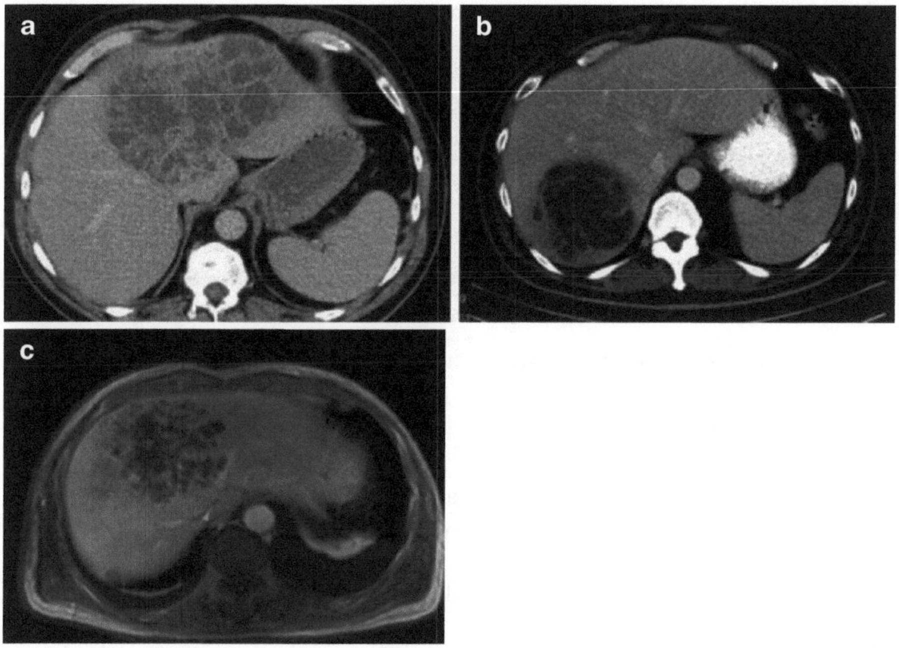

Fig. 17.1 (**a–c**) CT scan of three cases of liver abscesses by *Klebsiella pneumoniae* (Reprinted with permission from Moore et al. [5])

17.1.4 Therapy

Percutaneous drainage is required in addition to antibiotic therapy in the majority of cases, especially if the lesion is more than 3–5 cm in diameter [8, 9]. Surgical drainage is seldom required unless percutaneous approach is not feasible or a treatment for associated intra-abdominal infection is needed [7, 10].

Microbiologic tests are of capital importance for the identification of the etiologic agent and to help the choice of antibiotic: blood cultures are positive in half of the cases, and multiple sets (both aerobic and anaerobic) should be taken *before* the institution of empiric antibiotic therapy. In case of percutaneous or surgical drainage, samples for microbiologic examination (both Gram stain and culture) should be obtained. The importance of correct handling of the sample and its prompt dispatch to the lab, in order not to hamper the recovery of anaerobes, has to be stressed. The catheter usually is left in place for a few days until the drained volume becomes minimal.

The diagnosis of pyogenic abscess should be reevaluated if the drainage fails to give purulent material. In this case alternative differential diagnosis (amebic abscess, cyst, neoplasm) should be considered.

Empiric antibiotic therapy should be guided by the suspected origin of the abscess and may be started with an association of drugs (Table 17.1).

Table 17.1 Recommended antibiotic therapy for hepatic abscess [11]

First choice		Alternative	
Metronidazole +	Ceftriaxone *or* Cefoxitin *or* Tazobactam/piperacillin *or* Sulbactam/ampicillin *or* Ciprofloxacin *or* Levofloxacin	Metronidazole +	Imipenem *or* Meropenem *or* Doripenem

17.2 Amebic Liver Disease

17.2.1 Epidemiology

Amebiasis is the most aggressive intestinal human protozoan disease and is considered one of the leading causes of mortality from parasitic diseases worldwide, only surpassed by malaria, leishmaniasis, and African trypanosomiasis. The parasite is worldwide distributed; about 7–10 % of the world population is infected by one of the three human-infectious species: *E. histolytica*, *E. dispar*, and *E. moshkovskii* with mortality rates in excess of 100,000 annually. The nonsymptomatic form is ubiquitous (prevalence: 1–5 % in temperate countries, up to 50 % in tropical areas), while the clinical pathological one is mainly seen in India and Southeast Asia or in Africa. European and American patients with amebic liver abscess classically have a history of travel to endemic areas and are typically males in the third or fourth decade of life.

17.2.2 Etiology

The principal host and source of infection is the human. Amebic infection originates from ingestion of cysts (the dehydrated survival form) of *Entamoeba histolytica* with contaminated food or water; interhuman transmission is rare (dirty hands, oro-genital and oro-rectal practices) [12]. In the intestinal lumen, the excystation takes place and the trophozoites perpetuate the infection. In the majority of cases, the infection (*amebic infection*) does not evolve in the symptomatic clinical phase (*amebic illness*), and the trophozoite is found in (non-diarrheic) feces in its *minute* form (*E. histolytica minuta*); this ameba does not have invasive properties. Sometimes (10 %) the infection progresses and the vegetative form of the trophozoite in its pathogenic form (*E. histolytica histolytica*) invades the intestinal mucosa, causing its disruption with eventual dissemination to other organs (mainly the liver through the portal system). The parasite produces proteolytic enzymes and cytotoxins able to kill leukocytes, thus halting local inflammation response and causing multiple ulcerative lesions mainly in the cecum, ascending colon, and sigmoid. This usually stimulates peristalsis, causing dysentery (*amebic dysentery*) sometimes with severe evolution (fulminant hemorrhagic colitis). Sometimes (1 %), not related to the severity of intestinal disease, trophozoites reach the liver sinusoids through the portal blood flow, causing microinfarcts and focal areas of hepatocyte necrosis, and in a subsequent series of lyric steps, the abscess is formed. Since the majority of the portal blood flow reaches the right hepatic lobe, usually amebic abscesses are right sided. With time a fibrous connectival wall develops (capsule) which sharply demarcates the abscess from normal liver tissue. The cavity of the abscess is filled with a thick, acellular fluid, yellowish creamy often referred as "anchovy paste" or "like chocolate." Later calcification may develop as well as superinfection or extension to other organs: the pleura, lung, pericardium, peritoneum, spleen, and kidney (*amebic extraintestinal disease*).

17.2.3 Clinical Presentation

Hepatic amebiasis always needs a prior intestinal infection, but such an anamnestic element (diarrhea, gastrointestinal symptoms, abdominal pain or cramping) is present only in 15–35 % of cases. The main complaint may be irregular fever sometimes accompanied by malaise or vague digestive symptoms and right upper abdominal quadrant discomfort or even pain, possibly with posterior interscapular irradiation.

The onset of symptoms may be acute or may ensue months from a travel in an endemic area. Usually the abscess is single and right sided, but multiple lesions can also be observed.

The clinical presentation does not differ from the pyogenic liver abscess (see Sect. 17.1.3), and the differential diagnosis cannot be made on a pure clinical ground. Serology is of little help, since a positive result does not exclude other etiologies and a negative one does not rule out amebiasis [13]. Usually, however, the antibody titer is high. Stool examination is useless because cysts of *Entamoeba dispar* (a nonpathogen ameba) are indistinguishable from cysts of *Entamoeba histolytica*. US and CT scans reveal a cavity with liquid or mixed content with the lack of peripheral dense zone seen in pyogenic abscesses. Percutaneous aspiration of amebic abscess yields sterile chocolate-like or greenish material possibly without evidence of trophozoites (localized mainly in the peripheral wall). Eosinophilia usually is not present, and this can be used as a differential diagnosis criterion with hydatid disease (Fig. 17.2) (Table 17.2).

17.2.4 Therapy

Medical therapy is usually sufficient to eradicate amebic infection, and percutaneous or surgical drainage is seldom necessary. *Metronidazole* 750 mg thrice daily for 10 days is the first-line treatment. *Tinidazole* (2 g daily for 5 days) or *secnidazole* (500 mg TID for 5 days) may also be employed. A course of contact amebicidal agents like *paromomycin* (25–35 mg/kg/day p.o. divided in 3 doses × 7 days) or

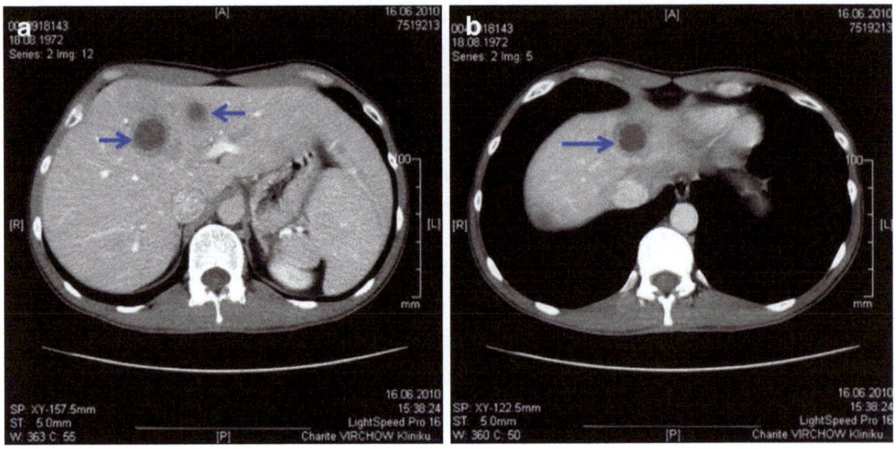

Fig. 17.2 Amebic abscesses on CT (Reprinted with permission by Marn et al. [13])

Table 17.2 Clinical symptoms of 104 cases of hepatic amebiasis [14]

Symptoms	%
Fever	98
Pain	100
Hepatomegaly	80
Jaundice	55
Vomiting	43
Diarrhea	35
Weight loss	31

iodoquinol (600 mg TID p.o. × 20 days) should follow in order to sterilize the intestinal colonization by *E. histolytica*.

Therapeutic aspiration associated with amebicidal therapy is a well-indicated alternative in patients with large abscesses (>5 cm). Superinfected abscesses may also benefit from percutaneous aspiration. Surgery is rarely used as a treatment alternative and may be needed in case of complicated abscess or abscess rupture.

17.3 Unusual Causes of Liver Abscess

17.3.1 Listeriosis

Infections from *Listeria monocytogenes* usually occur in the immunocompromised host. Frequently clinical manifestations include meningitis, meningoencephalitis, or bacteremia, but liver abscesses have also been described [15]. This rare condition may mimic a neoplastic disease. The antibiotic of choice is ampicillin +/– gentamicin; co-trimoxazole may be an effective alternative.

17.3.2 Brucellosis

Brucellosis is a common zoonosis with worldwide diffusion with more than 500,000 cases per year. The Mediterranean, Middle East, Latin America, and parts of Asia constitute areas of high endemicity. The disease occurs for occupational exposure, direct or indirect contact with the infected animal (sheets, goats, cattle, pork, domestic animals) or ingestion of contaminated product, especially fresh dairy products. Bacteria are phagocytized by macrophages and monocytes and directed to the spleen, liver, bone marrow, and lymph nodes, where tissue damage and granulomas progressively develop. After the acute febrile phase, which typically occurs 2 months after infection, in untreated (or undertreated) patients, chronic infection can develop.

Hepatic brucelloma is a rare localization occurring in the chronic phase of the disease and may be difficult to diagnose if not accompanied by symptoms typical of the systemic disease. Usually abscesses are single (but multiple abscesses also have been described) and hypoechoic, right sided, 3–10 cm in size, and with a central calcification. Abscesses show one or more loculi whose walls can show a contrast enhancement on TC scan.

Therapy of chronic brucellosis is still an object of debate: usually *rifampin*, doxycycline, *streptomycin*, and *co-trimoxazole* are used in various combinations and for long courses [16].

17.3.3 Tuberculosis

Tubercular liver abscess is a rare disease which occurs usually in the clinical setting of a pulmonary or intestinal tuberculosis. Together with fever and weight loss, ascites is the principal symptom. CA-125 is very high in almost all cases, and this can lead to misdiagnosis. Peritoneal fluid usually has an exudative appearance, the cellular component mostly constituted by lymphocytes. Acid-fast stain is usually negative. Cultures give positive results in about a third of cases, but they take as long as 6 weeks to grow. PCR can help the diagnosis in most cases [17].

17.3.4 Actinomycosis

Hepatic actinomycosis is a rare disease and usually originates from dissemination from other abdominal sites of infection. Symptoms are often nonspecific (nausea, malaise, weight loss, and fever). Alkaline phosphatase is usually elevated. The typical appearance is that of multiple hepatic abscesses often of small dimensions. Percutaneous aspiration may allow the diagnosis by detection of "sulfur granules" with Gram-positive acid-fast bacilli or by culture (provided that specimen is correctly handled and promptly placed in anaerobic conditions). Intravenous high-dose penicillin is the treatment of choice.

17.3.5 Bartonellosis

Bartonella henselae is the etiologic agent of cat-scratch disease, an infectious disease that can be acquired from infected cats, particularly in their first year of life, which causes a localized lymphadenopathy, usually spontaneously recovering. A systemic presentation may be possible both in immunocompromised and immunocompetent hosts (bacillary angiomatosis, hepatic peliosis, endocarditis). In the clinical picture of a disseminated infection, besides constitutional symptoms like fever, malaise, asthenia, and weight loss, hepatosplenic nodules may be found. They are 3–30 mm in diameter, hypoechoic, solid, and without contrast enhancement on CT. Since *Bartonella* is hard to grow in cultures, the diagnosis relies almost completely on serological tests and PCR. In disseminated bartonellosis or endocarditis, *macrolides*, *doxycycline*, *rifampin*, and *aminoglycosides* are employed.

17.3.6 *Candida*

Liver abscesses from *Candida* may sometimes occur, especially in immunocompromised hosts. The most common setting is patients with leukemia who can develop a systemic infection during the recovery phase from severe neutropenia. Clinical features include fever, nausea, vomiting, abdominal pain, and tender hepatomegaly. Liver function tests are usually abnormal, particularly an elevated serum alkaline phosphatase.

17.4 Hepatic Echinococcal Disease

17.4.1 Cystic Hydatid Disease

17.4.1.1 Epidemiology

Echinococcosis (or hydatid cystic disease) originates from the infestation with larvae of *Echinococcus granulosus*, a cosmopolitan tapeworm which sylvan strain is maintained in wolves and ungulates in Alaska, Canada, Scandinavia, and Eurasia and pastoral strain in dogs and domestic ungulates throughout the world. South America, the Mediterranean, Middle East, many parts of Africa, Russia, Central Asia, and China are endemic regions with an estimated 1.2 million people affected worldwide. The annual incidence in endemic areas varies from <1 to 220 per 100,000 persons per year.

17.4.1.2 Etiology

Dogs infected with *Echinococcus granulosus* (infestation is completely asymptomatic) pass cysts in the feces which can adhere to the hair, muzzle, and paws of the animal. Humans acquire the infection by contact with the infected animal: when the eggs reach the small intestine, an oncosphere is released, which can burrow the mucosa and migrate via the portal system to the liver. Metacestode (larva) then develops into a unilocular fluid-filled cyst. Sometimes the liver filter is trespassed and the cyst can develop in the lung.

The cyst is usually 1–15 cm in diameter and has a thick wall, the inner layer of which is the germinal zone; it forms small cellular masses projecting into the cyst cavity forming brood vesicles that contain many protoscolices (the head of the future worm). These protoscolices sometimes grow to form a daughter cyst within the mother cyst. The outer layer, called pericyst, is made of connective tissues that often become calcified with time.

17.4.1.3 Clinical Presentation

Infection usually occurs in childhood, while clinical manifestations typically affect adults in their third to fifth decade of life. Hepatic cyst may be completely asymptomatic and discovered thus incidentally, or symptoms related to the mass effect may be present, sometimes associated to those related to compression of the vessel or biliary system (Budd-Chiari syndrome, cholestasis). Common symptoms are upper abdominal discomfort and pain. On physical exam hepatomegaly can be found sometimes with the presence of a palpable mass. The rupture of the cyst into the biliary tree can provoke cholangitis, biliary colic, and pancreatitis. The rupture of the cyst into the peritoneum can cause a life-threatening anaphylaxis and peritoneal dissemination of the hydatidosis. Superinfected hydatid liver cysts can be indistinguishable from liver pyogenic abscesses.

Serological tests are available for the detection of specific antibodies, and even though false-positive results are possible, they can help the diagnosis especially in non-endemic areas (where serology is always positive) and are useful in monitoring the outcome of therapy.

Ultrasonography is of great help to diagnose echinococcal liver disease, and cysts may be well characterized (uni- or multilocular, with daughter cysts or not, presence of calcification, communication with the biliary tree), but sometimes CT scan is needed to better document the size, site, and structure of the cysts. An international classification has been proposed and universally adopted to define echinococcal cyst stage [18].

17.4.1.4 Therapy

The appropriate treatment depends on individual case characteristics. *Surgery* has the potential to remove cysts and lead to complete cure and for a long time has been considered the only treatment option. The operating procedure is the removal of the cyst together with the pericystic membrane. The residual cavity is filled with omentum (omentoplasty). Surgery is the treatment of choice in large cysts, in cysts with subcapsular location, complicated cysts, multiple cysts and cysts with daughter cysts, and cysts with communication with the biliary tree. A prophylaxis with albendazole, started before the operation and continued for 4 weeks after, is mandatory to prevent the risk of secondary peritoneal echinococcosis from intraoperative seeding of protoscolices.

The advent of US and TC imaging tools allowed the development of *percutaneous procedures* which are aimed to destroy the germinal layer with scolicidal agents

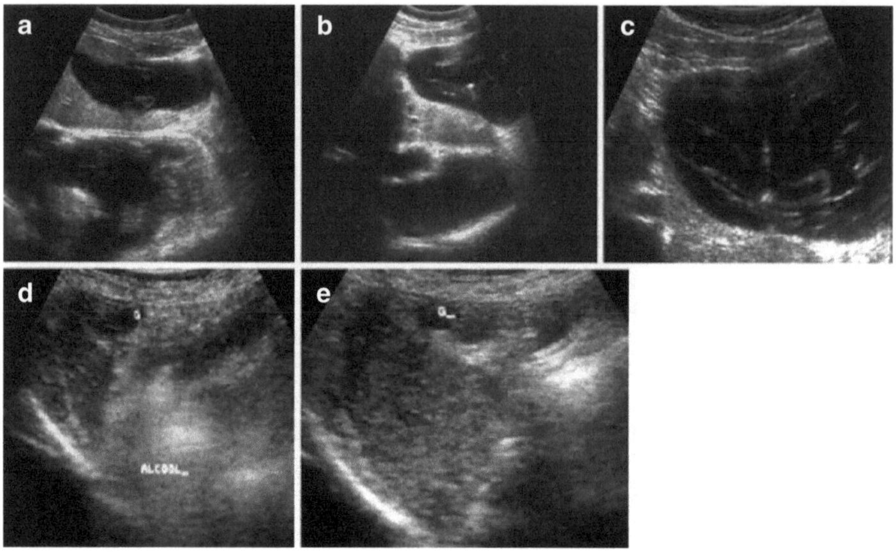

Fig. 17.3 (**a**) Young female patient 21 years old with two large cysts in the right lobe of the liver. (**b**) The needle tip is clearly visible during puncture of the anterior cyst. (**c**) Soon after the puncture of the cyst, detachment of the inner membrane is observed (*N*=needle). (**d**) Alcohol injected (250 ml) filled the entire cyst cavity. (**e**) Six months later, follow-up showed disappearance of the large cyst (Reprinted with permission of Giorgio et al. [21])

(namely, 20 % hypertonic saline and 95 % ethanol) and/or to completely evacuate the cyst. The most popular method is the PAIR (percutaneous aspiration injection reaspiration) technique [19], which has been demonstrated safe and effective, in specifically trained specialistic centers. Both in surgery and in percutaneous procedures, the use of scolicidal agents is not recommended without prior exclusion of a communication between the cysts and the biliary tree.

Chemotherapy may benefit from scolicidal agents like *mebendazole*, *albendazole*, *praziquantel*, and *isoquinoline* derivatives. *Albendazole* is better absorbed, especially if taken with fat-rich meal, and is thus preferred (10/15 mg per Kg divided in two daily doses). This regimen prolonged for 3–6 months can lead to a complete response in 30 % of cases and a partial response in another 40 %. *Watch and wait* approach can be applied in cases of asymptomatic and uncomplicated inactive cysts (Fig. 17.3) [20].

17.4.2 Alveolar Hydatid Disease

17.4.2.1 Epidemiology

The etiologic agent is *Echinococcus multilocularis*, a tapeworm with a distribution in the northern hemisphere (from northern tundra to regions around the 40–45° of northern latitude). Cases have been reported in Central Europe, Russia, Turkey, Iran, Afghanistan, India, Canada, and Japan. The annual incidence is low (0.03–1.2 per 100,000 persons per year).

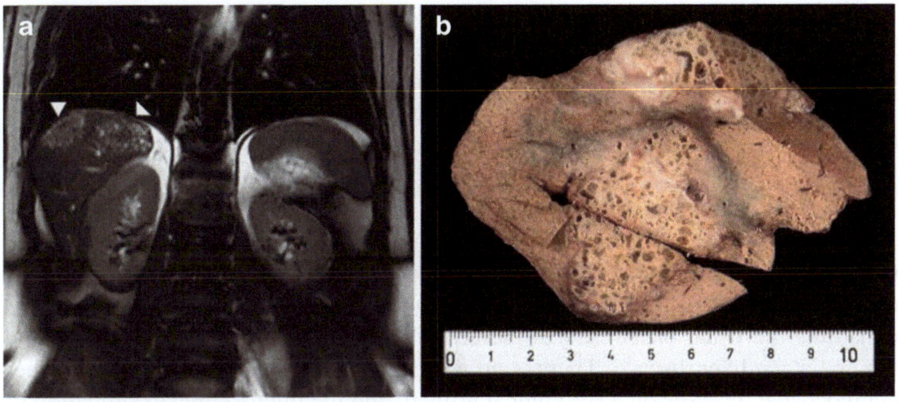

Fig. 17.4 Alveolar hydatids of the right hepatic lobe (Reprinted with permission from D. Tappe) *Arrowheads* indicate the two cysts

17.4.2.2 Etiology

Infection in humans occurs during manipulation of fox carcasses or by ingestion of contaminated wild berries. The parasite reaches the liver through the portal system, and vesicles are formed with surrounding intense inflammatory reaction which in the end causes the formation of a tumor which may cavitate. Calcification occurs in over 70 % of the cases with an irregular pattern. The disease invades bile ducts, portal and hepatic veins and inferior vena cava, and the surrounding organs (lung, liver, bone). The cysts keep growing during a long time (5–15 years) before becoming symptomatic.

17.4.2.3 Clinical Presentation

Fatigue, epigastric pain, abdominal mass, and abnormal liver function tests are the main symptoms and signs of the diseases, which are more common in an older age (fifth decade and beyond) and have a chronic progressive course toward hepatic decompensation due to extensive liver infiltration, jaundice, portal hypertension, and Budd-Chiari syndrome. Dissemination to the pleura, lung, pericardium, retroperitoneum, pancreas, and kidneys may occur. Serologic enzyme immunoassay with specific antigen allows diagnosis confirmation.

17.4.2.4 Therapy

Therapeutic options include surgical removal of the liver and extrahepatic localizations and long-term chemotherapy with mebendazole or albendazole (2 years after radical surgery, lifelong in nonsurgical cases). Liver transplant has been performed with a 6-year survival of 66 % (Fig. 17.4).

17.4.3 Polycystic Hydatid Disease

17.4.3.1 Epidemiology

This is a rare disease due to *Echinococcus vogeli* or *Echinococcus oligarthrus*. Sporadic cases have been described in Panama, Ecuador, Colombia, Venezuela, Suriname, Brazil, and India.

17.4.3.2 Etiology

Infection in humans occurs by exposure to hunt dogs fed on the raw viscera of infected pacas. The liver is the primary site of infection, with the formation of cysts of various size and grouped together, containing a gelatin-like substance. Calcification can occur, often in a bizarre fashion.

17.4.3.3 Clinical Presentation

While *E. vogeli* forms cysts in the liver, lungs, pericardium, heart, mesentery, and omentum, *E. oligarthrus* produces polycystic disease only in extrahepatic tissues (orbit, lower jaw, heart). Abdominal pain and distension, fever, and weight loss constitute the usual onset clinical picture. Evolution is slowly progressive toward the end-stage liver disease. There is no way to differentiate this disease from other echinococcal diseases on a serological ground, and the microscopic examination of scoleces is needed for the differential diagnosis.

17.4.3.4 Therapy

Radical surgical excision is the ideal treatment (Table 17.3).

Table 17.3 Human hydatid disease [22]

	Cystic hydatid disease	Alveolar hydatid disease	Polycystic hydatid disease	
Agent	*E. granulosus*	*E. multilocularis*	*E. vogeli*	*E. oligarthrus*
Species				
Adult size (mm)	2–7	4–11	2–4	2–3
Definitive hosts	Dog, wolf, jackal, lion	Foxes	Bush dogs	Wild felid
Intermediate hosts	Sheep, cattle	Rodents	Paca	Spiny rat
Human disease	Common	Uncommon	Rare	Extremely rare
Occurrence				
Mode of infection	Contact with infected dogs	Contact with fur from infected fox, ingestion of contaminated wild berries	Contact with hunting dog fed on paca	Contact with infected cats
Lesion	Fluid-filled unilocular cyst	Solid mass	Polycystic fluid filled	Polycystic fluid filled
Appearance				
Calcification	30 %, ring type	70 %, microcalcification or plaque-like foci	50 %, annular, bizarre, amorphous	Not known
Organs involved	Liver (65 %)	Liver (100 %)	Liver (100 %)	Extrahepatic (orbit others)
Primary	Lung (25 %)			

Table 17.3 (continued)

	Cystic hydatid disease	Alveolar hydatid disease	Polycystic hydatid disease	
Spread	By rupture	Contiguous, metastasis to the lung and brain	Contiguous	Contiguous
Presentation	No symptoms, mass effect, rupture, infection	Invasive liver mass, liver failure, cholestasis, Budd-Chiari's, portal hypertension, lung and brain involvement	Liver masses, liver failure, cholestasis, Budd-Chiari's, portal hypertension	Exophthalmos
Mortality	Unusual (<5 %)	High (75–100 %)	High (>75 %)	Not known

References

1. Johannsen EC et al (2000) Pyogenic liver abscesses. Infect Dis Clin North Am 14:547–563
2. Ferraioli G et al (2008) Percutaneous and surgical treatment of pyogenic liver abscesses: observation over a 21-year period in 148 patients. Dig Liver Dis 40:690–696
3. Garrido D et al (2013) Liver abscess as a complication of laparoscopic gastric banding bariatric surgery. Surg Infect (Larchmt) 14(5):464–468
4. Hyun Cheol K et al (2013) Should colonoscopy be performed in patients with cryptogenic liver abscess? Clin Res Hepatol Gastroenterol 37:86–92
5. Moore R et al (2013) Community-acquired Klebsiella pneumoniae liver abscess: an emerging infection in Ireland and Europe. Infection 41:681–686
6. Liu Y et al (2013) An increasing prominent disease of Klebsiella pneumoniae liver abscess: etiology, diagnosis and treatment. Gastroenterol Res Pract. Article ID 258514, 12 p
7. Mangukiya DO (2012) A prospective series case study of pyogenic liver abscess: recent trends in etiology and management. Indian J Surg 74(5):385–390
8. Yu-Meng T et al (2005) An appraisal of surgical and percutaneous drainage for pyogenic liver abscesses larger than 5 cm. Ann Surg 241(3):485–490
9. Lee-Won C et al (2014) Successful treatment of liver abscesses secondary to foreign body penetration of the alimentary tract: a case report and literature review. World J Gastroenterol 20(13):3803–3711
10. Tan L et al (2013) Laparoscopic drainage of cryptogenic liver abscess. Surg Endosc 27:3308–3314
11. Gilbert DN et al (2013) The Sanford guide to antimicrobial therapy, 43rd edn. Antimicrobial Therapy, Inc. Sperryville, USA
12. Hung C-C et al (2012) Entamoeba histolytica infection in men who have sex with men. Lancet Infect Dis 12:729–736
13. Marn H et al (2012) Amoebic abscess with negative serological markers for Entamoeba histolytica: mind the gap! Infection 40:87–91
14. Salles JM et al (2003) Hepatic amebiasis. Braz J Infect Dis 7(2):96–110
15. Onetto C et al (2013) Liver abscess due to Listeria monocytogenes. Cir Esp 91(4):264–276
16. Barutta L et al (2013) Hepatic brucelloma. Lancet Infect Dis 13:987–993
17. Uzunkoy A et al (2004) Diagnosis of abdominal tuberculosis: experience from 11 cases and review of the literature. World J Gastroenterol 10(24):3647–3549
18. WHO Informal Working Group (2003) International classification of ultrasound images in cystic echinococcosis for application in clinical and field epidemiological setting. Acta Trop 85:253–261

19. WHO Informal Working Group (2003) PAIR: puncture, aspiration, injection, re-aspiration. An option for the treatment of cystic echinococcosis, vol. WHO/CDS/CSR/APH/2001.6.2003. WHO, Geneva
20. Rinaldi F et al (2014) Cystic echinococcosis of the liver: a primer for hepatologists. World J Hepatol 6(5):293–305
21. Giorgio A et al (2008) Long-term results of percutaneous treatment of hydatid liver cysts: a single center 17 years experience. Infection 36(3):256–261
22. Tappe D et al (2008) Curative resection of hepatic alveolar hydatids. Infection 36(6):607–608

Part IV

Treatment of Benign Liver Tumors

18 Transplantation for Benign Liver Lesions

Vincenzo Scuderi, Federico Tomassini,
and Roberto Ivan Troisi

18.1 Introduction

Most cases of benign hepatic lesions (BHL) do not require any treatment and should be managed conservatively, but if it becomes symptomatic or malignant degeneration cannot be ruled out, resection is the standard approach.

To resect BHL even extended hepatectomy can be performed with acceptable risks, thanks to the improvements in technique and perioperative management in the tertiary referral centers for hepatobiliary surgery [1, 2].

Orthotopic liver transplantation (OLT) has become the standard treatment for chronic and acute liver disease because of its advances in technical skills, management of postoperative complications, and improvements in immunosuppressive drugs. From a review of the literature, OLT has been reported to treat BHL as shown in Table 18.1.

Published reports are limited and based on small case series or single case report with a consequent lack of data regarding optimal indications for OLT in case of BHL. The transplant is doubtless the definitive and curative therapy, but considering the shortage of donor grafts, the high morbidity, and the mortality risk (estimated to be 1–3 %), this indication remains not standard in this population for whom conservative approach and, if necessary, surgical resection are the gold standard. OLT is a valid therapeutic option in the case of the conditions reported in Table 18.2.

The European Register of Liver Transplants (ELTR) reports the data of 97,698 OLT carried out in the period 1988–2012 [3].

V. Scuderi, MD • F. Tomassini, MD • R.I. Troisi, MD, PhD, FEBS (✉)
Department of General, Hepatobiliary and
Liver Transplantation Surgery, Ghent University Hospital
Medical School, De Pintelaan 185, 2K12 IC, Ghent 9000, Belgium
e-mail: roberto.troisi@ugent.be

L. Aldrighetti et al. (eds.), *Benign Tumors of the Liver*,
DOI 10.1007/978-3-319-12985-3_18

Table 18.1 Benign hepatic tumors treated by OLT

Polycystic liver disease (PLD)
Liver Cell Adenoma (LCA) and Liver Adenomatosis (LA)
Hepatic Hemangioma (HH)
Hepatic epithelioid hemangioendothelioma (HEHE)
Other infrequent solid nodules (hepatic hydatid disease; nodular regenerative hyperplasia; lymphangiomatosis of the liver, mesenchymal hamartoma, focal nodular hyperplasia; biliary cystadenoma)

Table 18.2 Clinical indications for OLT in case of BHL

Severe symptoms with discomfort for abdominal encumbrance
Uncertain diagnosis or preneoplastic lesions
Increased risk of life-threatening complications, rupture, or malignant transformation
Lesions not amenable to resection due to wide diffusion in the hepatic parenchyma
Hepatic function impairment
Metabolic diseases and Kasabach–Merritt syndrome

A total of 994 (1.01 %) OLT due to Polycystic liver disease (PLD) are carried out and 324 OLT (0.33 %) for other benign tumor lesions.

Hepatic epithelioid hemangioendothelioma (HEHE) is instead classified to have a neoplastic etiology due to its borderline nature, and it represents 1.5 % of OLT performed for cancer (232/15,197) in the same period.

The survival rate of OLT performed in 1988–2012 for PLD and other benign liver lesions based on ELTR data is shown in Fig. 18.1.

The incidence of transplants for hepatic benign nodular disease is roughly the same in United Network for Organ Sharing (UNOS) area (0.9 %) [4] and ELTR (1.3 %). Among the different benign nodular diseases, although it is a cystic and not a solid tumor, PLD is by far the most common: 78 % in the UNOS area and 75 % in the ELTR; it takes therefore a prominent place also for the implications of renal failure due to polycystic kidney disease.

18.1.1 The Ghent University Hospital Experience

From 2002 to 2013, we performed 33 OLT for BLT (5.2 % of 633). PLD (Fig. 18.2) is the most common indication (29 pt; 87.8 %), and 7 (24.1 %) of these patients received combined liver kidney transplant (CLKT); other indications (3 pt; 9.1 %) were liver cell adenoma (LCA), liver adenomatosis (LA) (Fig. 18.3), and HEHE. The graft survival of OLT for PLD is reported in Fig. 18.4.

Two living donor liver transplantations (LDLT) were performed for LA and PLD. The retransplantation rate is 15 % (5/33): one late re-OLT for biliary cirrhosis

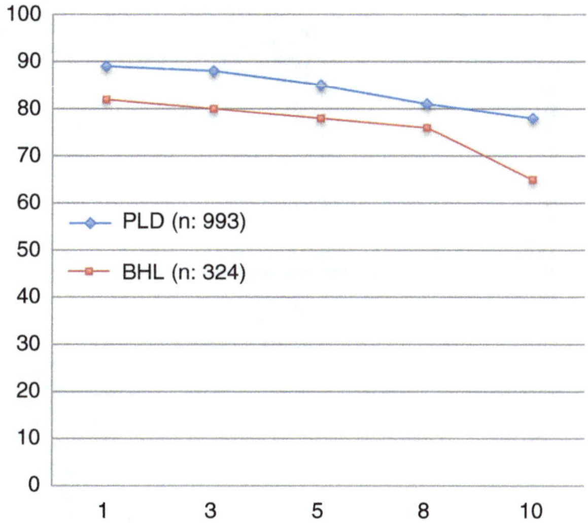

Fig. 18.1 Survival (1–10 years) after OLT for all benign hepatic lesions and polycystic liver disease (ELTR data 1988–2012)

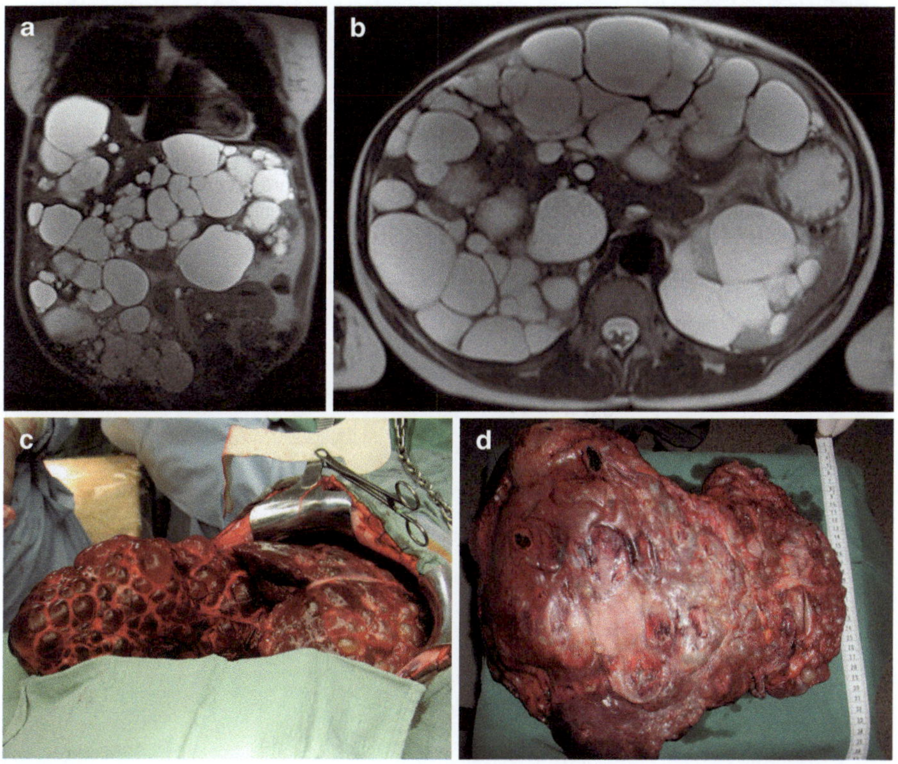

Fig. 18.2 (**a–d**) F 55 y.o. BMI 19. PLD in clinical follow-up (7 years). Impaired quality of life due to cachexia for severe malnutrition and recurrent cyst infection. MELD labo 13. Graft allocation: standard exception. OLT 9-1-2013. Donor: 53 y.o. intracerebral bleeding

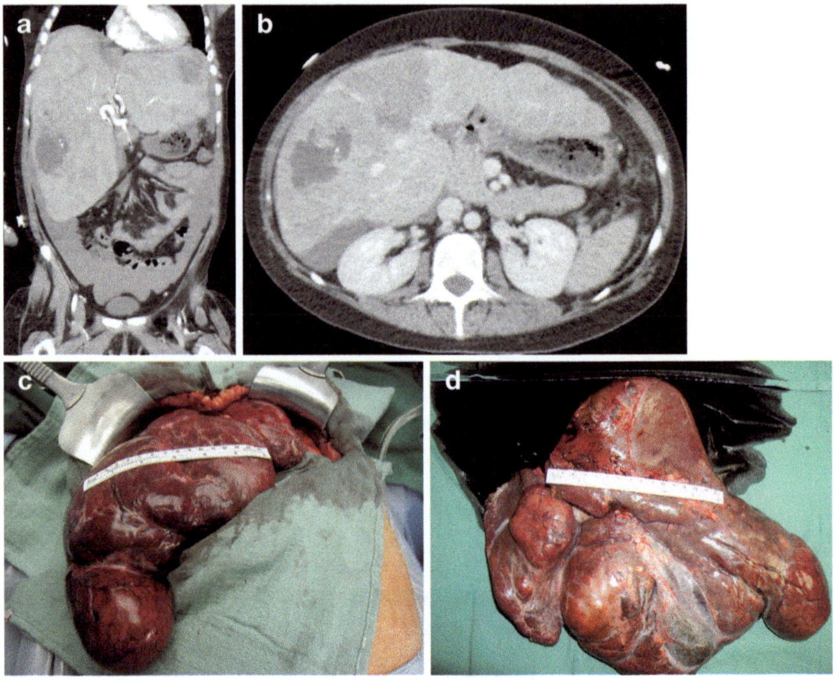

Fig. 18.3 (**a–d**) F 22 y.o. BMI 21. Maturity-onset diabetes of the young type 3. Liver adenomatosis in clinical follow-up (5 years) complicated by sudden hemoperitoneum due to spontaneous bleeding of the left lobe. MELD labo 9. Graft allocation: nonstandard exception. OLT 24-9-2013. Donor: F/63 y.o. intracranial bleeding. Native hepatectomy specimen: liver segments completely substituted by HNF1α non-activated adenomatous nodules

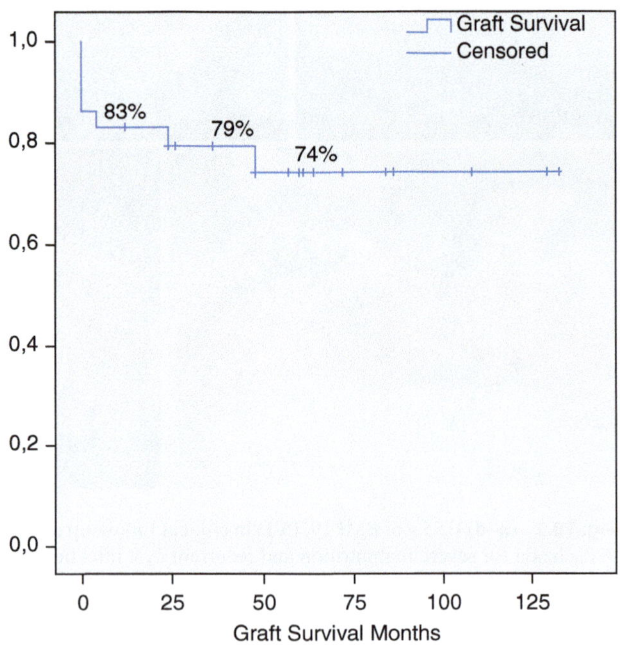

Fig. 18.4 Overall graft survival for PLD (Ghent University Hospital series)

4 years following the first OLT for PLD, three for early hepatic thrombosis, and the last for PNF. This last patient died 4 months after re-OLT due to septic complications.

The overall morbidity rate was of 33.3 % (11/33 pt), and this was concerning only patients transplanted for PLD.

Seven patients (21.2 %) had biliary anastomosis stricture after a mean of 4.2 months (range 3–6) post-OLT, and three were surgically treated. Hepatic artery thrombosis was recorded in four patients, three of them requiring urgent retransplantation.

18.2 Polycystic Liver Disease

PLD is a rare autosomal dominant benign disorder characterized by well-preserved liver function but can result in substantial morbidity, and this can increase mortality rates. Hepatic failure is uncommon, but quality of life (QoL) can be severely impaired with huge hepatomegaly causing abdominal distension accompanied with pain, dyspepsia or reduction of oral intake, malnutrition, weight loss, asthenia, dyspnea, and fatigue and physical and even psychological handicap. Symptoms develop when mass polycystic disease is already established or when the cyst/parenchyma ratio is above >1 [5].

Hepatic venous outflow impairment due to huge liver cysts causing a secondary Budd–Chiari syndrome for extrinsic compression of the hepatic veins and the inferior vena cava has been rarely reported also [6–8].

Although conservative therapy is the standard approach, in severe cases of PLD where conventional surgery (i.e., cyst fenestration) is not indicated [9], OLT might be considered.

The first OLT for PLD was a combined liver–kidney transplantation (CLKT) for massive organomegaly performed by Kwok and Lewin in 1988. Unfortunately, the patient died intraoperatively because of intractable bleeding [10]. Two years later, Starzl reported 4 CLKT in patients with polycystic disease with one patient died 5 months after transplantation [11].

Transplant can offer fully curative and radical treatment also if some controversies remain, considering the absence of liver failure, the relative organ shortage, the perioperative risks of mortality, and the need for lifelong immunosuppression. OLT should be considered as a valid therapeutic option in carefully selected patients with symptomatic PLD. Considering that the organ function is preserved until a late stage, the question of "when" the transplant is appropriate is challenging. Due to the absence of signs of liver failure, the Model for End-Stage Liver Disease (MELD) score is not representative for these patients. According to Arrazola et al. [12], patients with PLD should meet the criteria reported in Table 18.3 in order to be listed for LT.

In the MELD-driven system, he proposed that the eligibility for OLT should continue to be addressed by the regional review board in a case-by-case basis,

Table 18.3 Criteria for listing patients with PLD for OLT

Massive PLD (total cyst/parenchyma ratio >1)
Complication of the PLD that is likely to resolve after OLT
Clinically significant manifestations of liver disease that can be attributed to massive PLD *(cachexia, ascites, portal hypertension, hepatic venous outflow obstruction, biliary obstruction, cholestasis, or recurrent cyst infection)*
Not candidates for, or have disease that has failed to respond to, non-OLT interventions for relief of symptoms
Contraindication to non-transplant surgery: severe malnutrition
Hypoalbuminemia <2.2 mg/dL
Decreased lean body mass: decreased midarm circumference, measured in the nondominant arm midway between the acromion and the olecranon process (<23.1 cm in female patients and <23.8 cm in male patients)

suggesting that patients could be given 15 MELD points and MELD could be increased three points every 3 months [12].

The priority on the waiting list for patients with PLD is reasoned since results are clearly worse when OLT is delayed and malnutrition and severe compressive symptoms are present.

In the Eurotransplant area, the level of priority can be upgraded as *standard exception* after a waiting time of 12 months [12–14].

The unreliable representation by the MELD score, the increased perioperative risk in patients with severe cachexia and malnutrition, and the excellent long-term results after transplantation suggest the need for an earlier referral for transplantation.

The septic complications are indeed the main cause of a postoperative mortality up to 20–30 % of the earlier studies. The increased risk of sepsis might have been due to bacterial reservoirs in cysts and/or prolonged poor nutritional status, amplified by the immunosuppressive agents: it is therefore of paramount importance to adopt for these patients a tailored immunosuppressive regimen.

Except for this high postoperative risk, patients transplanted for PLD have a good long-term prognosis and excellent relief of symptoms, although in small case series [15].

In case of previous abdominal surgeries, a challenging total hepatectomy phase should be anticipated. According to the UNOS data, in 46 % of all PLD recipients surgical antecedents have been recorded [4]. Furthermore, the displacement of the vascular and biliary structures in the hilum alters the normal anatomical landmarks. In view of the encountered ntraoperative difficulties, iterative surgical approaches should be abandoned in favor of the more radical transplant procedure. Mainly the "wrapping" of the fenestrated parenchyma with omentum makes the transplant more difficult, hampering the subsequent OLT.

Laparoscopic cyst fenestration that leads to less morbidity compared to the open approach is strongly recommended in case of not numerous and huge cysts [9, 16, 17].

The best surgical approach during total hepatectomy is still under debate. Jiang et al. [18] sequential partial hepatectomy to reduce progressively the liver volume, while others believe this could involve a greater risk of hemorrhage. Cysts fenestration facilitates the IVC approach, reducing also hepatic venous congestion and subsequent bleeding. Considering that these are patients without severe portal hypertension, the portal vein is only clamped at the end of hepatectomy [18, 19].

In cases of PLKD, if the abovementioned symptoms are associated with renal failure requiring hemodialysis or with a glomerular filtration rate below 30 mL/min, CLKT is indicated. Indeed after OLT, the patients often get nephrotoxic calcineurin inhibitors as immunosuppressive agents, which often worsen the already deteriorated kidney function.

Liver cysts usually appear later than kidney cysts, often during the fourth or fifth decade of life [13, 20, 21].

The number and volume of renal cysts are correlated with age, severity of kidney disease, and decline of glomerular filtration rate. Structural and functional renal deterioration of polycystic disease is the fourth leading cause of end-stage renal failure in adults [22, 23].

For patients affected by a disease leading to both irreversible liver and kidney failures such as autosomal recessive polycystic kidney disease (ARPKD), combined liver–kidney transplantation is indicated.

CLKT is a two-step procedure, in which whole or partial liver and kidney from a donor are transplanted to a recipient in the same operation. Since kidney and liver manifestations progress differently, an individualized management is of paramount importance, mostly in the pediatric patient population. Most often isolated kidney transplant (KT) is performed first, followed by OLT or CLKT later in childhood or adulthood. Sometimes PLD proceeds quite fast, and OLT or CLKT should be regarded as the first option.

Srinath and Schneider [24] reported a survey of 116 transplanted ARPKD patients: 56 % KT, 34 % OLT, and 9 % CLKT.

The decision about the correct timing and type of transplant may be challenging. When isolated KT is performed, hepatic disease can worsen the outcome, especially by increasing the risk for cholangitis and sepsis [25].

Moreover, the post-KT QoL of children with ARPKD often remains impaired due to the hepatomegaly and the infectious complications.

There are no guidelines for CLKT in ARPKD patients: the higher morbidity and mortality associated with post-CLKT with respect to KT alone seem to favor the isolated KT as the first option; on the other hand, refractory complications of recurrent sepsis from large and infected biliary dilatations suggest CLKT as the first option (Table 18.4).

Simultaneous CLKT seems to provide better long-term kidney function than a sequential transplant [26].

Studies on adult patients report that recipients of simultaneous CKLT have a lower incidence of kidney rejection and allograft loss than patients with isolated KT or sequential transplantation [27].

Table 18.4 Indications for CLKT or isolated OLT in patients with ARPKD

Massive PLD (total cyst/parenchyma ratio >1)
Impaired liver function (low synthetic capacity of the liver, hyperammonemia)
Renal failure (hemodialysis or GFR <30 mL/m)
Complications of portal hypertension *(bleeding esophageal varices, splenomegaly and/or hypersplenism, refractory ascites)*
Complications of biliary tract dilatation *(repeated episodes of cholangitis or chronic cholangitis, large biliary dilatations)*
Severe liver cirrhosis in biopsy
"Severe" PKD1 mutations (truncating mutations)

According to the UNOS database, 21 % of adult CLKT patients had acute rejection episodes as compared to 30 % of patients with isolated KT [28, 29]. A suggestive hypothesis is that the liver "offers" immunological protection against rejection of the kidney graft, trapping with the Kupffer cells the preformed antibodies.

The study of Dar et al. [30] suggests that the liver may not be completely protective; preformed donor-specific antibodies seem to promote rejection as later confirmed in a large analysis [31] of over 2,484 CLKT recipients: pre-sensitization had a negative impact on survival of both the patient and the kidney graft.

The mechanism by which a liver simultaneously transplanted with a kidney would protect the kidney graft from rejection episodes, and prolonged renal allograft survival, is not known.

It has been suggested that CLKT results in microchimerism and donor-specific hyporesponsiveness. Soluble class I HLA antigens from the liver could neutralize cytotoxic T lymphocytes and anti-HLA antibodies. Similarly, regulatory HLA-G antigens produced by the liver might inhibit T-cell cytotoxicity [32].

Secretion by the liver of immunomodulatory cytokines has also been suggested. In a recent study of combined auxiliary liver–kidney transplantation, liver grafts strongly upregulated CCL20 lymphokine, which can recruit dendritic cells and regulatory T cells and thus prevent rejection [33].

Gedaly et al. [34] analyzed the data of the 357 OLT for PLD in the UNOS database from 1988 to 2010 (0.3 % of 107,411). A 10 % cohort of patients transplanted for a diagnosis other than PLD was randomly selected from the database and used as a comparison group. Perioperative mortality (<30 days) was higher in the PLD group (9 % vs 6 %), and survival was lower for the first months ($P<0.05$). Infectious morbidity was the most common cause of death, but a significant number of patients died also from intra- or early postoperative bleeding.

A direct relationship was also found between death and recipient's age showing that most patients dying in the early postoperative period were 69 years or older. At first year, the survival was the same to other diagnoses (85 %) and better at 3 (81 % vs 77 %) and 5 years (77 % vs 71 %; $P=0.006$).

Recently, van Keimpema et al. [35] published the largest retrospective analysis from ELTR demonstrating excellent long-term survival in patients undergoing transplantation for PLD. They reported a 5-year survival of 87.5 % in a series of 58 patients.

Kirchner et al. [13] published the largest single-center experience in 36 patients with PLD. They reported an excellent survival of 86 % and confirmed that infectious complications are the most common cause of death in PLD patients after OLT.

Assilou et al. [36] reported 85 % 5-year survival rates in their 27 PLD OLT also confirming high morbidity and perioperative mortality (15 %).

Due to severe cachexia and/or septic complications, for an indication so special and circumscribed is of great importance an earlier selection of the affected patients in order to reduce perioperative mortality.

This is in contrast to the fact that patients often have a normal metabolic liver function and usually do not feel affected by life-threatening disease.

In the early stages of PLD, symptoms such as abdominal pain, malnutrition, or reduced physical fitness may not be convincing enough for the patient to accept the risk and complications of organ transplantation.

Early referral and transplantation should be advised as malnutrition is usually associated with poor survival after OLT. Besides long-term survival, the changes in QoL after OLT or CLKT need to be addressed.

18.2.1 Liver Hemangioma

The vast majority of hepatic hemangiomas (HH) are small and asymptomatic but can also occur as a large lesion that in case of diffuse hemangiomatosis may almost completely replace the hepatic parenchyma.

Surgical treatment is the first choice in huge symptomatic lesions or in HH rapidly growing. The risk of bleeding is mainly correlated with the size, the relationships with the hepatic veins, and the lifestyle of the patient.

Considering the large incidence of HH in the adult population with prevalence in autopsy and imaging studies, up to 7 % OLT is an absolutely exceptional indication and in highly selected patients [37–40].

OLT is often needed due to the development of the Kasabach–Merritt syndrome (KMS), also known as "hemangioma with thrombocytopenia" that presents coagulopathy, thrombocytopenia, hypofibrinogenemia, and fibrinolysis [40–42].

Few cases of OLT using donor grafts affected by small HH have been reported [43, 44].

A completely different clinical condition is the infant hepatic single or multiple hemangiomas (hemangiomatosis). The incidence of infant HH is around 4–5 % of all pediatric neoplasm, and it is usually asymptomatic and diagnosed incidentally [45].

Pediatric HH can involve the entire liver or reveals itself with a diffuse-type hemangioma associated with a greater risk of death due to serious symptoms and KMS may possibly arise. The first-line approach in patients with significant arteriovenous shunts is represented by steroid therapy. However, 10–20 % of patients are refractory to medical therapies and can develop hepatomegaly and life-threatening hepatic complications. In such cases, a more aggressive treatment including liver resection, hepatic artery embolization, and OLT should be considered. Kuroda et al. [46] published in 2014 a Japan nationwide survey for pediatric critical hemangioma proposing OLT as an appropriate option for both acute and chronic phases of this disease.

However, it remains one of the latest options, which have to be considered after medical therapy failure or as a rescue therapy in emergency settings.

As reported by Zhong et al. [47], the use of living donor graft is a valid option in this scenario. Indeed, Markiewicz et al. [45] reported four OLT in newborn patients due to acute hemodynamic decompensation caused by a giant hemangioma and unresponsive to all other conventional therapies; in three cases, a living donor graft was used and all patients were alive between 9 and 37 months at the time of publication.

18.3 Hepatic Epithelioid Hemangioendothelioma

Hepatic epithelioid hemangioendothelioma (HEHE) is a soft tissue vascular tumor with an intermediate clinical course between benign hemangioma and malignant angiosarcoma. Due to its rarity and unpredictable behavior, it is difficult to standardize the treatment for the HEHE and a single therapeutic algorithm for all patients is not appropriate.

When a complete removal of the lesion is feasible, liver resection is the best treatment option, but palliative or incomplete resection is discouraged as aggressive tumor recurrence has been reported, probably due to the effects of resection-stimulated hepatotropic growth factor release on the neoplastic cells [48].

According the literature review of Mehrabi et al. [48] on 434 HEHE, the most common management was OLT (44.8 %) followed by no treatment (24.8 %), chemotherapy or radiotherapy (21 %), and liver resection (9.4 %). The 1-year and 5-year patient survival rates were 100 and 75 %, after liver resection; 96 and 54.5 % after OLT; 73.3 and 30 %, respectively, after chemotherapy or radiotherapy; and 39.3 and 4.5 %, respectively, after no treatment.

For the patients with extensive multifocal, bilobar disease, or anatomically difficult lesions, OLT is the most common and preferred treatment with 5-year survival rates ranging from 64 % in the UNOS area to 82 % in ELTR [49, 50].

Grotz et al. [51] reported the Mayo Clinic experience based on 30 patients with HEHE. OLT is a more appropriate treatment for diffuse disease pattern with more than ten nodules, more than four segments involved, and lesion size above 10 cm with 64 % of overall 5-year survival after OLT.

The post-OLT course is complicated by recurrence in approximately 30 % of the cases. In the study on 59 HEHE from ELTR, 96 % of the lesions were bilobar, and in 86 % of the cases, more than 15 lesions were detected in the liver specimen. Portal and/or hepatic vein thromboses were diagnosed in almost 50 % of the patients, and three patients presented an extrahepatic localization (2 pulmonary and 1 peritoneal) at the moment of OLT: 1 was treated with post-OLT lung resection and 1 with lung transplant, and the peritoneal lesion was resected during OLT followed by adjuvant chemotherapy.

At 3 months after OLT, two patients died for de novo lung lesion (21 and 70 months, respectively). The 23.7 % of the patients developed recurrent disease after a median time of 49 months, and the 15.3 % died of recurrent disease [50].

The mechanism of recurrence in the allograft is unclear: vascular invasion or extrahepatic disease demonstrated inconsistent influence on the clinical outcome after OLT. Lymph node invasion as well as limited extrahepatic invasion does not have to be considered a real contraindication for OLT: stability and regression of some extrahepatic metastases have been described. From the available data, only the macrovascular invasion affects the long-term outcomes [52].

Despite this good long-term survival, the incidence of HEHE recurrence rate, in and outside the graft, remains high, and currently, there is no consensus regarding the management of this recurrence. Efficacy of anti-VEGF [53] adjuvant therapies as well as other treatment modalities, including re-OLT, surgical resection, chemotherapy, chemoembolization, and radiotherapy, still remains debated due to the rare incidence of HEHE, which prevents large studies for reliable conclusions [51–56].

In conclusion despite satisfactory long-term results with 5-year survival close to 71 % and 5-year disease-free survival over 65 %, the role of OLT for HEHE is still debated and questioned on the basis of the high percentage of extrahepatic disease at the diagnosis, the risk of recurrence, and reports of long-term survival in non-treated patients.

OLT should be proposed at an earlier stage. The adjuvant therapy with anti-vascular endothelial growth factor agents has been advocated to decrease the risk of recurrence [53].

18.3.1 Liver Cell Adenoma and Liver Cell Adenomatosis

Liver cell adenoma (LCA) is a rare benign tumor of the liver often diagnosed, in asymptomatic patients, as an incidental finding during radiological procedures. The etiopathogenesis of LCA has not been fully clarified, although the relationship between the consumption of oral contraception or anabolic steroids containing androgens and the formation of LCA is obvious and dose dependent [57].

LCA is more frequent in patients with glycogenosis type Ia [58], III, and VI (with a greater risk of the cancer degeneration), tyrosinemias, galactosemia, b-thalassemias, steatohepatitis, hemochromatosis, familial polyposis, and Fanconi because of the use of androgens as treatment [59].

LCA has been recently classified into four different groups based on a combination of genetic aberrations and histological appearance [60, 61]:

1. Hepatocyte nuclear factor 1-alpha inactivation with phenotypic features of marked steatosis, lack of cytological atypia, and absence of inflammatory infiltrates (40–45 %)

2. β-catenin activation with atypical features such as pseudoglandular formation (15–19 %)
3. Inflammatory group with presence of acute inflammatory infiltrate (30–35 %)
4. Non-mutated HNF1α and β-catenin (unclassified) group without inflammatory infiltrate

LCA with β-catenin activation has a higher risk of malignant transformation, compared to other subtypes, and a subgroup of inflammatory LCA can harbor β-catenin mutation and consequently have an increased malignant risk [62].

A systematic review of literature on LCA found an incidence of malignant transformation of 4.2 % in the 1 617 LCA being studied [63].

The risk of cancer degeneration is superior in men (47 %), and the prevalence of malignancy is ten times more frequent in men than in women and in lesions larger than 5 cm [64].

The optimal management of LCA remains controversial, and any decision regarding the selection of conservative versus surgical approach will depend on the clinical context.

The molecular analyses of LCA have anyway contributed significantly, providing molecular characteristics that predict high risk of cancer degeneration. Surgical resection of LCA is indicated in case of [65]:

- Large size of HA (>5 cm) with the impending risk of rupture or hemorrhage
- Evidence of β-catenin activation
- Any HA in male patients
- Evidence of dysplasia or atypia within an adenoma
- Clinical features of malignant transformation in LCA (increasing size, malignant features on imaging)

Serum a-fetoprotein is not helpful as it is usually normal, and therefore, it is a poor indicator of HCC degeneration [66, 67].

The improvements of surgical techniques and perioperative management lead to reduced postoperative morbidity even after major hepatectomy for benign tumors from 10 to 25 % and the mortality rate from 0 to 3 % [1–68].

Surgical resection is therefore the standard approach for symptomatic and/or enlarging adenomas complicated by hemorrhage or malignant transformation, assuming the patient meets conventional criteria for resection as with any other liver tumor, including no extrahepatic disease and the ability to preserve >20 % of healthy parenchyma.

Despite a radical hepatic resection, even if LCA is a benign tumor, a close monitoring is mandatory because LCA has the tendency to recur (8 %) [57].

For recurrent and progressive LCA in highly selected patients, OLT is the last therapeutic option when hepatic resection is indicated but not technically feasible [69].

As mentioned, peculiar conditions that predispose to the development of LCA with high risk of neoplastic degeneration are metabolic diseases, in particular glycogenosis. Von Gierke disease (glycogen storage disease type Ia (GSD-Ia)) is a rare autosomal recessive metabolic disease caused by an abnormal accumulation of glycogen due to the deficiency of the glucose-6-phosphatase enzyme, involved in the last step of the production of glucose from liver glycogen stores [70, 71, 72].

OLT is the therapeutic approach for these patients not only for the functional impairment due to the storage disease but also when the presence of HCC in HA is confirmed without any evidence of metastatic disease for the multiple LCA.

In this decision-making model, about transplant for a BHL, the patient should always be informed and take into consideration the need of a lifelong immunosuppressive therapy and the high risk of morbidity and mortality related to the OLT to face also with the possibility of a hepatectomy specimen without any sign of neoplastic degeneration.

Multiple adenomas occur in 10–24 % of all patients with LCA, characterizing a clinical entity known as liver adenomatosis (LA) [73].

The typical findings of LA are [74, 75]:

- Presence of multiple adenomas (arbitrarily more than 10)
- Predominant in women but without sure correlation with oral contraceptives
- Unknown etiology and no history of glycogen storage disease

The management of liver adenomatosis remains problematic. Observation and strict follow-up are the basic requirements for management of LA. In most patients with tumors >5 cm or complicated by bleeding or when malignant transformation cannot be excluded, liver resection remains the treatment of choice.

According to the largest review reporting surgical management of 94 patients with LA after the initial surgical approach, around 25 % patients need a second operation and 43 % of the remaining adenomas continue to grow [75].

The only potential cure for LA is OLT but the benefit of this therapeutic approach to prevent bleeding or malignant transformation has to be balanced with the intrinsic potential risk of transplant.

The largest series of OLT for LA reported 17 patients with an overall survival at 5 and 8 years, about 66 and 61 %, respectively [74]. Three of 17 patients developed HCC in the transplanted liver (9 and 12 years after OLT) or developed lung metastasis; two of these three patients did not have any evidence of malignancy in their native liver.

These results although dated cause considerable doubt about the indication of OLT for LA to prevent malignant transformation, as malignant progression can still occur despite transplant.

Considering that the listing for OLT is based on priority criteria in accordance with the severity of the disease, the patients with LA that maintain normal hepatic function without portal hypertension, ascites, or other complications related to cirrhosis are poorly served. The long waiting time for these patients could be crucial in terms of malignant transformation and tumor progression. Alternatively, living donor liver transplantation has been advocated as a valid option [76].

18.4 Other Rare Indications for OLT in Case of BHL

18.4.1 Alveolar Echinococcosis

Alveolar echinococcosis (AE) of the liver is a rare parasitic disease characterized by the intrahepatic development of *Echinococcus multilocularis*, endemic in different parts of the world. The prognosis is generally poor and no parasitolytic medication is available to cure the patient by destroying the larvae: without appropriate treatment, most patients die within 10 years.

However, early diagnosis and long-term treatment with benzimidazole can slow the progression of the disease in inoperable cases [77]. For resectable lesions, liver resection is recommended with favorable results, but due to the high incidence of late diagnosis, it seems possible in only 40 % of cases [77].

Moreover, in severe not resectable cases, the patient can develop severe complication like cholangitis, abscesses and septic shock, Budd–Chiari syndrome, portal hypertension and biliary cirrhosis due to the biliary invasion, and possible necrosis of the core of the lesion. In these settings, in which liver failure can occur, LT may be the only treatment option [78].

OLT for AE was proposed first by Chapuis et al. [79] in 1987, and nowadays also the use of living donor is described in literature, even if it is limited to sporadic case report [80]. In 2003 Bresson et al. [81] published a review of 47 OLT performed in Europe from 1985 to 2002 for AE. Only two patients were treated with OLT after 2000, may be due to the introduction of benzimidazole and the improvement in early diagnosis and patient selection.

The two main indications in this population were biliary parasitic invasion of the hilum and bilobar disease with or without Budd–Chiari syndrome. The reported survival rates were 77, 71, and 49 % at 1, 5, and 10 years, respectively. Due to the high risk of recurrence, the authors suggest a minimum immunosuppressive regimen with continuous monitoring. In conclusion, the authors also report a decision-making algorithm for the management of this condition, in which OLT can be a choice in unresectable symptomatic patients not responding to high-dose albendazole therapy. The use of pre- and posttransplant benzimidazole is mandatory to stabilize the patient while on the waiting list and minimize the risk of recurrence.

The case described by Genzini et al. in 2013 in which a patient suffering from neotropical polycystic echinococcosis caused by *Echinococcus vogeli* was treated with LT is presented below [82].

This *Echinococcus* species is restricted to Central and South America (mainly in the Amazon region) and develops most commonly in the liver developing solitary or confluent cyst with vessel necrosis, biliary infection, and portal system involvement. In this case report, OLT was performed after 2 years of failed albendazole therapy and recurrent cholangitis.

The patient died 31 days following OLT due to pulmonary embolism, and the autopsy showed a healthy graft.

On the other hand, it is important to underline that, speaking about *Echinococcus granulosus*, also a few cases with the use of a marginal donor graft containing hydatid cyst is described in literature [83–85].

18.4.2 Hepatic Lymphangiomatosis

Hepatic lymphangiomatosis is a rare idiopathic disease characterized by abnormal lymphatic proliferation causing intrahepatic cyst or cavernous lesions that can also affect the spleen and lungs resulting in organ dysfunction for parenchymal substitution and/or symptoms from compression.

Liver resection and OLT can be both proposed as treatment for this disease. Miller et al. described first in 1988 a 41-year-old woman suffering of a massive hepatic and mediastinal lymphangiomatosis treated with OLT and successive mediastinal excision [86]. Sporadic cases (4 additional OLT) are reported in literature with good long-term results [87, 88].

Regarding pediatric patients, Ooi et al. described in 2011 a 12-year-old patient treated with OLT after 4 years of disease due to progression and liver failure; the authors reported a recurrence 9 months post-OLT [89].

Six years post-LT, the patient started systemic therapy due to the increased size and number of intrahepatic cystic lesions. Despite this the authors reported good long-term results prolonging significantly the life expectancy of the patient.

Conclusion

OLT for a benign, non-life-threatening liver disease can be justified only if morbidity and mortality are lower than that of conventional surgery and when long-term QoL would be improved [13] combining meticulous transplant surgery, reduction of the perioperative blood product use, and judicious use of immunosuppressive therapy.

Liver transplantation may therefore be considered cautiously a valid therapeutic option before patients become too sick.

The decision regarding the appropriateness and timely listing should usually be left to the multidisciplinary transplant team by judging the severity of disease and the complication rate to be anticipated related to the clinical state. Prioritization policy on the waiting list, especially in national or regional intercenter MELD-driven allocation, is a field of debate regarding which rare condition should be prioritized and how.

References

1. Belghiti J, Pateron D, Panis Y et al (1993) Resection of presumed benign liver tumours. Br J Surg 80:380–383

2. Cescon M, Vetrone G, Grazi GL et al (2009) Trends in perioperative outcome after hepatic resection: analysis of 1,500 consecutive unselected cases over 20 years. Ann Surg 249:995–1002
3. ELTR database, update to 31 Dec 20013. www.eltr.org
4. UNOS database, based on OPTN data as of 15 May 2014. www.unos.org
5. Everson GT, Scherzinger A, Berger-Leff N et al (1988) Polycystic liver disease: quantitation of parenchymal and cyst volumes from computed tomography images and clinical correlates of hepatic cysts. Hepatology 8:1627–1634
6. Buphalan A, Talbot K, Forbes A et al (1992) Budd-Chiari syndrome in association with polycystic disease of the liver and kidneys. J R Soc Med 85(5):296–297
7. Yaqoob M, Saffman C, Finn R et al (1990) Inferior vena caval compression by hepatic cysts: an unusual complication of adult polycystic kidney disease. Nephron 54(1):89–91
8. Torres VE, Rastogi S, King BF et al (1994) Hepatic venous outflow obstruction in autosomal dominant polycystic kidney disease. J Am Soc Nephrol 5(5):1186–1192
9. Gigot JF, Legrand M, Hubens G et al (1996) Laparoscopic treatment of nonparasitic liver cysts: adequate selection of patients and surgical technique. World J Surg 20(5):556–561
10. Kwok MK, Lewin KJ (1988) Massive hepatomegaly in adult polycystic liver disease. Am J Surg Pathol 12:321–324
11. Starzl TE, Reyes J, Tzakies A et al (1990) Liver transplantation for polycystic liver disease. Arch Surg 125:575–577
12. Arrazola L, Moonka D, Gish RG et al (2006) Model for end-stage liver disease (MELD) exception for polycystic liver disease. Liver Transpl 12:S110–S111
13. Kirchner G, Rifai K, Cantz T et al (2006) Outcome and quality of life in patients with polycystic liver disease after liver or combined liver-kidney transplantation. Liver Transpl 12:1268–1277
14. Eurotransplant Manual – version 4.4: July 2014. http://www.eurotransplant.org/cms/index.php?page=et_manual
15. Schwartz ME, Roayaie S, Konstadoulakis MM et al (2008) The Mount Sinai experience with orthotopic liver transplantation for benign tumors. Brief report and literature review: case reports. Transplant Proc 40:1759–1762
16. Ardito F, Bianco G, Vellone M et al (2013) Long-term outcome after laparoscopic fenestration of simple liver cysts. Surg Endosc 27(12):4670–4674
17. Gocho T, Misawa T, Suzuki F et al (2013) Single-incision laparoscopic surgery for giant hepatic cyst. Asian J Endosc Surg 6(3):237–240
18. Jiang WW, Zhang F, Pu LY et al (2009) Liver transplantation for polycystic liver with massive hepatomegaly: a case report. World J Gastroenterol 15:5112–5113
19. Lerut J, Ciccarelli O, Rutgers M et al (2005) Liver transplantation with preservation of the inferior vena cava in case of symptomatic adult polycystic disease. Transpl Int 18: 513–518
20. Everson GT (2008) Polycystic liver disease. Gastroenterol Hepatol 4(3):179–181
21. Ueno T, Barri Y, Netto G et al (2006) Liver and kidney transplantation for polycystic liver and kidney-renal function and outcome. Transplantation 82:501–507
22. Masoumi A, Reed-Gitomer B, Kelleher C et al (2008) Developments in the management of autosomal dominant polycystic kidney disease. Ther Clin Risk Manag 4(2):393–407
23. de la Piscina PR, Duca I, Estrada S et al (2014) Combined liver and kidney transplant in a patient with Budd-Chiari syndrome secondary to autosomal dominant Polycystic Kidney Disease associated with polycystic liver disease: report of a case with a 9-year follow-up. Case Rep Gastrointest Med 2014:585291. doi:10.1155/2014/585291, Epub 2014 Jun 1
24. Srinath A, Schneider BL (2012) Congenital hepatic fibrosis and autosomal recessive polycystic kidney disease. J Pediatr Gastroenterol Nutr 54:580–587
25. Davis ID, Ho M, Hupertz V et al (2003) Survival of childhood polycystic kidney disease following renal transplantation: the impact of advanced hepatobiliary disease. Pediatr Transplant 7:364–369

26. Chapal M, Debout A, Dufay A et al (2012) Kidney and liver transplantation in patients with autosomal recessive polycystic kidney disease: a multicentric study. Nephrol Dial Transplant 27:2083–2088
27. Creput C, Durrbach A, Samuel D et al (2003) Incidence of renal and liver rejection and patient survival rate following combined liver and kidney transplantation. Am J Transplant 3:348–356
28. Fong TE, Bunnapradist S, Jordan SC et al (2003) Analyses of the United Network for Organ Sharing database comparing renal allografts and patient survival in combined liver–kidney transplantation with the contralateral allografts in kidney alone or kidney–pancreas transplantation. Transplantation 76:348–353
29. Olausson M, Mjörnstedt L, Norder G et al (2007) Successful combined partial auxiliary liver and kidney transplantation in highly sensitized crossmatch positive recipients. Am J Transplant 7:130–136
30. Dar W, Agarwal A, Watkins C et al (2011) Donor-directed MCH class I antibody is preferentially cleared from sensitized recipients of combined liver/kidney transplants. Am J Transplant 11:841–847
31. Tait BD, Susal C, Gebel HM et al (2013) Consensus guidelines on the testing and clinical management issues associated with HLA and non-HLA antibodies in transplantation. Transplantation 95:19–47
32. Creput C, Le Friec G, Bahari R et al (2003) Detection of HLA-G in serum and graft biopsy associated with fewer acute rejections following combined liver-kidney transplantation: possible implications for monitoring patients. Hum Immunol 64:1033–1038
33. Ingelsten M, Karlsson-Parra A, Granqvist A et al (2011) Postischemic inflammatory response in an auxiliary liver graft predicts renal graft outcome in sensitized patients. Transplantation 91:888–894
34. Gedaly R, Guidry P, Davenport D et al (2013) Peri-operative challenges and long-term outcomes in liver transplantation for polycystic liver disease. HPB 15:302–306
35. van Keimpema L, Nevens F, Adam R et al (2011) Excellent survival after liver transplantation for isolated polycystic liver disease: an European Liver Transplant Registry study. Transpl Int 24:1239–1245
36. Aussilhou B, Douflé G, Hubert C et al (2010) Extended liver resection for polycystic liver disease can change liver transplantation. Ann Surg 252:735–743
37. Bioulac-Sage P, Laumonier H, Laurent C et al (2008) Benign and malignant vascular tumors of the liver in adults. Semin Liver Dis 28:302–314
38. Yildiz S, Katarci M, Kizrak Y (2014) Cadaveric liver transplantation for a giant mass. Gastroenterology 146:e10–e11
39. Ferraz A, Sette M, Maia M et al (2004) Liver transplant for the treatment of giant hepatic hemangioma. Liver Transpl 10:1436–1437
40. Lerut J, Weber M, Orlando G, Dutkowski P (2007) Vascular and rare liver tumors: a good indication for liver transplantation? J Hepatol 47:454–475
41. de la Longeville JH, Hall P, Dolan P et al (1997) Treatment of a giant haemangioma of the liver with Kasabach-Merritt syndrome by orthotopic liver transplant a case report. HPB Surg 10(3):159–162
42. Mora A, Cortés C, Roigé J et al (1995) Orthotopic liver transplant for giant cavernous hemangioma and Kasabach-Merritt syndrome. Rev Esp Anestesiol Reanim 1995;42:71–74
43. Sun B, Mu X, Wang S (2013) Successful adult-to-adult liver transplantation of an otherwise discharged partial liver allograft with a cavernous hemangioma: new strategy for expanding liver donor pool. Transpl Int 26(9):79–80
44. Aucejo FN, Ortiz WA, Kelly D et al (2006) Expanding the donor pool: safe transplantation of cadaveric liver allograft with a 10 cm cavernous hemangioma-a case report. Liver Transpl 12:687
45. Markiewicz-Kijewska M, Kasprzyk W, Broniszczak D et al (2009) Hemodynamic failure as an indication to urgent liver transplantation in infants with giant hepatic hemangiomas or vascular malformations-report of four cases. Pediatr Transplant 13:906–912

46. Kuroda T, Hoshino K, Nosaka S et al (2014) Critical hepatica hemangioma in infants: recent nationwide survey in Japan. Pediatr Int 56:304–308
47. Zhong L, Men TY, Yang G et al (2014) Case report: living donor liver transplantation for giant hepatic hemangioma using a right lobe graft without the middle hepatic vein. World J Surg Oncol 12:83–88
48. Mehrabi A, Kashfi A, Fonouni H et al (2006) Primary malignant hepatic epithelioid hemangioendothelioma. A comprehensive review of the literature with emphasis on the surgical therapy. Cancer 107:2108–2121
49. Rodriguez JA, Becker NS, O'Mahony CA et al (2008) Long-term outcomes following liver transplantation for hepatic hemangioendothelioma: the UNOS experience from 1987 to 2005. J Gastrointest Surg 12(1):110–116
50. Lerut JP, Orlando G, Adam R et al (2007) The place of liver transplantation in the treatment of hepatic epitheloid hemangioendothelioma: report of the European liver transplant registry. Ann Surg 246(6):949–957
51. Grotz TE, Nagorney D, Donohue J et al (2010) Hepatic epithelioid haemangioendothelioma: is transplantation the only treatment option? HPB 12:546–553
52. Mistry AM, Gorden DL, Busler JF (2012) Diagnostic and therapeutic challenges in hepatic epithelioid hemangioendothelioma. J Gastrointest Cancer 43:521–525
53. Emamaullee JA, Edgar R, Toso C et al (2010) Vascular endothelial growth factor expression in hepatic epithelioid hemangioendothelioma: implications for treatment and surgical management. Liver Transpl 16(2):191–197
54. Szymik-Kantorowicz S, Partyka L, Dembinska-Kiec A et al (2003) Vascular endothelial growth factor in monitoring therapy of hepatic haemangioendothelioma. Med Pediatr Oncol 40(3):196–197
55. Miller MA, Sandler AD (2005) Elevated plasma vascular endothelial growth factor levels in 2 patients with hemangioendothelioma. J Pediatr Surg 40(5):e17–e19
56. Demetris AJ, Minervini M, Raikow RB et al (1997) Hepatic epithelioid haemangioendothelioma: biological questions based on pattern of recurrence in an allograft and tumor immunophenotype. Am J Surg Pathol 21:263–270
57. Aseni P, Sansalone CV, Sammartino C et al (2001) Rapid disappearance of hepatic adenoma after contraceptive withdrawal. J Clin Gastroenterol 33:234–236
58. Cassiman D, Libbrecht L, Verslype C et al (2010) An adult male patient with multiple adenomas and a hepatocellular carcinoma: mild glycogen storage disease type Ia. J Hepatol 53(1):213–217
59. Colle I, Laureys G, Raevens S et al (2013) Living related liver transplantation in an adult patient with hepatocellular adenoma and carcinoma 13 years after bone marrow transplantation for Fanconi anemia: a case report. Hepatol Res 43:991–998
60. Bioulac-Sage P, Balabaud C, Zucman-Rossi J (2010) Subtype classification of hepatocellular adenoma. Dig Surg 27:39–45
61. Bioulac-Sage P, Laumonier H, Couchy G et al (2009) Hepatocellular adenoma management and phenotypic classification: the Bordeaux experience. Hepatology 50:481–489
62. Zucman-Rossi J, Jeannot E, Nhieu JT et al (2006) Genotype-phenotype correlation in hepatocellular adenoma: new classification and relationship with HCC. Hepatology 43:515–524
63. Stoot JHMB, Coelen RJS, de Jond MC et al (2010) Malignant transformation of hepatocellular adenomas into hepatocellular carcinomas: a systematic review including more than 1600 cases. HPB 12:509–522
64. Cho SW, Marsh JW, Steel J et al (2008) Surgical management of hepatocellular adenoma: take it or leave it? Ann Surg Oncol 15:2795–2803
65. Liau SS, Qureshi MS, Praseedom R et al (2013) Molecular pathogenesis of hepatic adenomas and its implications for surgical management. J Gastrointest Surg 17:1869–1882
66. Lin H, van den Esschert J, Liu C et al (2011) Systematic review of hepatocellular adenoma in China and other regions. J Gastroenterol Hepatol 26:28–35
67. Farges O, Ferreira N, Dokmak S et al (2011) Changing trends in malignant transformation of hepatocellular adenoma. Gut 60:85–89

68. Dokmak S, Paradis V, Vilgrain V et al (2009) A single center surgical experience of 122 patients with single and multiple hepatocellular adenomas. Gastroenterology 137: 1698–1705
69. Vennarecci G, Santoro R, Antonini M et al (2013) Liver transplantation for recurrent hepatic adenoma. World J Hepatol 5(3):145–148
70. Rake JP, Visser G, Labrune P et al (2002) Guidelines for management of glycogen storage disease type I. European Study on Glycogen Storage Disease Type I (ESGSD I). Eur J Pediatr 161 Suppl 1:S112–S119
71. Calderaro J, Labrune P, Morcrette G et al (2013) Molecular characterization of hepatocellular adenomas developed in patients with glycogen storage disease type I. J Hepatol 58(2): 350–357
72. Aparicio ACM, Bellido CB, González JT et al (2013) Fifteen years of follow-up of a liver transplant recipient with glycogen storage disease type Ia (Von Gierke Disease). Transplant Proc 45:3668–3669
73. Flejou JF, Barge J, Menu Y et al (1985) Liver adenomatosis. An entity distinct from liver adenoma? Gastroenterology 89:1132–1138
74. Barthelmes L, Tait I (2005) Liver cell adenoma and liver cell adenomatosis. HPB 7:186–196
75. Vetelainen R, Erdogan D, De Graaf W et al (2008) Liver adenomatosis: re-evaluation of aetiology and management. Liver Int 2008;28:499–508
76. Di Sandro S, Slim AO, Lauterio A et al (2009) Liver adenomatosis: a rare indication for living donor liver transplantation. Transplant Proc 41:1375–1377
77. Xia D, Yan LN, Li B et al (2005) Orthotopic liver transplantation for incurable alveolar echinococcosis: report of five cases from west China. Transplant Proc 37(5):2181–2184
78. Katarci M, Pirimoglu B, Aydinli B et al (2014) A rare reason for liver transplantation: hepatic alveolar echinococcosis. Transpl Infect Dis 16(3):450–452
79. Chapuis Y, Houssin D, Brouzes S et al (1987) Hepatic transplantation in alveolar echinococcosis. 3 attempts. Chirurgie 113:634–640
80. Hatipoglu S, Bulbuloglu B, Piskin T et al (2013) Living donor liver transplantation for alveolar echinococcus is a difficult procedure. Transplant Proc 45(3):1028–1030
81. Bresson-Hadni S, Koch S, Miguet JP et al (2003) Indications and results of liver transplantation for Echinococcus alveolar infection: an overview. Langenbecks Arch Surg 388:231–238
82. Genzini T, Ghiotti N, Noujaim HM et al (2013) Liver transplantation for neotropical polycystic echinococcosis caused by Echinococcus vogeli: a case report. Rev Soc Bras Med Trop 46(1):119–120
83. Eris C, Akbulut S, Sakcak I et al (2013) Liver transplantation with marginal donor graft containing a hydatid cyst-a case report. Transplant Proc 45:828–830
84. Bein T, Haerty W, Haller M et al (1993) Organ selection in intensive care: transplantation of a liver including a calcified cyst of Echinococcus granularis. Intensive Care Med 19(3):182
85. Jimenz Romero C, Moreno Gonzalez E, Garcia Garcia I et al (1995) Successful transplantation of a liver graft with a calcified hydatid cyst after back-table resection. Transplantation 60(8):883–888
86. Miller C, Mazzaferro V, Mokowka L et al (1988) Orthotopic LT for massive hepatic lymphangiomatosis. Surgery 103:490–495
87. Ra S, Bradley R, Fishbein M et al (2007) Recurrent hepatic lymphangiomatosis after orthotopic liver transplantation. Liver Transpl 13:1593–1597
88. Lee A, Rajanayagam J, Sarikwal A et al (2014) Hepatobiliary and pancreatic: liver transplantation for massive hepatic lymphangiomatosis. J Gastroenterol Hepatol 29(2):233
89. Ooi CY, Brody D, Wong R et al (2011) Liver transplantation for massive lymphangiomatosis in a child. J Pediatr Gastroenterol Nutr 52(3):366–369

Laparoscopic Liver Surgery in Benign Liver Lesions

19

Vishal G. Shelat, Federica Cipriani, and Mohammad Abu Hilal

19.1 Introduction

The first laparoscopic cholecystectomy was performed in the mid-1980s, and since then, laparoscopic surgery has replaced open surgery in some fields [1, 2]. It offers advantages of reduced postoperative pain and analgesia requirements, shorter hospital stay, more rapid return to social life, reduced overall cost, reduced postoperative adhesions, and improved cosmesis [3–6]. The first reported laparoscopic liver procedure was a laparoscopic drainage of an amebic liver abscess in 1985 [7]. Several reports of laparoscopic fenestration of symptomatic liver cysts then followed, but it was not until 1992 that the first laparoscopic liver resection (LLR) was performed [8–10]. This was a nonanatomical partial liver resection of a 6-cm focal nodular hyperplasia [11]. The majority of laparoscopic liver resections were originally performed for benign liver tumors. Up to 30 % of resections in the series of Buell et al. [12] and 60 % of resections in Koffron et al. [13] were for benign lesions. In a systematic review published in 2007, nearly half of LLR were done for benign lesions ($n = 281$, 44.4 %) [14]. This may be explained by the initial concerns that the new approach may compromise the oncological results by increasing cancer cell dissemination, affecting surgical margin clearance [15–17]. Further, technical challenges associated with localizing deeply seated

V.G. Shelat, FRCS, FICS • F. Cipriani, MD
HPB Surgery, Southampton General Hospital,
Tremona Road, Southampton SO16 6YD, UK
e-mail: vgshelat@gmail.com; cipriani.federica@mail.com

M. Abu Hilal, MD, PhD, FRCS, DocEur (✉)
Southampton General Hospital, University Hospital,
E Level, Tremona Road, Southampton SO166YD, UK
e-mail: abuhilal9@gmail.com

L. Aldrighetti et al. (eds.), *Benign Tumors of the Liver*,
DOI 10.1007/978-3-319-12985-3_19

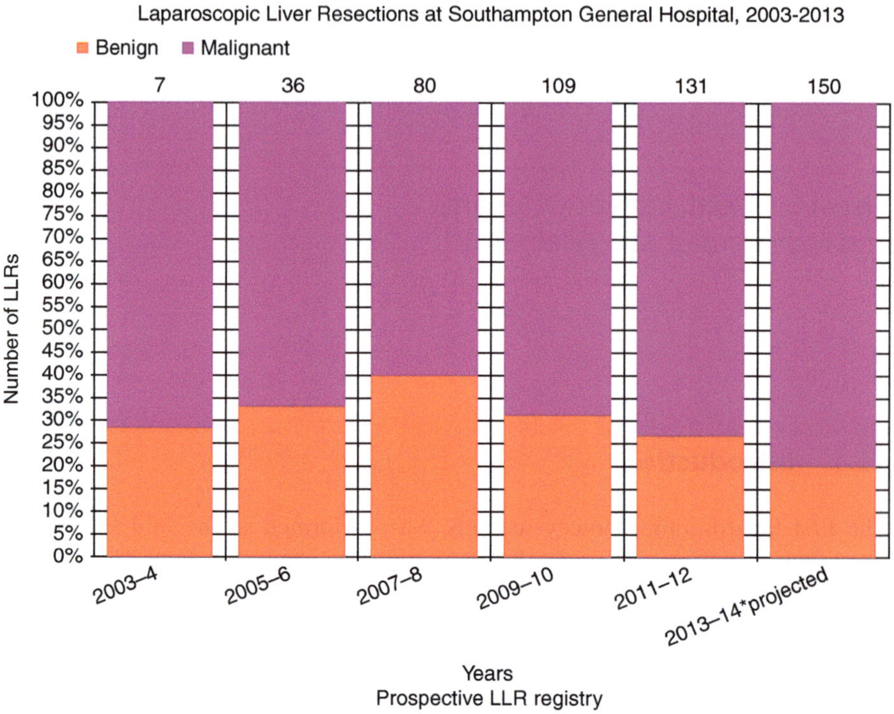

Fig. 19.1 Graph showing proportion of benign and malignant resections from a prospective Laparoscopic Liver Resection registry at Southampton General Hospital

tumors and controlling the hepatic inflow-outflow delayed the widespread implementation of laparoscopy in malignant liver tumors. With improved understanding of hepatic anatomy, better quality radiologic imaging, improved anesthetic and postoperative care, and technical advances in surgical devices, LLR has gained momentum. Safety, feasibility, and oncological efficiency of LLR have been proved by others and our team [18–24]. It is now a routinely used approach for the management of a variety of liver conditions with excellent results [25, 26]. In this chapter, we will discuss the general aspects of LLR with special dedication to benign liver lesions.

In our experience the percentage of LLR for malignant lesions has constantly increased year after year (Fig. 19.1). This is likely due to improved diagnosis of benign liver diseases and expansion of criteria of resectability for malignant lesions. The indications for LLR are no different than for open liver resection. Relative contraindications of LLR include lesion larger than 5 cm, multiple lesions, lesion adjacent to the hilum or inferior vena cava or major hepatic vessels, a need for vascular or biliary reconstruction, and resections that require an extensive portal lymphadenectomy. Absolute contraindications for LLR include patients unable to tolerate pneumoperitoneum, inability to obtain a surgical margin that could otherwise be achieved by open resection, laparoscopic approach requiring a larger parenchymal transection compared to open approach, hilar cholangiocarcinoma, and insufficient surgical training. Louisville statement [6] provides procedural definitions of *pure laparoscopy* where the liver resection is completed laparoscopically and the specimen removed via a remote incision (75 %), *hand-assisted laparoscopy* where the surgeon operates with his nondominant hand inside the abdomen, placed via an airtight device, through which the specimen is removed (17 %), *hybrid laparoscopy* where the liver is mobilized laparoscopically and most of the resection is done through a smaller than usual right upper quadrant incision (2 %), and *conversion* where the surgeon changes to an open operation from one of the above. One can also convert from pure laparoscopic to hand assist or hybrid[1]. All our LLR are performed by pure laparoscopy.

19.2 Benign Liver Lesions

A large percentage of benign liver lesions are identified incidentally during an imaging procedure performed for unrelated condition. In addition, with advances in imaging technology, previously undetected lesions are now identified. Cherqui D et al. have reported a sixfold increase in diagnosis of FNH over an 8-year period from 1985 to 1992 [27]. In order to recommend appropriate management, the surgeon must be aware of the different features of benign tumors, their natural history, and the diagnostic accuracy of various imaging techniques. Suspicious lesions represent a clinical management dilemma for the risk of missing a premalignant or malignant lesion or subjecting the patient to an unnecessary surgery [28–31]. In the absence of chronic liver disease or malignancy, most of these lesions are benign and will require no further treatment. A systematic approach for the work-up of a benign liver lesion is recommended. The importance of history taking and physical examination cannot be underestimated. The vast majority of benign cystic lesions of the liver do not require treatment. Rarer forms of these lesions may have an element of diagnostic uncertainty. The diagnostic dilemma is more pronounced in solid lesions as compared to cystic lesions.

19.2.1 Principles of Management

Principles of management of benign liver lesions are:

1. Confirmation that the lesion is benign
2. Determining whether the lesion requires surgical treatment
3. If not for surgical resection, to determine the optimal follow-up of these lesions, if needed

[1] The percentages do not add to 100 % as there would be some conversions from pure laparoscopy to hand-assisted laparoscopy, from hand-assisted laparoscopy to a laparotomy, and some primary thoracoscopic liver resections.

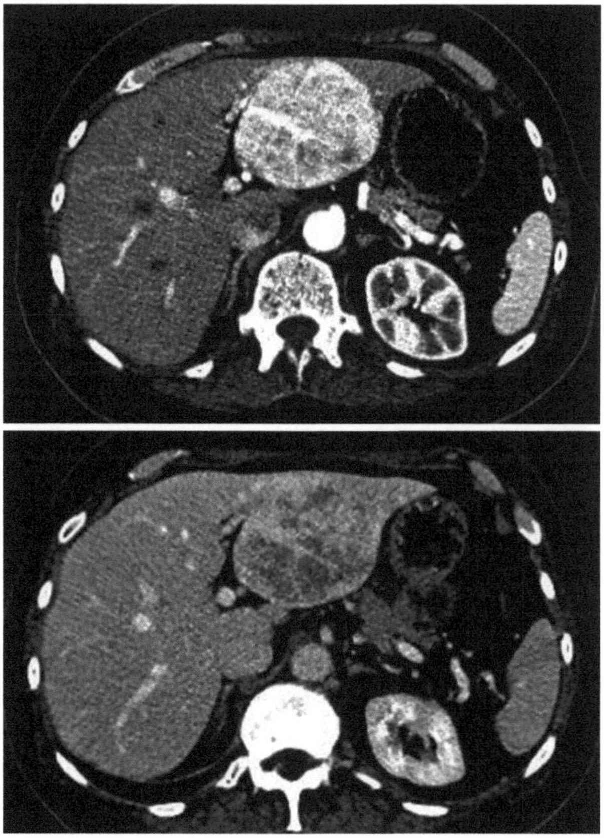

Figs. 19.2 and 19.3 Computerized tomography (CT) scan images of a 65-year-old female patient with abdominal pain and a 7.5 cm arterial avid lesion with washout. The radiological features were equivocal, and based on symptoms with diagnostic dilemma, surgical removal was recommended by the multidisciplinary team. She underwent a laparoscopic modified left hemihepatectomy, and postoperative histology confirmed this to be an angiomyolipoma of the liver

19.2.2 Indications for Surgery

Indications for surgery in benign liver lesions are:

1. Preoperative diagnosis of adenoma or cystadenoma.
2. Symptoms affecting quality of life. It is important to correlate that patients' symptoms are indeed related to the presence of the liver lesion. This may mandate further investigations, e.g., gastroscopy to evaluate upper abdominal symptoms. Cherny CK et al. in a study of 155 benign liver tumors concluded that symptomatic patients with a small focal nodular hyperplasia (FNH) or hemangioma can be observed because their symptoms are unlikely to be related to the liver tumor and percutaneous needle biopsy rarely changed management [32].
3. Diagnostic uncertainty. Figures 19.2 and 19.3 show a scan of a patient who presented with abdominal discomfort, and there was diagnostic uncertainty on imaging.
4. Complications of bleeding or rupture.
5. Fear of malignant transformation [33].

Weimann et al. [28] in a study involving observation of asymptomatic 157 benign liver tumors (103 hemangiomas and 54 with FNH) found a radiologic diagnostic accuracy of >90 % and no tumor-related rupture or malignant transformation during a median follow-up of 32 months. Also follow-up imaging showed that in 80 % of these patients, the size remained stable, and in 7 % of patients, the tumor regressed in size. They concluded that in asymptomatic benign liver tumors, as the size remains stable for many years, indications for surgery should be carefully evaluated. In the same series, 173 patients underwent surgery for benign liver tumors with a mortality of 0.6 %. In a study spanning over a 7-year period and involving 51 women of <50 years of age with a preoperative diagnosis of either FNH or hepatic adenoma (HA), 6 % of patients had a malignancy on histology [34].

19.2.3 Common Benign Liver Lesions

Hemangiomas, focal nodular hyperplasia (FNH), hepatic adenomas (HA), hepatic cysts, and hepatobiliary cystadenomas are common benign liver lesions, and we shall discuss them briefly [35]. Liver resection is also indicated in hepatolithiasis complicated with recurrent cholangitis, biliary strictures, liver atrophy, or secondary biliary cirrhosis [36].

19.2.3.1 Hemangioma

Hemangiomas are the most common benign liver tumors with an incidence of up to 20 % of the general population. These lesions have no malignant potential. Symptomatic hemangiomas often tend to be large, varying from 5 to 20 cm in diameter. Hemangiomas tend to grow by expansion and push liver tissue away as they grow. This creates a fibrolamellar plane of tissue that defines the border between a hemangioma and surrounding normal liver. Indications for resection have been a development of symptoms, consumptive coagulopathy, or Kasabach-Merritt syndrome [37]. Enucleation preserves normal parenchyma, limits blood loss, and has fewer complications than a segmental resection [38–40].

19.2.3.2 Focal Nodular Hyperplasia

Focal nodular hyperplasias (FNHs) are solid benign tumor of the liver and occur in 3 % of the population. FNH has no malignant potential and usually remains stable or decrease in size over time. Less than 20 % of patients develop symptoms or complications, and if so, may be resected [37].

19.2.3.3 Hepatic Adenoma

Hepatic adenomas (HAs) have an epithelial origin and are occasionally associated with the use of estrogen (contraceptive pills) and steroids. They are more frequently found as solitary lesions but sometimes can be multiple. The arguments in favor of the conservative approach are that discontinuation of oral contraceptive pills may induce HA regression; it is not always certain that abdominal symptoms are related to the HA; if bleeding occurs, this can be managed conservatively, and surgical resection has 10–27 % morbidity and up to 3 % mortality. Resolution of HA following cessation of oral contraceptive pills was uncommon in a Mayo Clinic series [41]. The arguments in favor of the surgical approach are difficulty of preoperative imaging in differentiating HA from hepatocellular carcinoma (HCC), the risk of malignant transformation (estimated around 5 %), the risk of rupture (estimated around 30 %) with potential fatal consequences, and the fact that surgical excision guarantees a definitive diagnosis and long-term cure [42]. In a study with 74 resections for benign tumors, Terkivatan et al. [30] have recommended a resection for large (>5 cm) HA to reduce risk of rupture and malignant transformations. Deneve et al. [43] in a multicenter pooled analysis of 119 patients with HA undergoing surgical treatment during a 10-year period showed that the laparoscopic approach was adopted in 3 % of ruptured adenomas and in 11 % of not ruptured hematomas. Cho et al. [44] reviewed a large single-center series of 41 patients who underwent surgical resection for HA. The laparoscopic approach was limited to 9 patients (22 %) who were admitted in an elective setting with non-ruptured HA. In our experience of 15 pure LLR for HA [42], the indications for surgery were symptoms ($n=12$), indeterminate character on imaging ($n=2$), and size >5 cm ($n=1$). The median tumor diameter was 85 mm (range 25–180), median length of stay was 4 days, and there was no mortality. Pure laparoscopic approach represents a safe and effective way for the surgical management of HA. Surgical resection ensures definitive diagnosis and treatment of HA with minimal risk of complications. This is particularly appealing for young individuals and for women who may worry about the risks of HA growth or rupture while using oral contraception or in future pregnancies.

19.2.3.4 Hepatic Cysts

Simple hepatic cysts are congenital hepatic lesions that are thought to result from progressive dilatation of biliary hamartomas, and they have no biliary communication. Their prevalence is estimated between 1.6 and 18 % [45]. Intracystic hemorrhage, secondary infection, and compression of the biliary tree are rare complications which may warrant a surgical intervention. If diagnosed with certainty, liver cysts must be managed conservatively regardless of their size. No follow-up is recommended because even if the cyst size increases, surgery will not be recommended if the patient remains asymptomatic.

19.2.3.5 Hepatobiliary Cystadenoma

Hepatobiliary cystadenomas are uncommon, benign cystic lesions of the biliary system and comprise less than 5 % of all hepatobiliary cystic masses. They can be serous or, more commonly, mucinous [46, 47]. Surgical resection is routinely indicated for fear of malignant transformation into a cystadenocarcinoma [48].

19.3 Preoperative Assessment

The evaluation of the patient undergoing LLR must include assessment of overall physical and functional fitness. LLR is an elective undertaking, and adequate optimization of patient's medical condition should be achieved. Planning an LLR needs to take into account the nature of the lesion, its location, expected margins, liver anatomy and function, and volume of the future liver remnant (FLR). Good quality imaging is important prior to operative planning as variations in arterial, portal venous, and biliary anatomy are a frequent occurrence. Various clinical scoring systems (Child-Pugh's score, Model for End-Stage Liver Disease score, etc.), dynamic liver tests (indocyanine green clearance, galactose elimination capacity, etc.), and volumetric assessments using imaging are helpful in preoperative planning. In high-risk surgical candidates, we routinely perform two dimensional echocardiography, pulmonary function test, and cardiopulmonary exercise test. Some patients (e.g., cirrhosis, nonalcoholic steatohepatitis [NASH], chemotherapy-associated steatohepatitis [CASH]) may have adequate volume but inadequate function and may experience liver failure if the FLR is too small [49]. In retrospective reviews evaluating outcomes of patients undergoing liver resection, the risk of death increases with decreasing volumes of the FLR [50, 51]. Therefore, assessment of operative risk prior to LLR includes establishing the severity of any possible ongoing liver disease. Patients with severe underlying functional liver disease or predicted low FLR are not surgical candidates. For patients who are candidates for LLR but who are deemed to have an inadequate FLR, strategies to induce FLR hypertrophy are to be considered (e.g., portal vein embolization). A frank conversation about the risk and benefits of LLR should be made with patients prior to any surgical plans.

19.4 Laparoscopic Liver Resections: Surgical Principles

19.4.1 Equipment and Manpower

Advanced laparoscopic surgery needs high-quality equipment and familiar operating room personnel to operate it. It is advisable that a trained scrub nurse and circulating nurse assistant dedicated to hepatobiliary surgery is available. A surgeon and an operating team should always ensure that a backup is handy in the event of equipment failure. A conventional instrument set for open hepatectomy should be handy as sometimes a conversion needs to be prompt. We prefer a 30° 10 mm camera and a pneumoperitoneum pressures up to 12–15 mmHg. We have had no problems of gas embolism with this strategy. We routinely use CUSA (Cavitron Ultrasonic Surgical Aspirator, Valleylab), intraoperative ultrasound, LOTUS (Laparoscopic Operation by Torsional Ultrasound, SRA Developments, Ashburton, Devon, UK), vascular clips, bulldog clamps, nylon slings, colored (red for arteries, blue for veins, and yellow for biliary structures) loops, disposable suction device, and disposable impermeable retrieval bags during LLR.

19.4.2 Preparation and Positioning

The patient is admitted on the day prior to surgery and reviewed by anesthetic and surgical teams. We maintain a dedicated LLR care pathway, and all the patients undergo standardized preparation. We do not administer intravenous hydration during

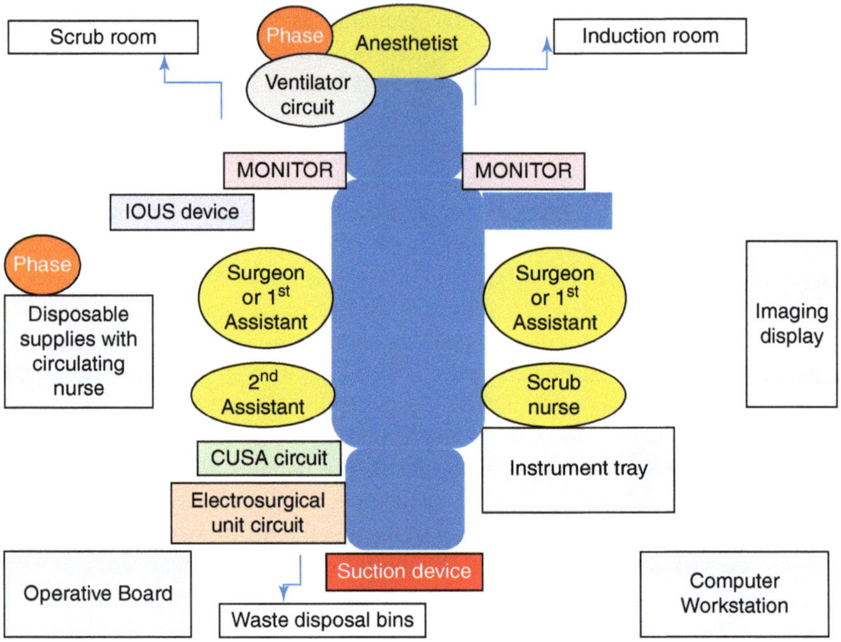

Fig. 19.4 Operating room setup for Laparoscopic Liver Resection at Southampton General Hospital

the preoperative fasting. On the day of surgery, following endotracheal intubation and insertion of invasive monitoring lines (arterial line and central line), the surgical team inserts a urinary catheter and does abdominal wall shaving. It is important to shave the suprapubic area as that is the specimen retrieval site. All the patients are positioned in supine position on an adjustable table which can achieve longitudinal or sideway tilts. Inflatable calf compressors for deep vein thrombosis prophylaxis and Bair's hugging forced-air warming blankets are routinely used. It is our preference to provide access to one of the arms, typically the left, to anesthetic team. Figure 19.4 explains our setup for a typical LLR case. It is important to ensure that all the ground wires are safely tapped to the floor to avoid accidental falls during movements.

19.4.3 Anesthetic Conduct

Mechanical ventilation, pneumoperitoneum, and surgical manipulation of the liver reduce the hepatic blood flow. Hypovolemia and hypotension could result from head-up tilt and restrictive fluid strategy. The resultant reduction in cardiac output also reduces the hepatic blood flow. The anesthetist should focus on optimizing the oxygen delivery/oxygen extraction ratio by mitigating the above effects. Low central venous pressure anesthesia (0–5 mmHg) reduces bleeding from the hepatic veins. In instances of hemodynamic instability, a 15° Trendelenburg position could provide a rapid physiological bolus to maintain cardiac output transiently. This position improves venous return, preserves renal function, and reduces risk of gas embolism [52, 53]. Fluid replacement ("filling up" or "catching up") is done after the resection is completed and hemostasis is achieved. Transesophageal echocardiography is sensitive to cardiac filling pressures and a useful adjunct.

19.4.4 Operative Technique

19.4.4.1 An Ideal Lesion

An ideal lesion for an LLR is solitary, small (<5 cm), and symptomatic and is located in the peripheral segments (II–VI) of the healthy liver. Pedunculated large lesions or lesions located in the segments II or III are also a good indication for LLR. However, one should question the indication of surgery when encountering such a patient with a benign disease, and surgery should only be considered when appropriate and after multidisciplinary team evaluation. When a hepatectomy is indicated in benign lesions, parenchyma-preserving surgery should be performed. Multiple lesions are suited if they can be resected en bloc with anatomical resection. Recently even lesions in the posterior section are approached laparoscopically; however, those are challenging resections and should be performed only by surgeons with advanced experience in LLR.

19.4.4.2 Basic Steps

The seven basic steps of LLR include:

1. Port placement and peritoneal exploration
   The number and position of ports will vary according to the type of resection which is planned, but it is our opinion that a surgeon should not hesitate to place an extra port if doing so facilitates the conduct of surgery.
2. Liver mobilization
   Once the ports are placed, the liver is mobilized along the falciform, triangular, and coronary ligaments as needed using ultrasonic dissectors or diathermy. It is important to have an astute assistant in order to avoid "manipulation injuries" or rupture of the lesions.
3. Deciding the transection plane
   Once the liver is mobile, the lesion is identified by correlating the preoperative imaging with intraoperative judgment. Intraoperative ultrasound is a useful adjunct, and we perform it routinely. This helps us in deciding the transection plane which is typically marked by electrocautery on the surface of the liver parenchyma (tattooing).
4. Vascular inflow control
   This is only needed in case of major anatomical resections and not in minor resections or left lobectomies. Selective inflow control may be achieved extrahepatically or intrahepatically. Extrahepatic control helps in demarcation of zone of

ischemia which dictates the plane of transection. A laparoscopic surgeon must be familiar with variations in the biliary and vascular anatomy, and we consider it always a safe practice to do test clamps prior to sacrificing any large structure. This is akin to the manual palpation which is performed during an open resection. It is important to note that the first short branches from the portal vein are supplied to the caudate lobe (and hence it is termed as segment I) and a delicate dissection, isolation, and clipping or preservation should be performed depending on the intent of surgery. Intrahepatic inflow control can be performed after a hepatotomy near the hilum in proximity to the gallbladder fossa. It is our practice to routinely counsel patients for a cholecystectomy during an LLR and perform cholecystectomy selectively where the gallbladder is grasped for mobilization and exposure. Intrahepatic inflow control approach prevents injury to contralateral inflow but can result in bleeding. When vascular inflow need not be compromised prior to transection, e.g., planning a segmental resection, we perform temporary clamping, i.e., Pringle's maneuver. Typically this is secured via the nylon sling via the left flank 5 mm port and controlled extracorporeally by the assistant. This helps us in reducing the blood loss. We perform Pringle's clamp in cycles of "10 min on" and "5 min off," and this time is typically maintained by anesthetic colleague. Compared to continuous clamping, intermittent clamping is shown to reduce ischemia/reperfusion injury and reduction in elevation of liver enzymes postoperatively [54]. In an attempt to reduce the ischemic insult associated with Pringle's maneuver, ischemic preconditioning is proposed [55]. It refers to the brief interruption of blood flow, followed by a short reperfusion interval, and then a more prolonged period of ischemia. Once the inflow is controlled, we aim for parenchymal transection.

5. Parenchymal transection
   Liver parenchymal transection can be performed safely by many tools, and we suggest that a surgeon should use the tool that he or she is most familiar with. We routinely use CUSA (Cavitron Ultrasonic Surgical Aspirator, Valleylab) and LOTUS (Laparoscopic Operation by Torsional Ultrasound, SRA Developments, Ashburton, Devon, UK) supported by clips and staplers. LOTUS dissection is performed for initial 1–2 cm of parenchymal depth and then CUSA dissection if preferred. CUSA dissection offers the possibility of a gentle dissection and identification of liver structures and hence their control and division accordingly. We do not use stapling devices for parenchymal transection and prefer to use them selectively for portal pedicles or hepatic veins after isolation [56–58].
6. Vascular outflow control
   This is again only needed in major anatomic hepatectomies. The understanding of hepatic venous drainage to the inferior vena cava on preoperative imaging is essential for this step. Readers are referred to Nakamura et al. to understand the variations in patterns of hepatic veins and their drainage to the inferior vena cava [59]. We do not attempt any extraparenchymal control of the outflow. This in our view may increase the risk of vascular injuries and subsequent bleedings and air embolus. After good parenchymal dissection the hepatic vein can be divided with a laparoscopic vascular stapler (white cartridges); for a better hemostasis of

the stapler, we prefer to thin the parenchyma around the vein but not to clean the vein completely. Bleeding around this area can be dangerous and should be dealt with carefully. A surgeon performing LLR should be able to perform laparoscopic suturing swiftly as a small delay would cause excessive bleeding. Increasing the pneumoperitoneum pressures could help reduce the flow of bleeding, albeit with increased risk of gas embolism. We find it very useful to place a small swab ("tonsil swab" or "paranasal sinus packs") in the operative field to maintain good vision.

7. Hemostasis, specimen retrieval, and closure
   The raw surface is carefully inspected for bile leaks and bleeding. All the bile leaks and bleeding spots are sutured. Once major leaks and bleeding spots are secured, white gauze is placed over the raw surface and specimen placed in the 15 mm impermeable disposable retrievable bag. The specimen is brought out via a 5 cm suprapubic incision unless there are previous scars (if so, we deliver specimen through existing scars). Our team has a routine policy to check the macroscopic margins ex vivo after specimen retrieval. The final check of the liver raw surface is performed and drains are placed in vicinity. At this stage we reduce the pneumoperitoneum to <8 mmHg and anesthetic team performs Valsalva maneuver for checking hemostasis. Oozing from the raw surface is secured by topical hemostatic agents. Major LLR patients are transferred to surgical high-dependency unit for an overnight monitoring. All the LLR patients receive standardized coordinated postoperative care with interprofessional and multidisciplinary involvement.

19.5 Our Results

We previously reported our experience in 178 LLR over a 6-year period of 2003–2009 [60]. Twenty-six percent of resections were done for benign liver lesions, and the common indications were presence of symptoms (50 %), hepatic adenoma or cystadenoma (28 %), and indeterminate lesions (22 %). One patient (2.2 %) in our series had a final malignant histology. It is important that the operative technique and conduct is not compromised during LLR for benign liver lesions as some lesions have a malignant potential. A laparotomy for liver resection in a young patient may be a devastating event with deleterious psychosocial consequences. Although quality of life after LLR is not studied, cosmetic results and early return to social life should not be perceived as surrogate parameters, but as relevant end points to pursue as long as safety is not compromised [61]. We reported a 28 % rate of major liver resections confirming that even when major hepatectomies are needed, these can be performed with a pure laparoscopic approach [60]. The extensive use of the pure laparoscopic approach may explain the short hospital stay we observed, which is one of the main benefits of the minimal access surgery. Longer hospital stays after major LLR for benign disease reported by other authors may be explained by their routine adoption of hand-assisted approach [62]. In a study of 208 patients spanning over a 20-year period from 1979 to 1999, 74 patients underwent resection for benign liver tumors, and 20 % of patients had persistent symptoms. The operative morbidity and mortality was 27 and 3 %, respectively, and authors cautioned about careful case selection [30]. A surgeon needs to maintain a balance in avoiding unnecessary surgery for asymptomatic benign tumors and risk treatment delay for malignant tumors. It is recommended that all the patients should be discussed at multidisciplinary meetings and patients themselves should also be involved in the decision process.

Conclusion

Laparoscopic liver surgery is expanding, and many studies have demonstrated the safety, feasibility, and advantages of the laparoscopic approach. More incidental and benign liver lesions are being diagnosed, and surgical indication should be evaluated carefully. It is important to note that more availability of expertise in laparoscopic liver surgery should not lead to relaxation in indications for benign liver lesions and that all the patients should be discussed in multidisciplinary team meeting prior to recommendation of surgery. We believe that whenever a liver resection is indicated for benign liver lesion, the laparoscopic approach should be considered if expertise is available.

References

1. Litynski GS (1998) Erich Mühe and the rejection of laparoscopic cholecystectomy (1985): a surgeon ahead of his time. JSLS 2:341–346
2. Blum CA, Adams DB (2011) Who did the first laparoscopic cholecystectomy? J Minim Access Surg 7:165–168
3. NIH Consensus Conference (1993) Gallstones and laparoscopic cholecystectomy. JAMA 269:1018–1024
4. Sain AH (1996) Laparoscopic cholecystectomy is the current "gold standard" for the treatment of gallstone disease. Ann Surg 224:689–690
5. Simillis C, Constantinides VA, Tekkis PP, Darzi A, Lovegrove R, Jiao L, Antoniou A (2007) Laparoscopic versus open hepatic resections for benign and malignant neoplasms: a meta-analysis. Surgery 141:203–211
6. Buell JF, Cherqui D, Geller DA et al (2009) The international position on laparoscopic liver surgery: the Louisville Statement, 2008. Ann Surg 250:825–830
7. Salky B, Finkel S (1985) Laparoscopic drainage of amebic liver abscess. Gastrointest Endosc 31:30–32
8. Klotz HP, Schlumpf R, Weder W, Largiadèr F (1993) Minimal invasive surgery for treatment of enlarged symptomatic liver cysts. Surg Laparosc Endosc 3:351–353
9. Katkhouda N, Fabiani P, Benizri E, Mouiel J (1992) Laser resection of a liver hydatid cyst under videolaparoscopy. Br J Surg 79:560–561
10. Wayand W, Woisetschläger R (1993) Laparoscopic resection of liver metastasis. Chirurg 64:195–197
11. Gagner M, Rheault M, Dubuc J (1992) Laparoscopic partial hepatectomy for liver tumor [abstract]. Surg Endosc 6:99
12. Buell JF, Thomas MT, Rudich S, Marvin M, Nagubandi R, Ravindra KV, Brock G, Mc-Masters KM (2008) Experience with more than 500 minimally invasive hepatic procedures. Ann Surg 248:475–486

13. Koffron AJ, Auffenberg G, Kung R, Abecassis M (2007) Evaluation of 300 minimally invasive liver resections at a single institution: less is more. Ann Surg 246:385–392
14. Laurence J et al (2007) Laparoscopic hepatectomy, a systematic review. ANZ J Surg 77:948–953
15. Johnstone PA, Rohde DC, Swartz SE, Fetter JE, Wexner SD (1996) Port site recurrences after laparoscopic and thoracoscopic procedures in malignancy. J Clin Oncol 14:1950–1956
16. Paolucci V, Schaeff B, Schneider M, Gutt C (1999) Tumor seeding following laparoscopy: international survey. World J Surg 23:989–995
17. Volz J, Koster S, Spacek Z, Paweletz N (1999) The influence of pneumoperitoneum used in laparoscopic surgery on an intra-abdominal tumor growth. Cancer 86:770–774
18. Cherqui D, Husson E, Hammoud R, Malassagne B, Stéphan F, Bensaid S, Rotman N, Fagniez PL (2000) Laparoscopic liver resections: a feasibility study in 30 patients. Ann Surg 232(6): 753–762
19. Aldrighetti L et al (2008) A prospective evaluation of laparoscopic versus open left lateral hepatic sectionectomy. J Gastrointest Surg 12:457–462
20. Rau HG et al (1998) Laparoscopic liver resection compared with conventional partial hepatectomy—a prospective analysis. Hepatogastroenterology 45:2333–2338
21. Dagher I, Proske JM, Carloni A, Richa H, Tranchart H, Franco D (2007) Laparoscopic liver resection: results for 70 patients. Surg Endosc 21(4):619–624
22. Abu Hilal M, Pearce NW (2008) Laparoscopic left lateral liver sectionectomy: a safe, efficient reproducible technique. Dig Surg 25(4):305–308
23. Abu Hilal M, Di Fabio F, Teng MJ, Lykoudis P, Primrose JN, Pearce NW (2011) Single-centre comparative study of laparoscopic versus open right hepatectomy. J Gastrointest Surg 15(5):818–823
24. Abu Hilal M, McPhail MJ, Zeidan B, Zeidan S, Hallam MJ, Armstrong T, Primrose JN, Pearce NW (2008) Laparoscopic versus open left lateral hepatic sectionectomy: a comparative study. Eur J Surg Oncol 34(12):1285–1288
25. Nguyen KT, Gamblin TC, Geller DA (2009) World review of laparoscopic liver resection-2,804 patients. Ann Surg 250:831–841
26. Abu Hilal M, Underwood T, Zuccaro M, Primrose J, Pearce N (2010) Short- and medium-term results of totally laparoscopic resection for colorectal liver metastases. Br J Surg 97(6): 927–933
27. Cherqui D, Rahmouni A, Charlotte F et al (1995) Management of focal nodular hyperplasia and hepatocellular adenoma in young women: a series of 41 patients with clinical, radiological, and pathological correlations. Hepatology 22(6):1674–1681
28. Weimann A, Ringe B, Klempnauer J, Lamesch P, Gratz KF, Prokop M, Maschek H, Tusch G, Pichlmayr R (1997) Benign liver tumors: differential diagnosis and indications for surgery. World J Surg 21:983–990
29. Kammula US, Buell JF, Labow DM, Rosen S, Millis JM, Posner MC (2001) Surgical management of benign tumors of the liver. Int J Gastrointest Cancer 30:141–146
30. Terkivatan T, de Wilt JH, de Man RA, van Rijn RR, Zondervan PE, Tilanus HW, IJzermans JN (2001) Indications and long-term outcome of treatment for benign hepatic tumors: a critical appraisal. Arch Surg 136:1033–1038
31. Liu CL, Fan ST, Lo CM et al (2004) Hepatic resection for incidentaloma. J Gastrointest Surg 8:785–793
32. Cherny CK, Jarnagin WR, Schwartz LH et al (2001) Management of 155 patients with benign liver tumours. Br J Surg 88(6):808–813
33. Choi BY, Nguyen MH (2005) The diagnosis and management of benign hepatic tumors. J Clin Gastroenterol 39(5):401–412
34. Belghiti J, Paterson D, Panis Y et al (1993) Resection of presumed benign liver tumours. Br J Surg 80(3):380–383
35. Buell JF, Tranchart H, Cannon R et al (2010) Management of benign hepatic tumors. Surg Clin North Am 90(4):719–735

36. Li SQ, Liang LJ, Peng BG et al (2012) Outcomes of liver resection for intrahepatic stones: a comparative study of unilateral versus bilateral disease. Ann Surg 255:946–953
37. Trotter JF, Everson GT (2001) Benign focal lesions of the liver. Clin Liver Dis 5(1):17–42
38. Baer HU, Dennison AR, Mouton W et al (1992) Enucleation of giant hemangiomas of the liver: technical and pathologic aspects of a neglected procedure. Ann Surg 216(6):673–676
39. Gedaly R, Pomposelli JJ, Pomfret EA et al (1999) Cavernous hemangioma of the liver: anatomic resection vs enucleation. Arch Surg 134(4):407–411
40. Yoon SS, Charny CK, Fong Y et al (2003) Diagnosis, management, and outcomes of 115 patients with hepatic hemangioma. J Am Coll Surg 197(3):392–402
41. Nagorney DM (1995) Benign hepatic tumors: focal nodular hyperplasia and hepatocellular adenoma. World J Surg 19(1):13–18
42. Abu Hilal M, Di Fabio F, Wiltshire DR et al (2011) Laparoscopic liver resection for hepatocellular adenoma. World J Gastrointest Surg 3(7):101–105
43. Deneve JL, Pawlik TM, Cunningham S et al (2009) Liver cell adenoma: a multicenter analysis of risk factors for rupture and malignancy. Ann Surg Oncol 16(3):640–648
44. Cho SW, Marsh JW, Steel J et al (2008) Surgical management of hepatocellular adenoma: take it or leave it? Ann Surg Oncol 15:2795–2803
45. Larssen TB, Rorvik J, Hoff SR et al (2005) The occurrence of asymptomatic and symptomatic simple hepatic cysts. A prospective, hospital-based study. Clin Radiol 60(9):1026–1029
46. Dixon E, Sutherland FR, Mitchell P et al (2001) Cystadenomas of the liver: a spectrum of disease. Can J Surg 44(5):313–376
47. Devaney K, Goodman ZD, Ishak KG et al (1994) Hepatobiliary cystadenoma and cystadenocarcinoma. A light microscopic and immunohistochemical study of 70 patients. Am J Surg Pathol 18(11):1078–1091
48. Ishak KG, Willis GW, Cummins SD et al (1977) Biliary cystadenoma and cystadenocarcinoma: report of 14 cases and review of the literature. Cancer 39(1):322–338
49. Truant S, Bouras AF, Petrovai G et al (2013) Volumetric gain of the liver after major hepatectomy in obese patients: a case-matched study in 84 patients. Ann Surg 258:696–702
50. Ferrero A, Viganò L, Polastri R et al (2007) Postoperative liver dysfunction and future remnant liver: where is the limit? Results of a prospective study. World J Surg 31:1643–1651
51. Kishi Y, Abdalla EK, Chun YS et al (2009) Three hundred and one consecutive extended right hepatectomies: evaluation of outcome based on systematic liver volumetry. Ann Surg 250:540–548
52. Cunningham JD, Fong Y, Shriver C et al (1994) One hundred consecutive hepatic resections: blood loss, transfusion, and operative technique. Arch Surg 129(10):1050–1056
53. Melendez JA, Arslan V, Fischer ME et al (1998) Perioperative outcomes of major hepatic resections under low central venous pressure anesthesia: blood loss, blood transfusion, and the risk of postoperative renal dysfunction. J Am Coll Surg 187(6):620–625
54. Belghiti J, Noun R, Malafosse R et al (1999) Continuous versus intermittent portal triad clamping for liver resection: a controlled study. Ann Surg 229:369–375
55. Clavien PA, Yadav S, Sindram D et al (2000) Protective effects of ischemic preconditioning for liver resection performed under inflow occlusion in humans. Ann Surg 232:155–162
56. McEntee GP, Nagorney DM (1991) Use of vascular staplers in major hepatic resections. Br J Surg 78(1):40–41
57. Schemmer P, Friess H, Hinz U et al (2006) Stapler hepatecomy is a safe dissection technique: analysis of 300 patients. World J Surg 30(3):419–430
58. Balaa FK, Tsung A, Gamblin TC et al (2008) Right hepatic lobectomy using the staple technique in 101 patients. J Gastrointest Surg 12(2):338–343
59. Nakamura S, Tsuzuki T (1981) Surgical anatomy of the hepatic veins and the inferior vena cava. Surg Gynecol Obstet 152(1):43–50

60. Abu Hilal M, Di Fabio F, Teng MJ et al (2011) Surgical management of benign and indeterminate hepatic lesions in the era of laparoscopic liver surgery. Dig Surg 28:232–236
61. Koller M, Lorenz W (2002) Quality of life: a deconstruction for clinicians. J R Soc Med 95:481–488
62. Ardito F, Tayar C, Laurent A et al (2007) Laparoscopic liver resection for benign disease. Arch Surg 142:1188–1193

Robotic Liver Resections

20

Alberto Patriti and Luciano Casciola

20.1 Introduction

Low morbidity, zero mortality, parenchyma-preserving resection is the main goal of liver surgery for benign conditions. This aim should be achieved in both open and minimally invasive liver surgery irrespectively to site and dimension of the liver mass [1]. When a minimally invasive approach is planned, every effort has to be taken to carry out a resection as safe as the open counterpart. Postoperative morbidity in laparoscopic liver resections is principally related to hemorrhage from cutting edge, ascites (especially in cirrhotic patients or, in case of deroofing, of biliary cysts), and intra-abdominal collections, with rates ranging from 11 to 34 % [1, 2].

Robotics (da Vinci Robotic System Intuitive Surgical Inc., Sunnyvale, CA), introducing the possibility of image integration and the "wrist-like" movements of the robotic tools, promises to overcome some of the limitations of laparoscopic surgery extending indications for a minimally invasive parenchyma-sparing surgery even to lesions located in the posterior segments or in contact with liver vessels [3]. In this chapter technical and technological features to carry out robotic liver resections will be discussed.

A. Patriti (✉)
Division of General Minimally Invasive and Robotic Surgery,
Department of Surgery, ASL2 Umbria – San Matteo degli Infermi Hospital,
Via Loreto, Spoleto, Perugia 06049, Italy
e-mail: albertopatriti@gmail.com

L. Casciola
Division of Minimally Invasive Surgery, Casa di Cura Città di Roma,
Via Francesco Maidalchini, 20, Rome 00152, Italy
e-mail: lucianocasciola@gmail.com

L. Aldrighetti et al. (eds.), *Benign Tumors of the Liver*,
DOI 10.1007/978-3-319-12985-3_20

20.2 The da Vinci Robotic System

The da Vinci robotic system has been gradually upgraded from the first three-arm system to the current lightweight da Vinci Si with four arms and a high-definition (HD) three-dimensional camera. Recently, a new system is going to be delivered to the market. The new da Vinci Xi is projected for complex multiquadrant surgeries. The main features of the new system are a new overhead instrument arm architecture designed to facilitate anatomical access from virtually any position. A new endoscope digital architecture that creates a simpler, more compact design with improved visual definition and clarity. The 8-mm diameter of the endoscope allows the ability to attach it to any arm, providing flexibility for visualizing the surgical site. Smaller, thinner arms with newly designed joints offer a greater range of motion in respect to the previous versions. Longer instrument shafts are designed to give surgeons greater operative reach.

All generations of the da Vinci robotic system is designed to detect, filter, and translate electromechanically the surgeon's finger movements into precise and scaled micro-movements of the instruments. Basically, three modules compose the da Vinci: the *surgeon console*, the *robotic cart*, and the *endoscopic column or vision cart*. The *robotic instruments*, connected to the robotic arms, are articulated with 7 degrees of freedom.

Surgeon Console The console contains the hardware, software, and human interfaces of the system. The latter are the binocular viewer, the master control, the control panels for system setup, and the foot control pedals. The surgeon operates sitting in front of the console viewing the operating field in a high-definition 3D-view screen. Two master controllers allow the surgeon to move robotic instruments using the thumb and index finger of each hand. The system translates the surgeon's wrist and finger movements into real-time movements to the surgical instruments. There are seven foot pedals in the da Vinci Si model: clutch pedal that disengages the instruments from the controllers, camera and focus pedals allowing adjustment of the surgical view, and bipolar and monopolar coagulation pedals. Camera and endoscopic calibration, motion scaling, and console setup are controlled by a touch pad.

Patient-Side Cart The console is connected to the cart by a cable carrying bidirectional information. The cart consists of four robotic arms: one for the camera and three for the instruments. Plastic drapes are necessary to cover the arms for sterility because these are the sole components of the robot reaching the surgical field. The robotic arms work into the patient's abdominal cavity through dedicated 8-mm trocars. Each arm moves likewise the human arm through a series of multiple joints and a terminal pivot joint, corresponding to the 8-mm trocar.

The *endoscopic column and camera system* have all the features of a standard laparoscopic column with a monitor, a CO_2 insufflator, a dual high-intensity light source, and a camera unit. The camera system, with 10× magnification, has a dual-lens system with two three-chip cameras. The spatial separation of these images projected to the surgeon's eyes in the binocular viewer allows true 3D image at the console.

Endo-wristed Instruments A wide range of dedicated instruments are available (forceps, hook, bipolar, grasper, etc.). Almost all the instruments have an articulated tip with seven degrees of freedom; the only exception is the ultrasonic dissector. Position sensing abolishes the human tremors. Almost all the instruments may be used ten times.

Imaging at the Console Both open and minimally invasive liver surgery largely depend on preoperative imaging (computer tomography and magnetic resonance) and intraoperative ultrasonography (IOUS) for the evaluation of vascular and biliary anatomy, identification of known and occult intrahepatic lesions, and operative planning. Actually, there are different solutions to allow the console surgeon to receive all these information during surgery. TilePro software (Intuitive Surgical Inc., Sunnyvale, CA), working with the da Vinci Si and Xi platforms, shows multiple data sources into the robotic operative view giving to the surgeon a more reliable system to integrate all the anatomical information. TilePro delivers information from up to two data sources simultaneously. Data are superimposed on the surgical view and could be delivered via s-video or Digital Visual Interface (DVI) input into the console. There can be a total of six data sources, which may be toggled to present any two at one time to the console surgeon. Additionally, the data can be broadcast to all monitors in the room so the assistants, nurses, and anesthesia teams can view the simulcast. The TilePro "inbox" in the console view may be scaled depending on surgeon preference, with a 50 % display dimension having a resolution of 512 × 384 pixels. The sources of data are limitless; static images, graphical data, or even dynamic video, LIOUS, can all be input. The console surgeon with one click of the camera foot pedal may perform changes or removal of the information.

20.3 Operating Room Setup and Patient and Trocar Position

The position of all the devices in the operating room, trocars, and patient has to be individualized according to tumor location. When approaching anterior segments and segment 1 (Spiegel lobe), a reversed Trendelenburg supine patient position is optimal. The on-table surgeon stands between the legs and the scrub nurse and instruments are positioned lateral to the left leg. The trocars are generally positioned along a bowl-shaped line passing through the umbilicus.

For lesions located in the right posterolateral sector (upper segment 6 and segment 7), the patient is rotated on the left flank in order to facilitate liver mobilization and inferior vena cava dissection, when necessary. The camera port and the left-sided trocars should be placed as close as possible to the right costal margin, whereas the right trocar can be inserted in the intercostal space between the 10th and 11th rib close to the scapular line. At this level the risk to accidentally injure the lung is very low, and a direct access to the posterolateral segments is provided [4].

For bilobar liver metastases with involvement of both anterior segments and S7–S8, two options are equally effective: re-docking the robot and changing patient position according to the tumor location and using a semi-left lateral patient position with the robot over the patient's head. The latter is that preferred in our institution since it does not require robot re-docking and changes during surgery of patient position with possible contamination of the surgical field.

20.4 Basic Maneuvers

20.4.1 Inflow Control

The availability of a system for intermittent inflow occlusion is of paramount importance when performing nonanatomical liver resections or when the planned parenchymal transection is close to a main liver vessel. Pringle maneuver is the easier and safer way to achieve inflow control, but its use in laparoscopic surgery has been neglected for years. An ideal system for laparoscopic Pringle maneuver should be cost-effective and as user-friendly as to permit intermittent inflow occlusion during parenchymal transection and guarantee a fast vascular control in case of bleeding. The device for inflow occlusion set in our institution is composed of a 20-Fr chest tube, an umbilical tape, and a plug used for occlusion of the Foley catheter [5].

The chest tube is inserted in the right upper abdominal quadrant and the umbilical tape is passed around the hepatoduodenal ligament with the use of endowristed Cadiere forceps (Intuitive Surgical Inc., Sunnyvale, CA) or an Endoflex (Surgical Innovations, Leeds, UK) [1]. The umbilical tape is then exteriorized through the chest tube with the use of 5-mm laparoscopic forceps. The chest tube is finally closed with the plug in order to avoid air loss. When inflow occlusion is needed, the on-table surgeon removes the plug and pulls the umbilical tape. When the desired tape tension is achieved, the chest tube is closed with the plug. With this technique, the console surgeon can proceed in parenchyma transection, while the on-table surgeon performs the intermittent pedicle clamping. The technique resulted to be safe when compared to the open counterpart in terms of postoperative bilirubin and liver enzyme blood levels [6].

20.4.2 Parenchymal Transection

The Kelly-clamp-crushing technique associated to intermittent Pringle maneuver is considered the safer and more cost-effective method for parenchymal division in open liver surgery [7]. The major advantages of the Kelly-clamp-crushing technique are the low costs and the ability to fragment the parenchyma preserving the vascular structures that can be ligated and divided or preserved according to the resection plan. This economic and ingenious technique is not performed laparoscopically on a routine basis due to the inherent difficulties to perform the Pringle maneuver and the lack of dedicated instruments. Actually, robotics has renewed the interest for this technique. Using the endo-wristed bipolar PreCise forceps (Intuitive Surgical Systems, Sunnyvale, CA, USA), the parenchyma can be easily fragmented exposing the inner vessels as in open surgery. The on-table surgeon uses to perform the intermittent inflow occlusion, thereby allowing the console surgeon to focus his/her attention only on the transection line. The wristed instruments took back to the laparoscopic surgeon the possibility to perform curved and angled resections in all the liver segments, an ability lost with the rigid laparoscopic tools. Therefore, the robotic clamp-crushing technique allows parenchymal preservation even for deeply located lesions, widening the indications for a minimally invasive approach even to lesions in the posterior segments and located close to major liver vessels. Hemostasis of small vessels is obtained with monopolar or bipolar cautery. To secure larger vessels on the transection line, we use Hem-o-lok® clips or ligatures with Vicryl® and Prolene®. The hepatic veins are usually divided with the laparoscopic linear stapler or sutured with Prolene®. Biliostasis is assessed by observation and the bile leaks controlled with sutures as in open surgery.

20.4.3 Liver Retraction

Retraction and tension have a great role in all aspects of surgery including liver resections. For resections on anterior segments, left lateral sectionectomy included, some stay sutures can be useful to retract the specimen using the fourth robotic arm or the assistant grasper. A vessel loop held by the fourth arm around the left lobe can be used to stretch the parenchyma along the transection plane facilitating the effect of the Kelly-clamp-crushing technique. For deeply located lesions or when the tumor is close to a major vessel, the "corkscrew technique" can be reproduced. After identification of the lesion by inspection and intraoperative ultrasound, Glisson capsule is marked with electrocautery 1–2 cm away from the tumor margin. According to the location of the tumor, the marked area is anchored by stitches with caution in order to prevent the needle from entering the tumor. The suture is held together by clips, and upward traction is performed, facilitating the transection of the parenchyma and correct identification of vascular and biliary structures. The stitch can be also exteriorized using an Endo Close Trocar Site Closure Device (Covidien, USA) in order to avoid the use of the fourth robotic arm (Fig. 20.1). Parenchymal transection is performed with the monopolar shears for the first liver layer (1 cm from the Glisson capsule) and then with the Kelly-clamp-crushing technique. For steady exposure of the parenchymal transection plane in major hepatectomies, the "rubber band technique" can be used. Two sterile rubber bands are introduced into the abdominal cavity. One end of each rubber band is anchored with stay sutures at the right and left resection margins. The other end is pulled outside and fixed with appropriate tension.

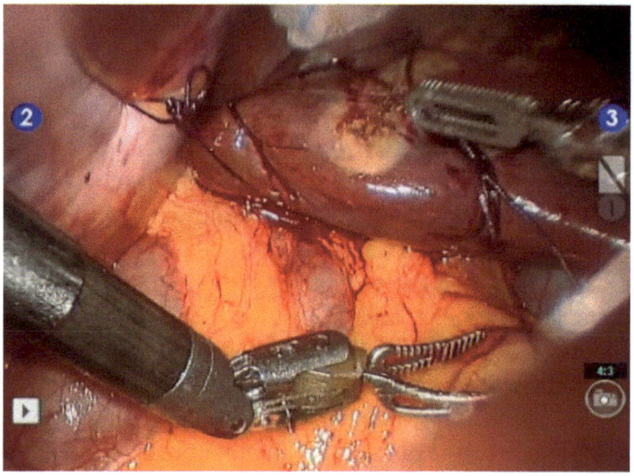

Fig. 20.1 Liver resection using two stay sutures for retraction. One of them is exteriorized (the right one)

20.5 Robotics for Benign Liver Tumors

The da Vinci robotic system can be used for all the spectrum of benign liver conditions. From a technical perspective, the robot can be used for:

- Deroofing of nonparasitic liver cysts (NPLC)
- Enucleation of benign solid tumors and parasitic and nonparasitic liver cysts
- Liver resection for benign tumors

A real advantage of robotics over traditional laparoscopy to carry out such procedures is not clearly demonstrated [3]. Therefore, the authors' choice is to limit a robotic approach to most complex cases for location, dimensions, and relationship with the main liver vessels.

20.5.1 Deroofing of Nonparasitic Liver Cysts

Deroofing of NPLC consists in the aspiration and cutting out the more external portion of the cystic wall. Laparoscopically this procedure is considered a simple task that can be carried out with electrocautery or the Harmonic ACE (Ethicon Endosurgery, OH, USA). Robotics seems to have nothing more to add. Since aspiration of the cystic fluid is an important step of the procedure, a fourth accessory trocar is required for the robotic procedure in respect to the three trocars required by laparoscopy. We suggest to limit deroofing of NPLC for teaching purposes at the beginning of the surgeon's learning curve.

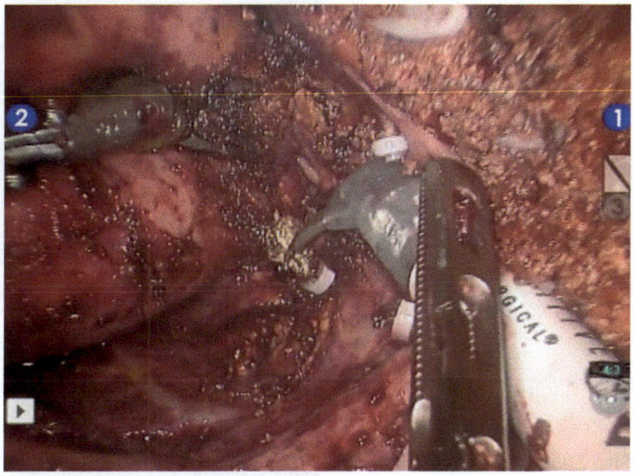

Fig. 20.2 Pericystectomy of a large hydatid cyst in segments 6 and 7. Portal branches for segments 6, 7, and 8 are exposed on the cutting surface

20.5.2 Enucleation of Benign Solid Tumors and Parasitic and NPLC

Enucleation is considered a safe parenchyma-preserving option for liver hemangiomas and hydatid cysts.

In 1988, Alper et al. described the technique for hemangioma enucleation by dissecting the fibrous cleavage plane between the capsule of the liver mass and the surrounding liver tissue.

This technique resulted in a lower morbidity rate than liver resection, avoiding unnecessary sacrifice of healthy liver parenchyma and damage to blood vessels and bile ducts.

Later, studies demonstrated that complication rate and blood loss were lower for hemangioma enucleations in respect to liver resections [8].

Therefore, enucleation is the treatment of choice for giant hemangiomas when technically feasible, confining liver resection to large, deeply located lesions and to lesions encasing liver great vessels [9]. A hydatid cyst presents technical challenges very similar to those of liver hemangioma. Enlarging hydatid cyst determines formation of an enclosing fibrous wall around the cyst called "pericyst." Therefore, the hydatid cyst can be removed along with its pericyst dissecting the surrounding compressed liver parenchyma. This procedure is associated to a low rate of recurrence and is named pericystectomy [10]. Endowristed fine movements of the robot allow bloodless dissection along the compressed parenchyma of both hydatid cyst and hemangioma (Figs. 20.2 and 20.3). Hook cautery and monopolar scissors are equally effective for this purpose. For giant liver hemangiomas and hydatid cysts in close relation with a liver vessel, the Pringle maneuver has a tremendous role to reduce blood loss and to carry out a safe dissection (Figs. 20.4 and 20.5).

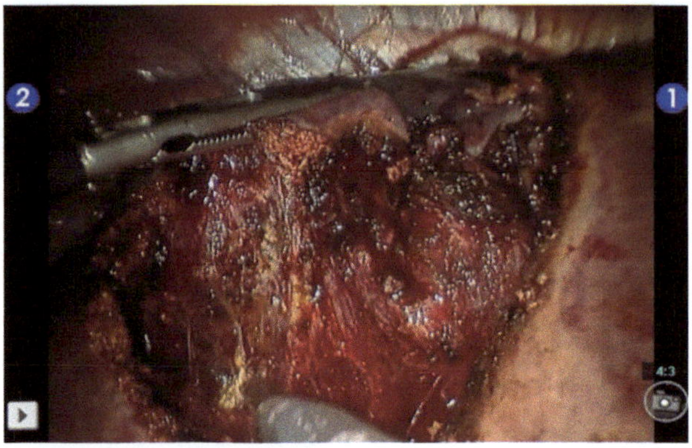

Fig. 20.3 Enucleation of a giant hemangioma in segment 8

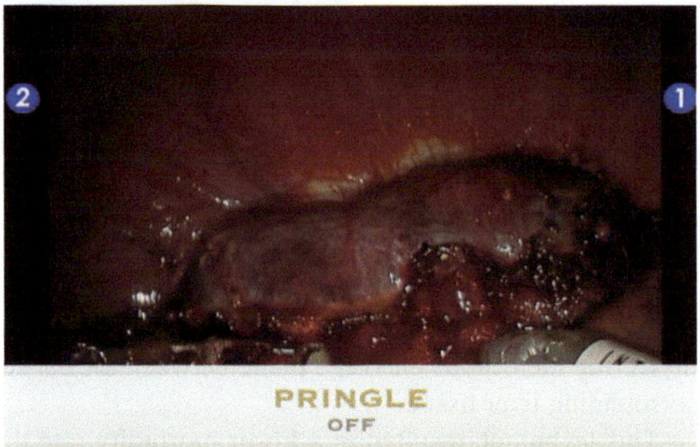

Fig. 20.4 Hemodynamic effect of inflow control. The hemangioma is completely distended when Pringle maneuver is off

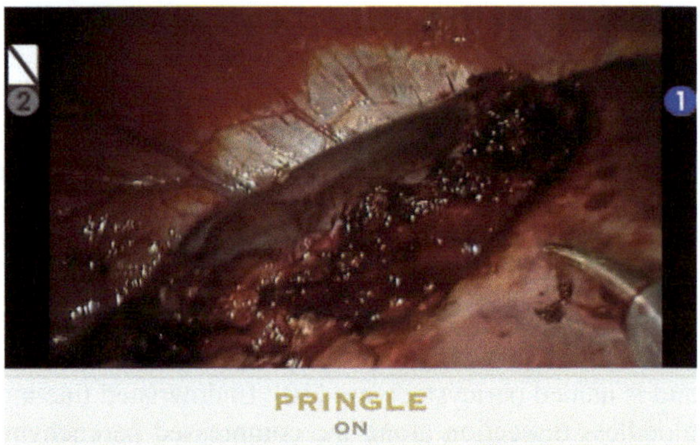

Fig. 20.5 The hemangioma is collapsed during the Pringle maneuver

20.5.3 Liver Resections: Technical Aspects of Segmentectomies and Sub-segmentectomies

For segmentectomies and sub-segmentectomies, patient positioning and trocar placement should be individualized according to the tumor location. Pneumoperitoneum induction with the Veress needle can help to tailor trocar position, limiting the use of an umbilical port to the cases where it is really necessary. Anatomical and nonanatomical liver resections of peripheral (segments 2-3-4b-5-6), superficial lesions are generally feasible and can be done with minimal morbidity and mortality rates. Pedicle clamping is optional or can be applied only in case of bleeding, and liver division can be performed with all the available transection devices. Generally 3–4 trocars disposed at the level of the umbilical line are adequate. For lesions located in the posterolateral sector (upper segment 6, segments 7–8), the patient is rotated on the left flank in order to facilitate liver mobilization and inferior vena cava dissection, when necessary. The camera port and the left-sided trocars should be placed as close as possible to the right costal margin, whereas the right trocar can be inserted in the intercostal space between the 10th and 11th rib along the scapular line. Due to the higher risk of bleeding, intermittent pedicle clamping is advisable when approaching posterosuperior segments. Careful ultrasonographic exploration with demarcation on the Glisson capsule of the right hepatic vein can avoid major bleeding during parenchymal transection. For deeply located lesions or when the tumor is close to a major vessel, even in case of lesions located in the anterior segments, the "corkscrew technique" can be useful. After identification of the lesion by inspection and intraoperative ultrasound, Glisson capsule is marked with electrocautery 1–2 cm away from the tumor margin. According to the location of the tumor, the marked area is anchored by stitches with caution in order to prevent the needle from entering the tumor. Metallic clips hold the suture together, and upward traction is performed, facilitating the transection of the parenchyma and correct identification of vascular and biliary structures. The control of the surgical margin can be verified by intraoperative ultrasonography during parenchymal transection. Generally, small specimens can be extracted by endoscopic bag through any port site; otherwise, enlarging the umbilical port or rarely a Pfannenstiel incision could be necessary. Robot assistance is particularly useful to perform parenchymal-preserving resections especially in the posterosuperior segments and when the tumor is in contact with a portal branch and hepatic vein and when both are close to the tumor mass. In fact, the endo-wristed instruments allow fine movements and complex transection planes reducing the discomfort coming from the use of rigid tools. Principles of patient and trocar positions in conventional laparoscopic surgery are applicable also for the robot-assisted approach. For liver surgery the robot is docked over the patient's head.

All liver resections should be guided by the ultrasound performed by the on-table surgeon. The console surgeon can view the ultrasound screen in a picture-in-picture modality directing the dissection plane, which appeared as an echogenic line between the cut surfaces. Parenchyma is usually transected with the harmonic scalpel for straight-line resections. The Kelly-clamp-crushing technique with the endo-wristed bipolar Precise forceps (Intuitive Surgical Systems, Sunnyvale, CA, USA) is preferred for curved and angulated section lines and tumor dissection close to a major liver vessel. Hemostasis of small vessels is obtained with monopolar or bipolar cautery. To secure larger vessels on the transection line, we use Hem-o-lok® clips or ligatures with Vicryl® or Prolene®. The hepatic veins are usually divided with the laparoscopic linear stapler or sutured with Prolene®. Biliostasis is assessed by observation and the bile leaks controlled with sutures as in open surgery.

20.6 Results of Robotic Liver Surgery

Interests in robotic liver resections date back to 2008 when Choi et al. published their first series of four liver left lobectomies [11]. After this report, several series have been published investigating different aspects of robotic liver surgery.

Actually, two lines of research can be drawn in the current literature. The first aims to investigate the possibilities of robotics to perform major hepatectomies, even with biliary reconstruction. The other tries to delineate the technical aspects to carry out a robot-assisted parenchyma-sparing surgery. Casciola et al. demonstrated that robotics allows an easy access to the posterosuperior segments to carry out parenchymal-saving resections instead of a major hepatectomy even when the tumor is in close contact with a great liver vessel. The use of endo-wristed instruments for parenchymal transection was the main technical tip evidenced in this study. Reproducing a traditional Kelly-clamp-crushing technique for curved resection planes made possible to perform liver resections with a maximal parenchymal preservation even for lesions deeply located and in contact with the main liver vessels [3, 4, 12]. Giulianotti et al. recently described the applications of robotics in major liver surgery. A total of 24 right hepatectomies were carried out with zero mortality and with a low conversion rate (4.2 %). Postoperative morbidity was acceptable (25 %) as well as blood loss. After a mean follow-up of 34 months, no port-site metastases were described among the oncologic cases [13]. In the same center, the da Vinci robotic system was used to complete complex biliary reconstructions with curative and palliative intent. Asian surgeons achieved the same results, reporting series with a high rate of major hepatectomies [14, 15]. Finally, possible advantages of robotics in hepatobiliary surgery are going to be delineated, but prospective controlled studies involving a large number of patients are required for definitive results.

References

1. Troisi R, Montalti R, Smeets P, Van Huysse J, Van Vlierberghe H, Colle I, De Gendt S, de Hemptinne B (2008) The value of laparoscopic liver surgery for solid benign hepatic tumors. Surg Endosc 22(1):38–44. Epub 2007 Aug 21
2. Descottes B, Glineur D, Lachachi F, Valleix D, Paineau J, Hamy A, Morino M, Bismuth H, Castaing D, Savier E, Honore P, Detry O, Legrand M, Azagra JS, Goergen M, Ceuterick M, Marescaux J, Mutter D, de Hemptinne B, Troisi R, Weerts J, Dallemagne B, Jehaes C, Gelin M, Donckier V, Aerts R, Topal B, Bertrand C, Mansvelt B, Van Krunckelsven L, Herman D, Kint M, Totte E, Schockmel R, Gigot JF (2003) Laparoscopic liver resection of benign liver tumors. Surg Endosc 17(1):23–30. Epub 2002 Oct 8
3. Troisi RI, Patriti A, Montalti R, Casciola L (2013) Robot assistance in liver surgery: a real advantage over a fully laparoscopic approach? Results of a comparative bi-institutional analysis. Int J Med Robot 9:160–166
4. Casciola L, Patriti A, Ceccarelli G, Bartoli A, Ceribelli C, Spaziani A (2011) Robot-assisted parenchymal-sparing liver surgery including lesions located in the posterosuperior segments. Surg Endosc 25:3815–3824

5. Patriti A, Ceccarelli G, Bartoli A, Casciola L (2011) Extracorporeal pringle maneuver in robot-assisted liver surgery. Surg Laparosc Endosc Percutan Tech 21:e242–e244
6. Patriti A, Ceribelli C, Ceccarelli G, Bartoli A, Bellochi R, Casciola L (2012) Non-cirrhotic liver tolerance to intermittent inflow occlusion during laparoscopic liver resection. Updates Surg 64:87–93
7. Castaldo E, Earl TM, Chari R, Gorden DL, Merchant N, Wright JK, Feurer I, Pinson CW (2008) A clinical comparative analysis of crush/clamp, stapler, and dissecting sealer hepatic transection methods. HPB (Oxford) 10:321–326
8. Patriti A, Graziosi L, Sanna A, Gullà N, Donini A (2005) Laparoscopic treatment of liver hemangioma. Surg Laparosc Endosc Percutan Tech 15:359–362
9. Lerner SM, Hiatt JR, Salamandra J, Chen PW, Farmer DG, Ghobrial RM, Busuttil RW (2004) Giant cavernous liver hemangiomas: effect of operative approach on outcome. Arch Surg 139:818–821; discussion 821–823
10. Safioleas MC, Misiakos EP, Kouvaraki M, Stamatakos MK, Manti CP, Felekouras ES (2006) Hydatid disease of the liver: a continuing surgical problem. Arch Surg 141:1101–1108
11. Choi SB, Park JS, Kim JK, Hyung WJ, Kim KS, Yoon DS, Lee WJ, Kim BR (2008) Early experiences of robotic-assisted laparoscopic liver resection. Yonsei Med J 49:632–638
12. Tranchart H, Ceribelli C, Ferretti S, Dagher I, Patriti A (2014) Traditional versus robot-assisted full laparoscopic liver resection: a matched-pair comparative study. World J Surg 38:2904–2909
13. Giulianotti PC, Sbrana F, Coratti A, Bianco FM, Addeo P, Buchs NC, Ayloo SM, Benedetti E (2011) Totally robotic right hepatectomy: surgical technique and outcomes. Arch Surg 146:844–850
14. Chan OCY, Tang CN, Lai ECH, Yang GPC, Li MKW (2011) Robotic hepatobiliary and pancreatic surgery: a cohort study. J Hepatobiliary Pancreat Sci 18:471–480
15. Wakabayashi G, Sasaki A, Nishizuka S, Furukawa T, Kitajima M (2011) Our initial experience with robotic hepato-biliary-pancreatic surgery. J Hepatobiliary Pancreat Sci 18:481–487

Interventional Radiology in Benign Liver Tumors

21

Massimo Venturini and Claudio Sallemi

Transcatheter arterial embolization (TAE) and radiofrequency ablation (RFA) are interventional radiological techniques widely used in the locoregional treatment of malignant, unresectable lesions confined to the liver.

Although surgical resection is the gold standard treatment for symptomatic-enlarging benign liver lesions, TAE and RFA can represent a valid, less invasive alternative in selected cases, with low morbidity/mortality rate and shortening hospitalization.

A conservative approach with a radiologic surveillance for asymptomatic or small benign liver lesions is usual, but in case of symptomatic-enlarging tumors, high-risk bleeding, or malignant degeneration, a surgical resection or an interventional radiological treatment can be necessary.

Myriad benign tumors may be found in the liver, and, according to their cell of origin, they can be classified into hepatocellular tumor (adenoma, focal nodular hyperplasia, regenerative/dysplastic nodules in cirrhosis, nodular regenerative hyperplasia), cholangiocellular tumor (hepatic cyst, biliary hamartomas, peribiliary cyst, biliary cystadenoma, Caroli disease, biliary papillomatosis), and mesenchymal tumor (cavernous hemangioma, focal fat, angiomyolipoma, lipoma, peliosis hepatis, paraganglioma, inflammatory pseudotumor) [1].

Most of them are small asymptomatic lesions, but others, due to their nature or large dimension or sub-glissonian position, present variable risk of hemorrhage, infection, hepatic insufficiency, and malignant degeneration: for example, giant cavernous hemangioma [2] or adenoma [3] presents high risk of bleeding, hepatic

M. Venturini, MD (✉) • C. Sallemi, MD
Department of Radiology, San Raffaele Hospital,
Vita-Salute University, Milan, Italy
e-mail: venturini.massimo@hsr.it; sallemi.claudio@hsr.it

L. Aldrighetti et al. (eds.), *Benign Tumors of the Liver*,
DOI 10.1007/978-3-319-12985-3_21

cyst may have an infection risk [4], and Caroli disease [5] or polycystic liver [6] can lead to hepatic insufficiency. Malignant degeneration is described for adenoma in hepatocellular carcinoma [7], cystadenoma in cystadenocarcinoma [8], and Caroli disease in cholangiocarcinoma [9].

When a nonconservative approach becomes necessary, TAE can be used either as less invasive alternative to surgery, for example, in symptomatic-enlarging masses located centrally in the liver in order to determine a size reduction or as a presurgical treatment in bleeding masses to temporarily stop hemorrhage.

RFA is usually indicated in lesions of diameter less than 4 cm, neither sub-glissonian nor adjacent to the main hepatic vessels.

21.1 Embolization

The embolization of benign liver tumors is a well-known less invasive therapeutic alternative to surgery in case of particular conditions which make a surgical approach difficult and hazardous.

The young age or the general conditions of the patient, the large volume, or the peculiar position of the mass can contraindicate an open and also a laparoscopic surgery.

Usually hepatic embolization means TAE, or TACE (transarterial chemoembolization) in case of associated chemotherapeutic agent for the treatment of primary [10] or secondary [11, 12] malignant liver tumors. In case of benign liver tumors, the aim of TAE is to significantly reduce the blood flow of the feeding arteries to determine a shrinkage of the mass or to stop a hemorrhage of a bleeding lesion allowing a safer surgical treatment.

However hepatic embolization can be more rarely used in liver benign tumors to occlude the veins. For example, portal and hepatic vein can be embolized, respectively, in case of extensive hepatectomy as presurgical treatment to prevent hepatic insufficiency [13] and in case of neonatal cavernous hemangiomas with extended arteriovenous shunting conditioning a cardiac output insufficiency [14].

TAE is indicated in different benign liver tumors, not only hypervascular, because they are mainly fed by the hepatic artery (focal nodular hyperplasia, adenoma), but also relatively hypovascular (hemangioma, polycystic liver).

TAE can be performed with different materials to occlude the main feeding arteries (coils, Amplatzer vascular plugs), their medium size branches (glue, nonpolymerized liquid agents), or their intratumoral capillaries (PVA particles, gelatin microspheres).

Embolizing material can be carried through standard 4 (or 5)-French angiographic catheters into the main branches of the hepatic artery, although the advancement of microcatheters (3 French or less) into its peripheral branches permits a more precise deposition of the embolization particles in the lesion microcirculation. The routine use of microcatheters allows a more selective embolization avoiding the occlusion of the main arterial branches and reducing the risk of nontarget vessel embolization.

21.1.1 Indications

The main benign tumors which, in selected cases, can be treated by TAE are the following.

Cavernous Hepatic Hemangioma It represents the most common benign tumor of the liver and consists of multiple large, blood-filled vascular channels [15]. Most of them are solitary, small (<4 cm), and asymptomatic and are typically found incidentally on ultrasound scanning [16].

In contrast, giant cavernous hemangiomas, those whose diameter exceeds 4 cm and may be greater than 20 cm, can be symptomatic and present with pain, abdominal fullness, or an upper abdominal mass [17]. In some rare cases, severe complications such as jaundice, Kasabach–Merritt syndrome [18], or intra-abdominal hemorrhage, due to their rupture, occur [19]. The likelihood of spontaneous bleeding is unknown, but large subcapsular lesions can be considered at greater risk [20]. Interventions should be performed only in case of symptomatic, progressively growing, and at high risk of bleeding hemangiomas [19, 20].

Treatment options for symptomatic liver giant hemangiomas have included steroids [21], radiation therapy [22], surgical resection [23], hepatic arterial ligation [24], RFA, and TAE. Several reports have demonstrated the value of percutaneous TAE in treating infantile hepatic hemangioendotheliomas [25] and diffuse hemangiomatosis [26].

In giant cavernous hemangiomas of the adults, TAE has been used in case of ruptured hemangiomas [27] and symptomatic hemangiomas [28] and as presurgical treatment [29] and associated with medical therapy [30].

Some authors have expressed reluctance to interrupt arterial circulation by TAE or arterial ligation for the fear of causing ischemia, intracavitary bleeding, or infection.

Focal Nodular Hyperplasia (FNH) It is the second most common benign liver tumor, predominantly solitary, usually detected as incidental finding in young healthy women [31]. A clear association with the use of oral contraceptives and adenomas [32] has been demonstrated. FNH is a hypervascular benign nodule, usually with a typical central scar corresponding to a central feeding artery [33]. A conservative approach for asymptomatic lesions is well established in consideration of a poor predisposition to hemorrhage, necrosis, or malignant transformation. Nevertheless large lesions (>4 cm) may be responsible for abdominal complaints due to liver capsule distension and pressure on the surrounding organs. In order to establish the best clinical approach, it is crucial to differentiate tumor-related symptoms from symptoms caused by extrahepatic pathology [34]. Treatment should be considered when a growing lesion with compressive symptoms is diagnosed or in cases of suspected increased risks of traumatic hemorrhage. Surgical resection is currently the first-choice treatment [35, 36], despite the potential bleeding risk due to the hypervascular nature of FNH [37].

Usually TAE is performed in case of symptomatic [38] or enlarging lesions [39], as alternative to surgery.

Hepatocellular Adenoma (HCA) It is a rare benign liver tumor that occurs more frequently in young women with a history of prolonged use of oral contraceptives. HCA is a heterogeneous disease comprising three subtypes with distinct molecular and complication profiles: the inflammatory or telangiectatic subtype is at increased risk of hemorrhage, the b-catenin-activated subtype is at increased risk of malignant transformation, and the hepatocyte nuclear factor-1a-inactivated or steatotic subtype is at the least risk of complications. One-third of patients with HCA have multiple tumors on imaging with no increased risk of complications. Surgical resection is indicated because of the risk of hemorrhage in 25 % of patients and malignant transformation in 5 % of patients [40].

In males, systematic resection of HCA is recommended owing to the higher incidence of malignant transformation, while in females surgical excision should be reserved for tumors 5 cm or larger associated with high bleeding risk. Radiologic surveillance of women with HCA tumors smaller than 5 cm, who have dropped hormonal therapy, has shown that the majority of HCA remains stable or undergoes spontaneous regression [41]. TAE can be performed as emergent treatment in case of bleeding lesion [42] or as elective treatment in order to determine the shrinkage of a single large HCA [43] or of a multiple adenomatosis [44]. Considering the possible degeneration in HCC, also treatments with TACE were performed [45].

Polycystic Liver Disease (PLD) It is the most common extrarenal manifestation of autosomal dominant polycystic kidney disease (ADPKD), presenting in 78.4 % of all ADPKD patients. Most ADPKD patients with PLD are asymptomatic and require no treatment [46]. Symptoms, mainly related to a marked hepatomegaly, can include abdominal distension, discomfort, nausea, loss of appetite, constipation, and shortness of breath [47]. In symptomatic patients, several interventions have been tried including percutaneous cyst aspiration with or without injection of a sclerosing solution, internal drainage with cystojejunostomy, laparoscopic fenestration, open surgical cyst fenestration, partial hepatectomy, and hepatic transplantation [48]. Because the hepatic cysts in ADPKD patients are mostly supplied from hepatic arteries but not from portal veins, TAE can lead to shrinkage of the cysts and reduction of liver volume [49]. After TAE, the cystic segments become less tense and begin to shrink, allowing the decompressed hepatic parenchyma to expand its volume.

21.1.2 Technical Aspects

After local anesthesia with Seldinger technique, TAE is usually performed using standard 4 (or 5)-French catheters/introducers through a transfemoral approach. Other approaches can be used (transbrachial, transaxillary), in case of unfavorable conditions (stenosis/obstructions or previous surgical bypass at the level of the iliac–femoral axis).

A preliminary diagnostic digital subtraction angiography (DSA) with selective catheterization of the celiac trunk and the superior mesenteric artery is mandatory before TAE.

In arterial phase, the presence of anatomic hepatic artery anomalies must be evaluated. Hepatic artery course and the lesion-feeding arteries must be accurately assessed in order to choose adequate guidewires, catheters, microcatheters, and embolizing material. In some cases an intrahepatic mass can also be vascularized by extrahepatic vessels, as, for example, phrenic, intercostal, or adrenal arteries, often hypertrophic and well visible with aortography.

In parenchymal phase, the grade of hyper- (or hypo-)vascularization of the lesion with respect to the adjacent liver and the angiographic pattern of the lesion must be evaluated. FNH shows a typical hypervascular pattern, with a single major feeding artery, which divides into smaller radiating branches with the appearance of a spoke wheel at DSA [39, 50] (Fig. 21.1).

Cavernous hemangioma usually shows contrast-containing vascular spaces orderly in their configuration which persist into the venous phase [51] (Fig. 21.2). HCA appears usually hypervascular [53] (Fig. 21.3), while PLD shows arteries and portal veins coursing not parallel, as usual, but in a different fashion: almost all hepatic arterial branches are well developed, whereas portal venous branches in the cystic segments are obstructed and replaced by multiple cysts [49] (Fig. 21.4). Arteriovenous shunting with early opacification of the hepatic veins or of the portal system must be considered to avoid an accidental embolization of nontarget vessels [14].

In venous phase, a preserved opacification of the portal vein represents an essential condition to perform a TAE: an unknown portal vein thrombosis can potentially contraindicate a TAE due to the potential risk of a hepatic insufficiency.

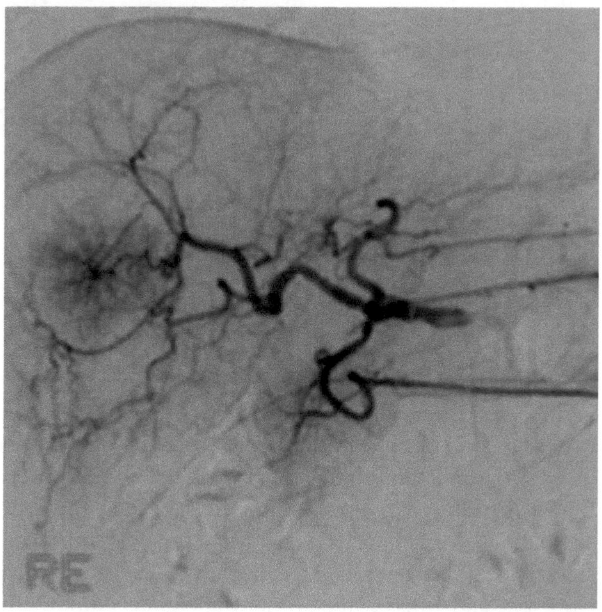

Fig. 21.1 Celiac angiography shows the typical appearance of FNH as a hypervascular lesion with a central feeding artery radiating in a spoke-wheel manner into the lesion (Reprinted with permission from Terkivatan et al. [50])

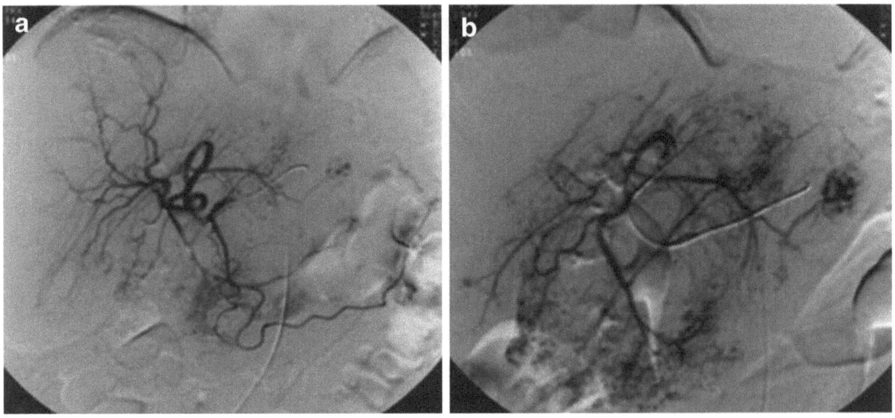

Fig. 21.2 DSA of a giant cavernous hemangioma in the right liver lobe. (**a**) Right hepatic arteriogram. (**b**) Superselective catheterization of the feeding artery (Reprinted with permission from Giavroglou et al. [52])

Fig. 21.3 Selective angiogram of the common hepatic artery shows a large adenoma in the right liver lobe. Pathological branches and splaying of normal branches by the adenoma are observed (Reprinted with permission from Erdogan et al. [53])

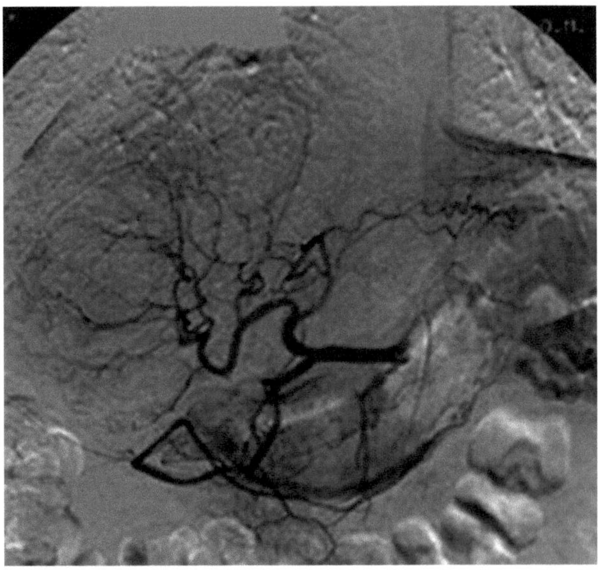

While the goal of an elective TAE in benign liver tumors is to obtain a significant shrinkage of the lesion, minimizing its related symptoms, in emergency the aim of TAE is to stop an active arterial bleeding. The risk of concomitant ischemic damage of liver parenchyma remains low because of the portal vein tributaries accounting for 70 % of the total blood supply of the liver. However caution is necessary to preserve the major liver arteries avoiding unnecessary liver damage. Selective or superselective catheterization of the hepatic artery and its distal branches using dedicated catheters and microcatheters and adequate embolizing material is essential. The

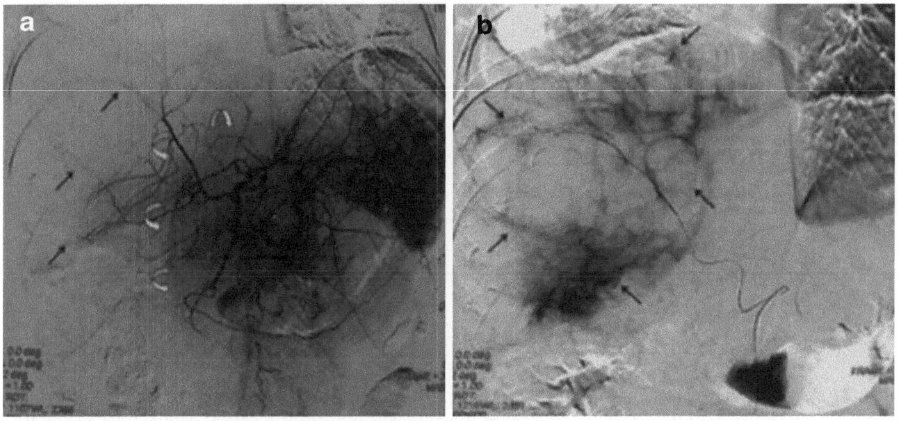

Fig. 21.4 Symptomatic polycystic liver disease: (**a**) Celiac arteriography shows that the right hepatic arterial branches are well developed and stretched (*arrows*), representing cystic regions. The left hepatic arterial branches are relatively normal (*curved arrows*), representing nearly intact hepatic parenchyma. (**b**) Superselective right hepatic angiography shows the multiple right lobe liver cysts (*arrows*) (Reprinted with permission from Wang et al. [47])

current use of flexible microcatheters of small caliber (less than 3 French) but with adequate diameter of their internal lumen (0.025–0.028 in.) determines several advantages: it allows great trackability, distal superselective catheterization, good diagnostic capacity (adequate quantity/flow of contrast agents can be injected), and low rate of microcatheter subocclusion due to embolizing material passage. Various embolizing materials can be used to occlude the feeding vessels of a lesion. The materials for embolization should be easy to use and capable of occluding the supplying vessel without compromising the flow of the main liver arteries [53]. Different materials, to perform proximal or distal TAE, are available: devices, as coils or Amplatzer plugs, which are pushed and released adjacently to the (micro) catheter tip and particles or solutions, as polyvinyl alcohol (PVA) particles, microsphere, gelatin sponge, glue, N-butyl cyanoacrylate (NBCA), liquid polymeric embolic system, and ethanol, which are injected and carried with the blood flow in the lesion microcirculation. Metallic coils of different diameters (0.035, 0.025, and 0.018 in.) and lengths, if used alone, often prove insufficient in blocking the peripheral arterial flow due to recanalization and collateral formation (Fig. 21.5); sometimes the use of Amplatzer plug [14] can represent a good solution in case of arteriovenous shunting or to avoid a nontarget vessel embolization. However metallic coils have been previously used in TAE of HCA [53] and PLD [54]. Gelatin sponge has been commonly used for embolization of arterial bleeding [53], but its temporary nature leaves a high risk of collateralization. PVA particles of different sizes (150–250; 250–350; 300–500 μm) have been largely used in TAE of giant hepatic hemangiomas [51, 52, 55], FNH [39, 50], and HCA [53]. The wide use of PVA particles in TAE of benign liver tumors is due to their long-term occlusive properties, efficacy in occluding small arteries, and biocompatibility [52] (Fig. 21.6).

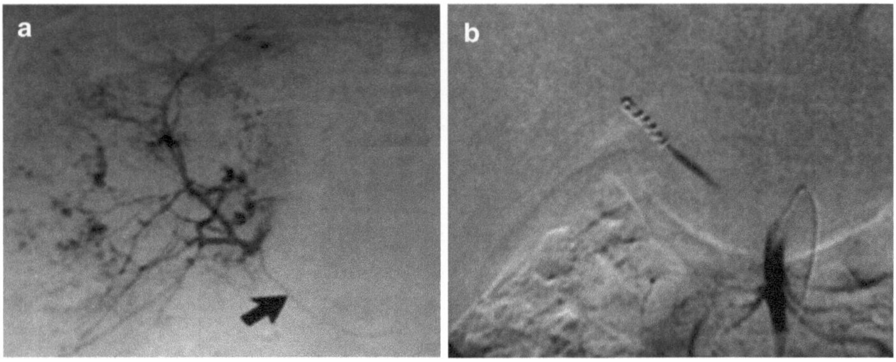

Fig. 21.5 Large cavernous hemangioma in the right lobe of the liver. (**a**) The angiographic catheter (*arrow*) in the hepatic artery arising from the superior mesenteric artery shows a large cavernous hemangioma supplied by the right hepatic artery. (**b**) The tumor was embolized with multiple steel coils and, successively, polyvinyl alcohol particles (Reprinted with permission from Srivastava et al. [28])

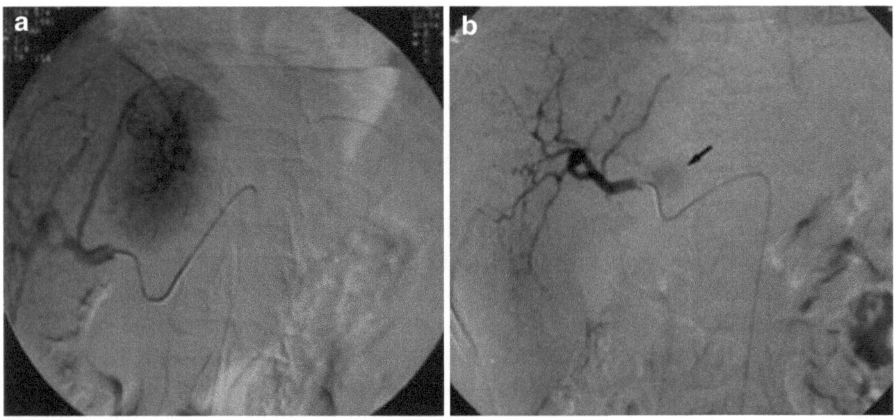

Fig. 21.6 (**a**) DSA shows a hypervascular lesion (FNH) with a microcatheter placed in the left hepatic artery, which supplied the tumor. (**b**) Angiographic image after the embolization procedure of the lesion by using embolization particles (contour; diameter 150–250 μm). After the procedure a small part of the lesion remains (*arrow*) (Reprinted with permission from Terkivatan et al. [50])

NBCA mixed with iodized oil [47] has been used to reduce hepatomegaly in PLD: unlike coils, which are solid, NBCA is deployed in a liquid form before polymerization, and this feature is beneficial in occlusion of smaller vessels.

The association of two embolizing materials, for example, coils and PVA particles, can be useful in selected cases to simultaneously perform a proximal and a distal embolization.

Finally, the choice of the embolizing material depends on many factors: lesion characteristics, angiographic evidence, interventional radiologist experience, and elective or emergent procedure (Fig. 21.7).

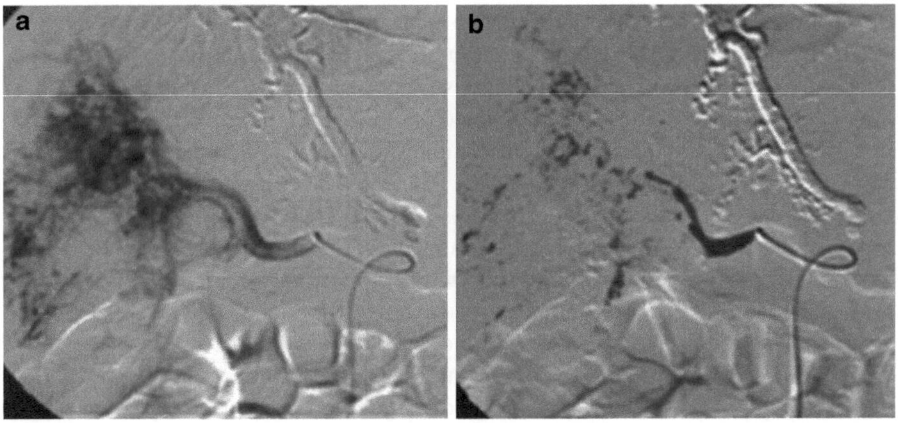

Fig. 21.7 Catheter embolization in infantile hepatic hemangioma. (**a**) DSA with coaxial technique with microcatheters shows a large hemangioma in the right lobe. (**b**) Especially when intrahepatic macroshunts are present, proximal embolization of feeding vessels with glue is effective (Reprinted with permission from Temple and Marshalleck [49])

21.1.3 Complications

Complications of vascular embolization include the use of intra-arterial contrast medium, procedure-related complications, and postembolization syndrome. The postembolization syndrome usually occurs within 24–48 h of embolization and lasts 3–7 days. It is characterized by pain at the site of embolization, nausea and vomiting, malaise, fever, and leukocytosis. Severity depends on the size of the embolized tissue [39]. The main procedure-related complications are represented by liver abscess, developing in the necrotized tissue [56], biliary damage [57], and systemic infections [58]. Therefore, a strict aseptic approach is essential, and, if necessary, prophylactic antibiotics can be discussed. Prophylactic antibiotics should be administered in case of previous bile duct surgery or systemic disorders. Further complications are accidental tissue necrosis of adjacent organs due to either reflux of embolizing material or permeation of liquid embolic material into the capillary bed. Renal failure may occur if a large mass of tissue is infarcted due to toxic radical release [39]. Other possible complications are pneumonia, pleural effusion, ascites, increased serum transaminases, and hepatic insufficiency.

21.2 Ablation

Basing on the mechanism to cause injury, local ablation techniques can be divided as follows: thermal therapies such as radiofrequency ablation, percutaneous cryoablation, microwave ablation, and interstitial laser chemotherapy and chemical ablative techniques such as percutaneous ethanol injection and electroporation, which alters the electrical conductivity and permeability of the cell membrane [59].

Radiofrequency ablation (RFA) is one of the main local treatment strategies that can be used for the destruction of a variety of unresectable malignant (and benign) liver tumors. Hepatic RFA is less invasive than surgery and carries a low risk of major complications [60]. RFA has gained universal acceptance as a safe and effective method to treat unresectable liver tumors showing excellent local tumor control and survival in different liver tumors [61, 62]. The use of RFA determines hyperthermia-induced coagulation necrosis of the hepatic lesion which typically exits as an area (RFA zone) demonstrating a defect in contrast enhancement at CT, MR, and CEUS [63]: according to the *American Heritage Medical Dictionary,* the term coagulation necrosis is defined as "necrosis in which the affected cells or tissue are converted into a dry, dull, fairly homogeneous eosinophilic mass as a result of coagulation of proteins" [64]. This definition is a description of the microscopic tissue change; in the case of RFA-induced coagulation necrosis, the protein coagulation is induced by hyperthermia. With the use of current RFA technologies, the area of coagulation necrosis, the RFA zone, is oval or round and can measure approximately 5 cm in diameter. However, the size and the shape can vary according to many factors, including the electrode type, the duration of ablation, and hepatic perfusion [65]. The clinical role of RFA of the liver has been well established, and its overall therapeutic efficacy, especially in cases of hepatocellular carcinoma (HCC), is known to be comparable to that of surgical resection as long as the tumor size is sufficiently small [66]. The role of RFA in the management of benign liver tumors has been more recently described in adults and children in selected cases [67]. RFA can be performed using a laparoscopic approach [68] or a percutaneous approach, with ultrasonographic guidance [69] or, more rarely, with CT guidance [70]. In the treatment of large benign liver tumors, as, for example, symptomatic hepatic hemangiomas with diameter over 10 cm [68–70], large and separate ablation sessions with clustered electrodes and multiple overlapping treatment zones can be useful to reduce the prevalence of postablation syndrome and risk of treatment failure.

21.2.1 Indications

RFA represents an emerging interventional procedure increasingly used in the treatment of malignant and benign liver tumors as valid alternative to surgery.

Indications to RFA for treatment of benign liver tumors are represented by symptomatic nodules or at high risk of malignant degeneration or rupture.

The main benign liver tumors treated with RFA are hepatic hemangiomas [69–71], HCA [72, 73], and, more rarely, also FNH [74].

Cavernous Hepatic Hemangioma Differently from small and asymptomatic hepatic hemangiomas, hepatic cavernous hemangiomas of diameter superior to 5 cm can be symptomatic with abdominal discomfort, swelling, abdominal pain, jaundice, and thrombocytopenia [68]. Giant hepatic hemangiomas can also have high risk of rupture [75]. Besides surgical resection [23], management of symptomatic, increasing in volume, large hepatic hemangiomas has been based on RFA, TAE [27–29], steroid treatment [21], radiation therapy [22], and hepatic arterial ligation [24]. The RFA mechanism of action in the treatment of hepatic hemangiomas is still not completely clear. Most of hepatic hemangiomas are of the cavernous type, composed of widely dilated nonanastomotic vascular spaces lined by flat endothelial cells and supported by fibrous tissue. RFA is a localized thermal technique designed to destroy tumors by using radiofrequency energy to heat tumor tissue to temperatures exceeding 90 °C. Damage to the endothelium lining the vascular structures may promote thrombosis [68]. The site of the hepatic hemangioma determines different approaches: laparoscopic approach in case of subcapsular lesion or percutaneous approach for deeper tumors. Ultrasonography represents the main standard method of guidance of RFA, but also CT guidance, in case of ultrasonographic poor visibility, has been described [70]. Most of hepatic hemangiomas show hyperechoic pattern at ultrasonography.

In case of giant hepatic hemangiomas, the RF electrode is repositioned to fully cover the hemangioma without ablating the surrounding liver tissue according to the overlapping ablation method. The total number of puncture of RFA can exceed 5 until 8 [68]. The benign biologic nature and high vascular properties of hepatic hemangiomas determine more advantages than disadvantages. The advantages include the following three aspects. First, differently from malignant tumors, RFA for hepatic hemangiomas does not require an ablative margin of the normal hepatic parenchyma surrounding the tumor. Second, one well-performed RFA can lead to an obvious collapse of tumor tissue around the ablation zone, making RFA for hepatic hemangiomas be more efficient and easier than for malignant tumors. Third, the residual hepatic hemangioma tissue after RFA does not necessarily need a prompt further treatment due to the slow tumor progression and the inability to metastasize.

The main disadvantage, especially for giant hepatic hemangiomas with diameter more than 10 cm, is their generous blood supply which is responsible for hemolysis and subsequent hemoglobinuria, hemolytic jaundice, anemia, and, in severe cases, renal damage [70].

Hepatocellular Adenoma (HCA) HCA is a benign liver tumor histologically characterized by closely approximated cords of hepatocytes which have vacuolated sinusoidal borders. They are usually solitary nodules variable in size. HCA occurs primarily in young women; it is associated with oral contraceptive use, diabetes, and type 1 glycogen and can develop during pregnancy. Treatment is recommended in selected patients due to the risk of life-threatening hemorrhage and malignant transformation [40]. TAE and RFA are less invasive therapeutic options than surgical resection, which remains the gold standard treatment. Usually percutaneous RFA for HCA is performed in children [72, 73] and adults [76, 77] under ultrasonographic guidance. Most HCAs show hypoechoic pattern at ultrasound. RFA can be performed safely with a good local tumor control and low morbidity. In case of liver adenomatosis, RFA can have an important role as concurrent treatment with surgical resection [78]. As limit, RFA is not able to make large-volume ablations in a single session.

Focal Nodular Hyperplasia (FNH) FNH is a hypervascular benign nodule with a typical central scar corresponding to a central feeding artery [33]. It can be rarely treated with RFA, in case of symptomatic, unresectable nodule [74].

21.2.2 Technical Aspects

Image-guided percutaneous RFA is a minimally invasive, relative low-risk procedure for the treatment of malignant and benign liver tumors. Local recurrence and survival rate depend on complete ablation of the entire tumor including a sufficient margin of surrounding healthy tissue. Currently a variety of different RFA devices are available. Tumors may currently be approached either via use of an expandable needle electrode that deploys multiple hooks into a lesion or via a straight-tip internally cooled electrode. In RFA, the high-frequency alternating current from the electrode generates marked agitation of the ions in the tissue that surrounds the uninsulated tip of the probe. The frictional heat results in thermal coagulation necrosis of the surrounding tissue. The size of ablation correlates with the intensity and duration of energy deposition. In order to achieve an effective heating throughout the tumor, a temperature of 60–100 °C has to be maintained throughout the entire target volume at least for 4–6 min, but the duration of application may increase to 10–30 min. The flow of current and heat absorption depend on tissue characteristics and perfusion [79]. Thus, the coagulation size may be increased by reduction of the hepatic perfusion during RFA by temporary occlusion of the portal vein or the hepatic artery [80, 81]. Another key component for successful tissue destruction involves the technique of overlapping ablations, as, for example, in RFA treatment of giant hepatic cavernous hemangioma. Treatment of even larger lesions may be attempted via creation of spherical zones of overlapped ablation to create a cylinder ("thermal cylinders"). These cylinders are then overlapped to systematically ablate a larger tumor [82]. Differently from HCC, in the RFA of HCA, the ablation zone can be limited to the nodule without extending to the surrounding healthy hepatic tissue. Accurate planning and execution of RFA according to the size and geometry of the tumor is essential. In order to minimize complications, individualized treatment strategies may be necessary for tumors close to vital structures [83].

Liver tumor RFA can be carried out by a percutaneous, laparoscopic, or laparotomic approach. The guidance system is generally represented by ultrasound [84] (Fig. 21.8). In case of unsatisfactory sonographic window, recent alternatives to ultrasound guidance are CEUS [85] and CT fusion-imaging guidance [86, 87]. CEUS, CT, and MR examinations are the most sensitive test for assessing therapeutic results [88].

Percutaneous RFA can be performed with local anesthesia and mild sedation; deep sedation or general anesthesia is also used. The skin is pricked with a small lancet, and the active electrode needle tip is introduced into the tumor under imaging guidance. The access is intercostal or subcostal. If an expandable electrode is used, the hooks are deployed after needle placement and retracted before withdrawing it. If a cooled electrode is employed, the pump is switched on, and chilled sterile

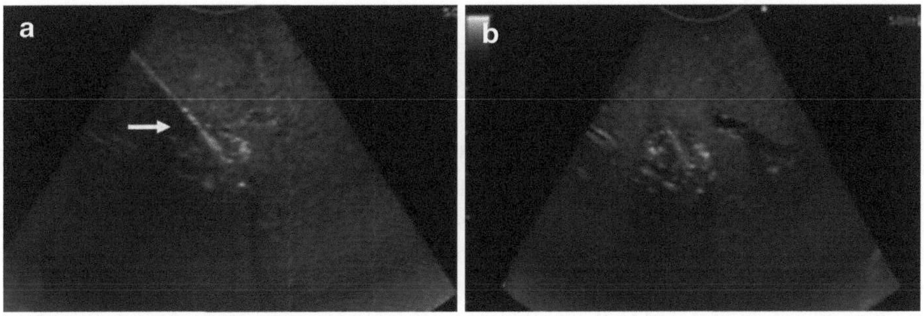

Fig. 21.8 US-guided radiofrequency ablation of a small HCA. (**a**) The needle tip (*arrow*) is in the center of the lesion to be ablated. (**b**) Ablation in progress: tumor and surrounding tissue are going through tissue necrosis and coagulation. As the tissue is undergoing severe heat conditions, the bleeding vessels are seared, and microbubble formation appears as a hyperechoic cloud around the needle tip

saline circulates through the needle. At the end of the procedure, the RFA generator is reactivated to obtain a hot withdrawal so as to prevent oozing and tumor seeding. For RFA of very large tumor as giant hepatic cavernous hemangiomas with diameter more than 10 cm, the application of bipolar RFA can be useful to obtain a significant shrinkage of the mass: an important disadvantage of the bipolar RFA system is the relative unsafeness of the percutaneous approach (asymmetrical axis of 8 × 14 gauge instead of the traditional 15–18 gauge) which makes an open approach preferable [89].

In addition to size, tumor location is one of the most important factors influencing efficacy and complication rate of RFA. For example, if the tumor lies in the subcapsular area, no safety margin along the capsule is possible. In addition tumor in the central zone of the liver near the hepatic hilum is almost always surrounded by large vessels that, because of the heat-sink effect of flowing blood, make it difficult to ablate the periphery of the tumor and the cuff of normal hepatic tissue [82]. In these situations, which can potentially contraindicate RFA, different strategies are needed to obtain successful treatment and minimize complications, for example, the creation of an artificial ascites with saline solution local injection before RFA of a subcapsular lesion [90].

21.2.3 Complications

Complications of RFA can be classified in two general categories: those related to imaging-guided electrode placement and those related to thermal treatment itself [60]. Complications in both categories can be major or minor. A major complication, as defined by Society of Interventional Radiology, is any post RFA complication that (a) requires therapy with minor hospitalization (<48 h); (b) requires major therapy, an unplanned increase in the level of care, or prolonged hospitalization (>48 h); (c) results in permanent adverse sequelae; or (d) leads to death [91]. All other complications are considered minor and include anything that either (a) does not require therapy or (b) requires nominal therapy, with overnight admission for observation only. In a large study of 3,554 treated hepatic tumors, Livraghi et al. [92] reported major complications in 2.2 % of cases and minor complications in less than 5 % of cases, with a death rate of 0.3 %.

Complications related to imaging-guided electrode placement are the following: intraperitoneal or intrahepatic bleeding; vascular complications, including arteriovenous fistula, pseudoaneurysm, thrombosis, stenosis, and infarction; pneumothorax; hemobilia; and grounding pad burns.

Complications related to thermal treatment include injury to nontarget organs as bowel, gallbladder, bile ducts, and diaphragm.

Other eventual complications are represented by infection, postablation syndrome, fulminant liver failure, tumor seeding, and treatment failure.

Bleeding, often self-limiting, represents one of the most common complications and occasionally can require endovascular or surgical management, in case of hemodynamic instability of the patient.

Another common complication of RFA liver ablation is infection which can vary from a transient postablation fever to intrahepatic abscess or fluid collections managed with antibiotics and percutaneous drainages. A high-risk factor for septic complication due to ascending bile duct colonization seems to be represented by previous biliary surgery with hepaticojejunostomy or sphincterectomy: in this situation, an antibiotic prophylaxis is mandatory.

Postablation syndrome is defined as a combination of flulike symptoms, including fever, malaise, pain at the ablation side, nausea, and vomiting [93, 94].

References

1. Anderson SW, Kruskal JB, Kane RA (2009) Benign hepatic tumors and iatrogenic pseudotumors. Radiographics 29:211–229
2. Shimoji K, Shiraishi R, Kuwatsuru A et al (2004) Spontaneous subacute intratumoral hemorrhage of hepatic cavernous hemangioma. Abdom Imaging 29:443–445
3. Bieze M, Phoa SS, Verheij J et al (2014) Risk factors for bleeding in hepatocellular adenoma. Br J Surg 101:847–855
4. Ihara K, Naito S, Yamaguchi W et al (2014) Hepatic cyst infection in an autosomal dominant polycystic kidney disease patient diagnosed by right pleural effusion. Intern Med 53:1355–1359
5. Zahmatkeshan M, Bahador A, Geramizade B et al (2012) Liver transplantation for Caroli disease. Int J Organ Transplant Med 3:189–191
6. Morgan DE, Lockhart ME, Canon CL et al (2006) Polycystic liver disease: multimodality imaging for complications and transplant evaluation. Radiographics 26:1655–1668
7. Farges O, Dokmak S (2010) Malignant transformation of liver adenoma: an analysis of the literature. Dig Surg 27:32–38
8. Kubota E, Katsumi K, Iida M et al (2003) Biliary cystadenocarcinoma followed up as benign cystadenoma for 10 years. J Gastroenterol 38:278–282
9. Totkas S, Hohenberger P (2000) Cholangiocellular carcinoma associated with segmental Caroli's disease. Eur J Surg Oncol 26:520–521

10. Yoshimitsu K (2014) Transarterial chemoembolization using iodized oil for unresectable hepatocellular carcinoma: perspective from multistep hepatocarcinogenesis. Hepat Med 6:89–94
11. Gruber-Rouh T, Naguib NN, Eichler K et al (2014) Transarterial chemoembolization of unresectable systemic chemotherapy-refractory liver metastases from colorectal cancer: long-term results over a 10-year period. Int J Cancer 134:1225–1231
12. Venturini M, Pilla L, Agostini G et al (2012) Transarterial chemoembolization with drug-eluting beads preloaded with irinotecan as a first-line approach in uveal melanoma liver metastases: tumor response and predictive value of diffusion-weighted MR imaging in five patients. J Vasc Interv Radiol 23:937–941
13. Madoff DC, Hicks ME, Vauthey JN et al (2002) Transhepatic portal vein embolization: anatomy, indications, and technical considerations. Radiographics 22:1063–1076
14. Kretschmar O, Knirsch W, Bernet V (2008) Interventional treatment of a symptomatic neonatal hepatic cavernous hemangioma using the Amplatzer vascular plug. Cardiovasc Intervent Radiol 31:411–414
15. Ishack KG, Rabin L (1975) Benign tumors of the liver. Med Clin North Am 59:995–1013
16. Xu HX, Liu GJ, Lu MD et al (2006) Characterization of small focal liver lesions using real-time contrast-enhanced sonography: diagnostic performance analysis in 200 patients. J Ultrasound Med 25:349–361
17. Taitelbaum G, Hinchey EJ, Herba MJ et al (1982) Giant hemangioma of the liver. Can J Surg 25:652–654
18. Malagari K, Alexopoulou E, Dourakis S et al (2007) Transarterial embolization of giant liver hemangiomas associated with Kasabach-Merritt syndrome: a case report. Acta Radiol 48:608–612
19. Jr MA, Papaiordanou F, Gonçalves JM et al (2010) Spontaneous rupture of hepatic hemangiomas. A review of the literature. World J Hepatol 2:428–433
20. Griffa B, Basilico V, Bellotti R et al (2005) Spontaneous rupture of giant subcapsular hemangioma of the liver with hemoperitoneum and hemorrhagic shock: a case report. Chir Ital 57:389–392
21. Schmitz R, Heinig J, Klockenbusch W et al (2009) Antenatal diagnosis of a giant fetal hepatic hemangioma and treatment with maternal corticosteroid. Ultraschall Med 30:223–226
22. Biswal BM, Sandhu M, Lal P et al (1995) Role of radiotherapy in cavernous hemangioma liver. Indian J Gastroenterol 14:95–98
23. Choi J, Lee YJ, Hwang DW et al (2011) Surgical treatment of giant hepatic hemangiomas: technical point of view. Am Surg 77:48–54
24. Peveretos P, Panoussopoulos D (1986) Giant cavernous hepatic hemangioma: treatment by ligation of the hepatic artery. J Surg Oncol 31:48–51
25. Komatsu S, Iwasaki T, Demizu Y et al (2014) Two-stage treatment with hepatectomy and carbon-ion radiotherapy for multiple hepatic epithelioid hemangioendotheliomas. World J Gastroenterol 20:8729–8735
26. Stratte EG, Tope WD, Johnson CL et al (1996) Multimodal management of diffuse neonatal hemangiomatosis. J Am Acad Dermatol 34:337–342
27. Jain V, Ramachandran V, Garg R et al (2010) Spontaneous rupture of a giant hepatic hemangioma – sequential management with transcatheter arterial embolization and resection. Saudi J Gastroenterol 16:116–119
28. Srivastava DN, Gandhi D, Seith A et al (2001) Transcatheter arterial embolization in the treatment of symptomatic cavernous hemangiomas of the liver: a prospective study. Abdom Imaging 26:510–514
29. Suzuki H, Nimura Y, Kamiya J et al (1997) Preoperative transcatheter arterial embolization for giant cavernous hemangioma of the liver with consumption coagulopathy. Am J Gastroenterol 92:688–691
30. Yamashita S, Okita K, Harada K et al (2013) Giant cavernous hepatic hemangioma shrunk by use of sorafenib. Clin J Gastroenterol 6:55–62
31. Wanless IR, Mawdsley C, Adams R (1985) On the pathogenesis of focal nodular hyperplasia of the liver. Hepatology 5:1194–2000

32. Nagorney DM (1995) Benign hepatic tumors: focal nodular hyperplasia and hepatocellular adenoma. World J Surg 19:13–18
33. Dohan A, Soyer P, Guerrache Y et al (2014) Focal nodular hyperplasia of the liver: diffusion-weighted magnetic resonance imaging characteristics using high b values. J Comput Assist Tomogr 38:96–104
34. Weimann A, Ringe B, Klempnauer J et al (1997) Benign liver tumors: differential diagnosis and indications for surgery. World J Surg 21:983–990
35. Ortega G, Price M, Choo S et al (2013) Multidisciplinary management of focal nodular hyperplasia in children: experience with 10 cases. JAMA Surg 148:1068–1070
36. Perrakis A, Demir R, Müller V et al (2012) Management of the focal nodular hyperplasia of the liver: evaluation of the surgical treatment comparing with observation only. Am J Surg 204:689–696
37. Demarco MP, Shen P, Bradley RF et al (2006) Intraperitoneal hemorrhage in a patient with hepatic focal nodular hyperplasia. Am Surg 72:555–559
38. Birn J, Williams TR, Croteau D et al (2013) Transarterial embolization of symptomatic focal nodular hyperplasia. J Vasc Interv Radiol 24:1647–1655
39. Vogl TJ, Own A, Hammerstingl R et al (2006) Transarterial embolization as a therapeutic option for focal nodular hyperplasia in four patients. Eur Radiol 16:670–675
40. Deneve JL, Pawlik TM, Cunningham S et al (2009) Liver cell adenoma: a multicenter analysis of risk factors for rupture and malignancy. Ann Surg Oncol 16:640–648
41. Agrawal S, Agarwal S, Arnason T et al (2014) Management of hepatocellular adenoma: recent advances. Clin Gastroenterol Hepatol. doi:10.1016/j.cgh.2014.05.023
42. Stoot JH, van der Linden E, Terpstra OT et al (2007) Life-saving therapy for haemorrhaging liver adenomas using selective arterial embolization. Br J Surg 94:1249–1253
43. Deodhar A, Brody LA, Covey AM et al (2011) Bland embolization in the treatment of hepatic adenomas: preliminary experience. J Vasc Interv Radiol 22:795–799
44. Lee SH, Hahn ST (2004) Treatment of multiple hepatic adenomatosis using transarterial chemoembolization: a case report. Cardiovasc Intervent Radiol 27:563–565
45. Kim YI, Chung JW, Park JH (2007) Feasibility of transcatheter arterial chemoembolization for hepatic adenoma. J Vasc Interv Radiol 18:862–867
46. Drenth JP, Chrispijn M, Nagorney DM et al (2010) Medical and surgical treatment options for polycystic liver disease. Hepatology 52:2223–2230
47. Wang MQ, Duan F, Liu FY et al (2013) Treatment of symptomatic polycystic liver disease: transcatheter super-selective hepatic arterial embolization using a mixture of NBCA and iodized oil. Abdom Imaging 38:465–473
48. van Keimpema L, Drenth JP (2013) Polycystic liver disease: a critical appraisal of hepatic resection, cyst fenestration, and liver transplantation. Ann Surg 253:419–420
49. Temple M, Marshalleck FE (eds) (2014) Pediatric interventional radiology: 177 handbook of vascular and non-vascular interventions. Springer, New York. doi:10.1007/978-1-4419-5856-3_14
50. Terkivatan T, Hussain SM, Lameris JS et al (2002) Transcatheter arterial embolization as a safe and effective treatment for focal nodular hyperplasia of the liver. Cardiovasc Intervent Radiol 25:450–453
51. Vassiou K, Rountas H, Liakou P et al (2007) Embolization of a giant hepatic hemangioma prior to urgent liver resection. Case report and review of the literature. Cardiovasc Intervent Radiol 30:800–802
52. Giavroglou C, Economou H, Ioannidis I (2003) Arterial embolization of giant hepatic hemangiomas. Cardiovasc Intervent Radiol 26:92–96
53. Erdogan D, van Delden OM, Busch OR et al (2007) Selective transcatheter arterial embolization for treatment of bleeding complications or reduction of tumor mass of hepatocellular adenomas. Cardiovasc Intervent Radiol 30:1252–1258
54. Hoshino J, Ubara Y, Suwabe T et al (2014) Intravascular embolization therapy in patients with enlarged polycystic liver. Am J Kidney Dis 63:937–944
55. Althaus S, Ashdown B, Coldwell D et al (1996) Transcatheter arterial embolization of two symptomatic giant cavernous hemangiomas of the liver. Cardiovasc Intervent Radiol 19:364–367

56. de Baère T, Roche A, Amenabar JM et al (1996) Liver abscess formation after local treatment of liver tumors. Hepatology 23:1436–1440
57. Huang XQ, Huang ZQ, Duan WD et al (2002) Severe biliary complications after hepatic artery embolization. World J Gastroenterol 8:119–123
58. Miller FJ Jr, Mineau DE (1983) Transcatheter arterial embolization of major complications and their prevention. Cardiovasc Intervent Radiol 6:141–149
59. Goldberg SN, Grassi CJ, Cardella JF et al (2009) Image-guided tumor ablation: standardization of terminology and reporting criteria. J Vasc Interv Radiol 20:S377–S390
60. Mendiratta-Lala M, Brook OR, Midkiff BD et al (2010) Strategies for anticipating and reducing complications and treatment failures in hepatic radiofrequency ablation. Radiographics 30:1107–1122
61. Solbiati L, Livraghi T, Goldberg SN et al (2001) Percutaneous radio-frequency ablation of hepatic metastases from colorectal cancer: long term results in 117 patients. Radiology 221:159–166
62. Tateishi R, Shiina S, Teratani T (2005) Percutaneous radiofrequency ablation of hepatocellular carcinoma: an analysis in 1000 cases. Cancer 103:1201–1209
63. Kim Y, Rhim H, Lim HK et al (2011) Coagulation necrosis induced by radiofrequency ablation in the liver: histopathologic and radiologic review of usual to extremely rare changes. Radiographics 31(2):377–390
64. Houghton Mifflin Harcourt. American Heritage medical dictionary. Houghton Mifflin Company (2010) Boston
65. Ng KK, Lam CM, Poon RT et al (2005) Porcine liver: morphologic characteristics and cell viability at experimental radiofrequency ablation with internally cooled electrodes. Radiology 235:478–486
66. Livraghi T, Meloni F, Di Stasi M et al (2008) Sustained complete response and complications rates after radiofrequency ablation of very early hepatocellular carcinoma in cirrhosis: is resection still the treatment of choice? Hepatology 47:82–89
67. Gomez FM, Patel PA, Stuart S et al (2014) Systematic review of ablation techniques for the treatment of malignant or aggressive benign lesions in children. Pediatr Radiol. doi:10.1007/s00247-014-3001-5
68. Fan RF, Chai FL, Xe GX et al (2006) Laparoscopic radiofrequency ablation of hepatic cavernous hemangioma. A preliminary experience with 27 patients. Surg Endosc 20:281–285
69. Park SY, Tak WY, Jung MK et al (2011) Symptomatic-enlarging hepatic hemangiomas are effectively treated by percutaneous ultrasonography-guided radiofrequency ablation. J Hepatol 54:559–565
70. Gao J, Ke S, Ding X et al (2013) Radiofrequency ablation for large hepatic hemangioma: initial experience and lessons. Surgery. doi:10.1016/j.surg.2012.06.004
71. Cui Y, Zhou LY, Dong MK et al (2003) Ultrasonography guided percutaneous radiofrequency ablation for hepatic cavernous hemangioma. World J Gastroenterol 9:2132–2134
72. Rocourt DV, Shiels WE, Hammond S et al (2006) Contemporary management of hepatic adenoma using percutaneous radiofrequency ablation. J Pediatr Surg 41:1149–1152
73. Mc Daniel JD, Kukreja K, Ristagno RL et al (2013) Radiofrequency ablation of a large hepatic adenoma in a child. J Pediatr Surg 48:E19–E22
74. Hedyati P, Van Sonnemberg E, Shamos R et al (2010) Treatment of symptomatic focal nodular hyperplasia with percutaneous radiofrequency ablation. J Vasc Interv Radiol 21: 582–585
75. Corigliano N, Mercantini P, Amodio PM et al (2003) Hemoperitoneum from a spontaneous rupture of a giant hemangioma of the liver: report of a case. Surg Today 33:459–463
76. Atwell TD, Brandhagen DJ, Charboneau JW et al (2005) Successful treatment of hepatocellular adenoma using percutaneous radiofrequency ablation. Am J Roentgenol 84:828–831
77. Rhim H, Lim HK, Kim Y et al (2007) Percutaneous radiofrequency ablation of hepatocellular adenoma: initial experience in 10 patients. J Gastroenterol Hepatol 23:e422–e427
78. Fugita S, Kushihata E, Herrmann G et al (2006) Combined hepatic resection and radiofrequency ablation for multiple hepatic adenomas. J Gastroenterol Hepatol 12(8):1351–1354.

79. Venkatesan AM, Gervais DA, Mueller PR (2006) Percutaneous radiofrequency thermal ablation of primary and metastatic hepatic tumors: current concepts and review of the literature. Semin Intervent Radiol 23:73–84
80. Rossi S, Garbagnati F, Lencioni R et al (2000) Percutaneous radiofrequency thermal ablation of nonresectable hepatocellular carcinoma after occlusion of tumor blood supply. Radiology 217:119–126
81. Yamasaki T, Kurokawa F, Shirahashi H et al (2002) Percutaneous radiofrequency ablation therapy for patients with hepatocellular carcinoma during occlusion of hepatic blood flow. Comparison with standard percutaneous radiofrequency ablation therapy. Cancer 95:2353–2360
82. Rhim H, Goldberg SN, Dodd GD et al (2001) Essential techniques for successful radiofrequency thermal ablation of malignant hepatic tumors. Radiographics 21:S17–S35; discussion S36–S39
83. Widmann G, Bodner G, Bale R (2009) Tumor ablation: technical aspects. Cancer Imaging 9:S63–S67
84. Buscarini E, Savoia A, Brambilla G et al (2005) Radiofrequency thermal ablation of liver tumors. Eur Radiol 15:884–894
85. Dong Y, Wang WP, Gan YH et al (2014) Radiofrequency ablation guided by contrast-enhanced ultrasound for hepatic malignancies: preliminary results. Clin Radiol. doi:10.1016/j.crad.2014.06.016
86. Xu ZF, Xie XY, Kuang M et al (2014) Percutaneous radiofrequency ablation of malignant liver tumors with ultrasound and CT fusion imaging guidance. J Clin Ultrasound 42:321–330
87. Song KD, Lee MW, Rhim H et al (2013) Fusion imaging-guided radiofrequency ablation for hepatocellular carcinomas not visible on conventional ultrasound. Am J Roentgenol 201:1141–1147
88. Minami Y, Nishida N, Kudo M (2014) Therapeutic response assessment of RFA for HCC: contrast-enhanced US, CT and MRI. World J Gastroenterol 20:4160–4166
89. Van Tilborg AA, Nielsen K, Scheffer HJ et al (2013) Bipolar radiofrequency ablation for symptomatic giant (>10 cm) hepatic cavernous haemangiomas: initial clinical experience. Clin Radiol 68:e9–e14
90. Kang TW, Lim HK, Lee MW et al (2013) First-line radiofrequency ablation with or without artificial ascites for hepatocellular carcinomas in a subcapsular location: local control rate and risk of peritoneal seeding at long-term follow-up. Clin Radiol 68:e641–e651
91. Sacks D, McClenny TE, Cardella JF et al (2003) Society of Interventional Radiology clinical practice guidelines. J Vasc Interv Radiol 14:S199–S202
92. Livraghi T, Solbiati L, Meloni MF et al (2003) Treatment of focal liver tumors with radiofrequency ablation: complications encountered in a multicenter study. Radiology 226:441–451
93. Wah TM, Arellano RS, Gervais DA et al (2005) Image-guided percutaneous radiofrequency ablation and incidence of post-radiofrequency ablation syndrome: prospective survey. Radiology 237:1097–1102
94. Dodd GD 3rd, Napier D, Schoolfield JD et al (2005) Percutaneous radiofrequency ablation of hepatic tumors: postablation syndrome. Am J Roentgenol 185:51–57

Intraoperative Ultrasound in Liver Surgery for Benign Tumors

22

Fabio Procopio and Guido Torzilli

22.1 Introduction

Intraoperative ultrasound (IOUS) has gained an important role in liver surgery, becoming mandatory in the clinical practice of the hepatic surgeon: it plays a relevant role in providing additional diagnostic elements as lesion characterization, anatomical details, and more accurate staging of disease. Based on these findings, IOUS is central for establishing the surgical strategy.

On the other hand, the role of IOUS in diagnosing benign liver lesions is marginal since the indication for surgery in such patients is limited [1, 2]. Indeed, many of these lesions are asymptomatic and do not grow and/or degenerate so that they do not need surgery; advances in imaging modalities as well as progress in immunohistochemistry have greatly improved the accurate recognition of these lesions [3]. However, IOUS not rarely faces with lesions discovered intraoperatively or lesions which coexist with malignancies and for which should be in differentiated form. Furthermore, in those patients with benign tumors, surgery plays a crucial role for their removal in a parenchyma-sparing fashion.

22.2 Technical Equipment

High-frequency probes (7.5–10 MHz) are generally recommended in the IOUS application since they allow a higher spatial resolution than those working at lower frequencies (2.5–5 MHz). However, these last warrantee more panoramicity.

F. Procopio • G. Torzilli (✉)
Department of Hepatobiliary and General Surgery, Humanitas Research Hospital, University of Milan-School of Medicine, via Manzoni, 56, 20089 Rozzano, Milan
e-mail: guido.torzilli@humanitas.it

L. Aldrighetti et al. (eds.), *Benign Tumors of the Liver*,
DOI 10.1007/978-3-319-12985-3_22

Different shapes of probes are available for intraoperative use: linear T-shaped probe, interdigital probe, microconvex probe, and, more recently, T-shaped probes with trapezoid scanning window. The optimal probe, however, is the one that ensures the best compromise between the volume, which should be minimal to allow an easy handling, the scanning window, which should be largest to provide a widest area in a single view, and the stability once in contact with liver surface. Microconvex probes and linear probes with trapezoid scanning represent the optimal solutions (Fig. 22.1).

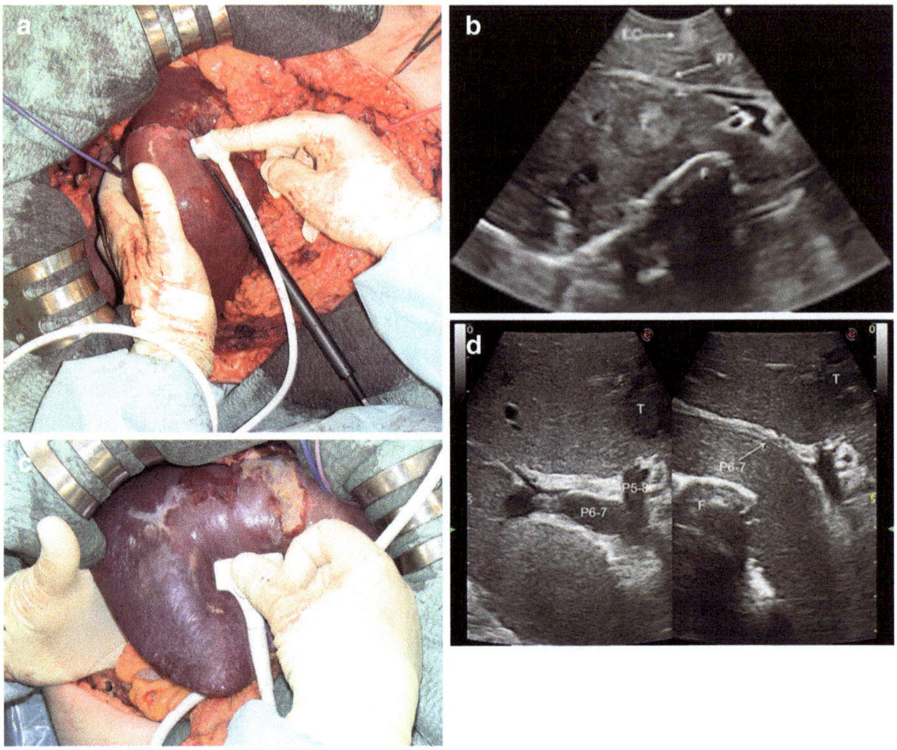

Fig. 22.1 (**a**, **b**) The microconvex probe handled by the surgeon during resection area demarcation and the corresponding ultrasound imaging with a large scanning window, (**c**, **d**) a new T-shaped probe with trapezoid scanning window designed by the surgeon to be easily handled and to allow surgical maneuvers, electrocautery (*EC*), tumor (*T*), finger (*F*), portal branch to the segment 7 (*P7*), portal branch to the right posterior section (*P6-7*), portal branch to the right anterior section (*P5-8*)

22.3 Technical Tricks of Liver Exploration

The ultrasound machine should be placed in front of the first operator with the aim to simultaneously check the screen and the operation field. The screen must be large enough for an optimal visibility at that distance, and the assistants should then control the machine's keyboard that can be covered with a sterile drape. The liver exploration should always start with the inspection and palpation of the entire peritoneal cavity: this should not be avoided even with IOUS because inspection and palpation still play a relevant role [4]. Liver mobilization starts with the division of the round and falciform ligaments as well as of adhesions to free the liver surfaces in order to get enough space for handling of the probes for exploration by IOUS. Thus, pulling the round ligament, the liver surface is widely exposed, and following the examination of the portal branches and hepatic veins, the whole liver can be studied.

22.4 Diagnosis and Staging of Benign Lesion

The two main targets of IOUS explorations are represented by detection and differentiation. Particular attention has to be paid in those patients with multinodular malignant disease in which some benign lesions could be misdiagnosed as part of the neoplastic involvement or in those patients who are going to be resected for liver neoplasms which at preoperative imaging resulted as carrier of benign lesions which have to be confirmed intraoperatively as really benign.

Proper interpretation of the echo pattern of a lesion is of paramount importance. Simple hepatic cysts are frequently encountered, and they appear typically as well-defined anechoic (black) lesion, with very tiny or unapparent wall, and a posterior acoustic shadow which exists also when they are very small (Fig. 22.2). Inversely, this phenomenon is absent if the lesion is a solid one as in the case of tiny liver

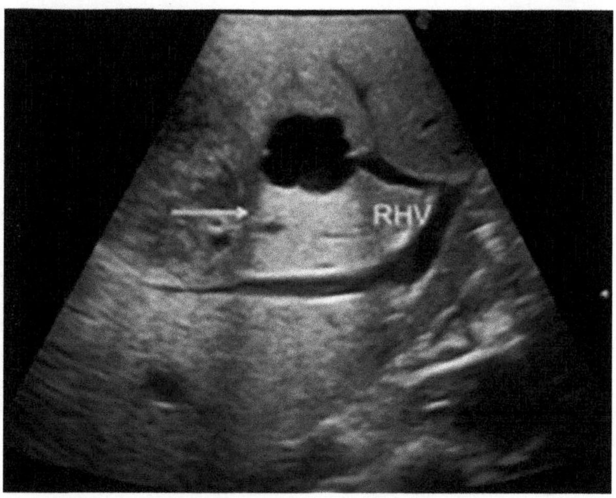

Fig. 22.2 Ultrasound appearance of a simple hepatic cyst with anechoic content and its posterior wall echo (*arrow*), right hepatic vein (*RHV*)

metastasis (Fig. 22.3). However, it should be noted that the misinterpretation may result if the IOUS image is not properly set and in particular the gain and the focus are not correctly adjusted. Therefore, the gain of the gray scale should not be too high, and the focus level should not be positioned distant from the level of the target; otherwise, a cystic lesion may appear as a solid one (Fig. 22.4).

Furthermore, occasionally the round ligament may be unexpectedly prominent, raising the suspicion of a solid hepatic mass appearing in a transverse scan as a hyperechoic target lesion: shifting to a sagittal scan helps in disclosing its linear shape (Fig. 22.5).

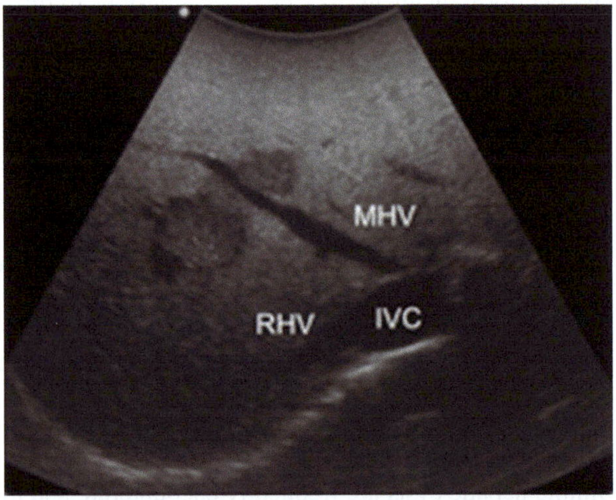

Fig. 22.3 Two small colorectal liver metastases with hypoechogenic pattern, right hepatic vein (*RHV*), middle hepatic vein (*MHV*), inferior vena cava (*IVC*)

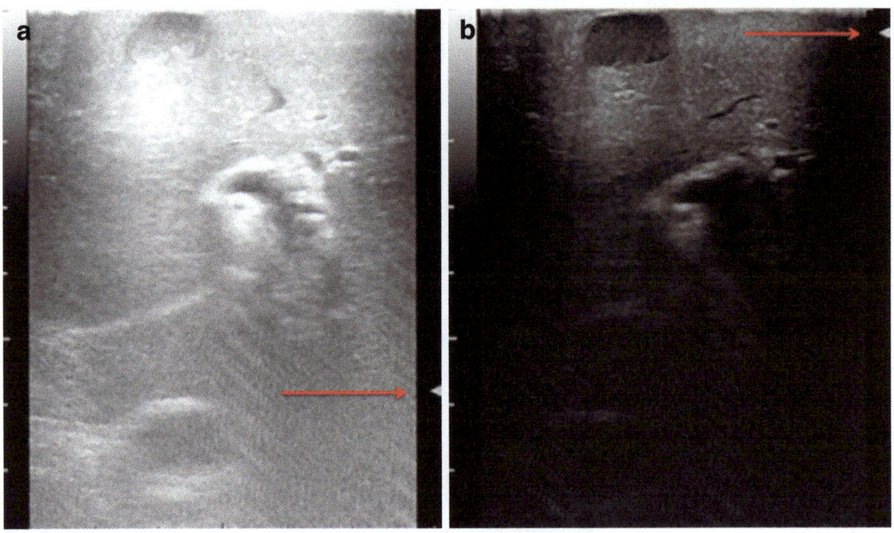

Fig. 22.4 (**a**) Example of ultrasound image not adequately set with focus (*arrow*) level incorrectly positioned (deep) in accordance to the lesion location (superficial) and with high gain regulation (high brightness level) where a typical hepatic cyst mimics a solid lesion, (**b**) the typical ultrasound appearance of the hepatic cyst is here revealed once the image equalization is adequately set and the focus correctly located based on the location of the target lesion

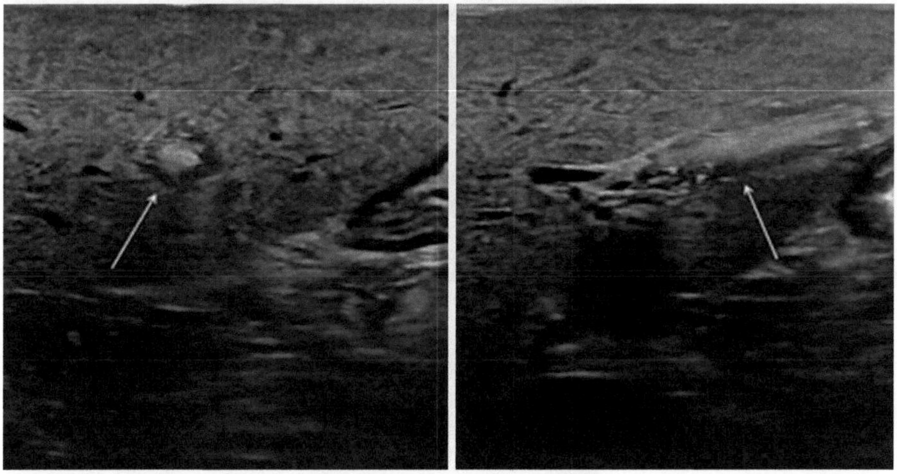

Fig. 22.5 (*left*) Particularly prominent round ligament (*arrow*) simulating an intrahepatic echogenic mass, (*right*) changing the transducer axis of the origin of the ligament from the umbilical portion and its linear shape is revealed

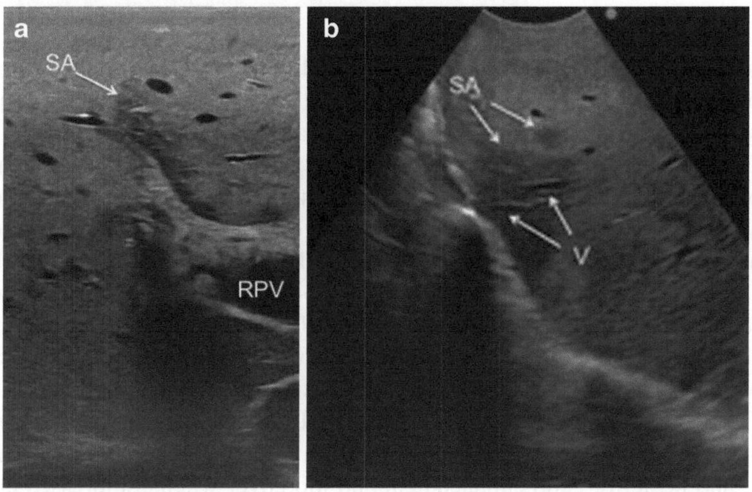

Fig. 22.6 Focal fatty infiltration area, also called "skip area," typically located around the main portal pedicles (**a**) and featured as irregularly shaped with vessels running through without structural distortion or interruption (**b**); skip area (*SA*), vessel (*V*), right portal vein (*RPV*)

A frequent source of misinterpretation is also represented by the focal steatosis areas, consisting in portions of the liver with localized accumulation of hepatocytes with abnormal distribution of cytoplasmatic lipid shell [5], resulting in areas with different echogenicity. In some cases this focal accumulation can assume a nodular shape which could be misleading. However, there are some features which should secure from misinterpretation: indeed, these areas are typically located around the gallbladder or around the main portal pedicles, have an irregular shape, and present vessels passing through without distortions (Fig. 22.6).

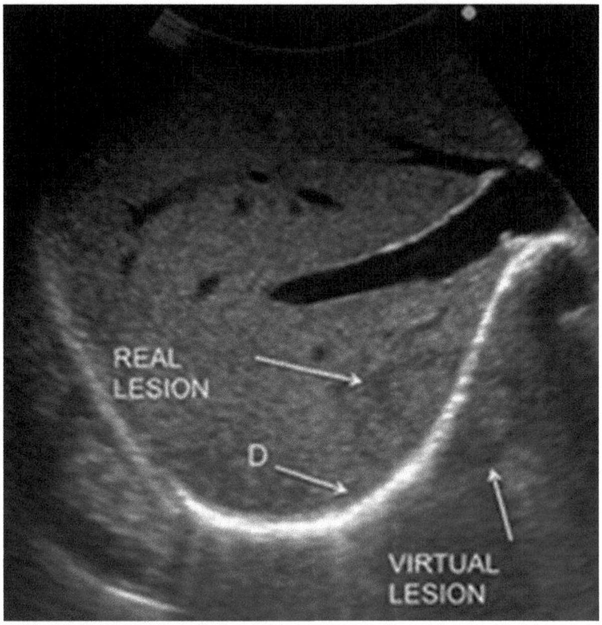

Fig. 22.7 Typical appearance of the so-called mirror effect obtained for a lesion just adjacent to the diaphragm in which a duplicated lesion is visualized; diaphragm (*D*)

Finally, there is an artifact being a true optical illusion which is called the mirror effect and can mimic an additional lesion generally outside the organ. This typically happens when a lesion is just superficial and adjacent to the diaphragm (Fig. 22.7).

IOUS allows the detection of new lesions in around 30 % of cirrhotic patients: most of the nodules, however, detected in these patients are nonneoplastic with thereby the risk of overestimating the tumor stage. Indeed, excluding those nodules with mosaic ultrasonographic patterns, typical of hepatocellular carcinoma (HCC), which are malignant in 84 % of cases, only 24–30 % of hypoechoic nodules and 0–18 % of those hyperechoic are malignant [6, 7]. To overcome this problem, even biopsy may not be adequate. The only nodule which can be easily differentiated intraoperatively from an HCC or a liver metastasis is the tiny hemangioma which is not infrequently encountered primarily during IOUS exploration: it has a typical ultrasonographic pattern including a uniform hyperechogenicity, well-defined margin, and posterior echo enhancement and moreover when compressed changes its size and shape (Fig. 22.8). This feature is based essentially on the different stiffness of the hemangioma compared to other lesions. Stiffness measurements are advantageous in this respect. Recently, intraoperative elastography has been applied to the clinical practice as promising imaging method for differential diagnosis of hepatic tumor. In fact, elastography can provide information about the lesion differentiation based on tissue elasticity expressed on the IOUS screen by differences in colors. As reported, some authors have introduced a classification for differentiating HCC from metastatic lesions based on their tissue elasticity at intraoperative elastography (Fig. 22.9) [8].

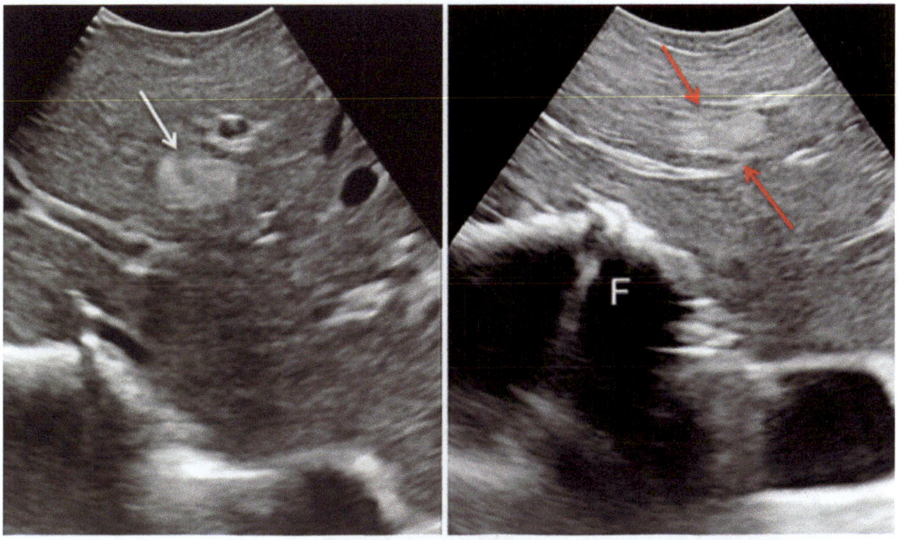

Fig. 22.8 (*left*) A hemangioma with typical uniform hyperechogenicity (arrow); (right) the diagnosis of hemangioma is here confirmed since once compressed under IOUS guidance, the lesion changes its shape and thickness (*arrows*); finger (*F*)

Focal lesions which liver surgeons now more frequently should need to address in patients affected by colorectal liver metastases are the focal nodular hyperplasia (FNH). FNH is a benign condition that occurs in normal liver with prevalence up to 3 %, as reported in autoptic studies [9, 10]. Recently, the extensive use of oxaliplatin-based systemic chemotherapy to treat patients who are carriers of colorectal cancer has been observed to be associated with the development of liver FNHs with a prevalence up to 15 % of the cases [11]. As reported, small FNHs arising during systemic treatment may have preoperative imaging appearance which overlaps with those of metastatic lesions [12]: in this way, the preoperative diagnostic modalities introduce the risk of overestimating the disease or postoperatively the incidence of recurrences in patients resected of CLM. Thus, IOUS exploration of the liver remains crucial. In this sense, if a strict parenchyma-sparing approach is attempted, the attention paid to discriminate eventual new lesions is probably more pronounced than in case of preference of a conventional surgical approach such as major or extended hepatectomy.

Indeed, larger FNH are less problematic for diagnosis because the capability of diagnostic imaging is higher, with proven sensitivity greater than 90 % [13, 14], in detecting the typical central scar which is distinctive of this liver entity. Sometimes, however, the central scar is so small in size to be easily detected by ultrasound (Fig. 22.10): the use of color Doppler, providing the presence of the central feeding artery, improves the detection and the characterization of this kind of lesion (Fig. 22.11).

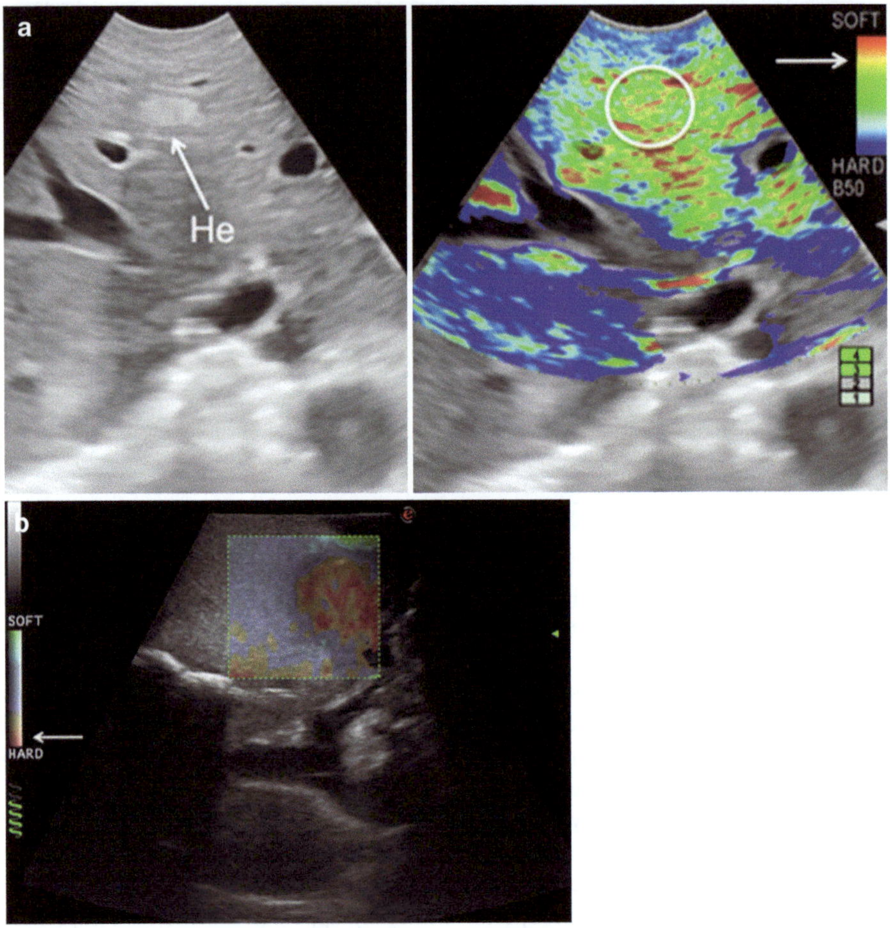

Fig. 22.9 (**a**) Comparison of elastogram (*right*) and B-mode ultrasound scan (*left*) in a patient with small hemangioma (*circle*): the real-time intraoperative elastography confirmed the lesion softness according to the color scale (*arrow*); (**b**) hardness of a colorectal liver metastasis is here confirmed by the real-time elastography based on its predominantly red color according to the color scale (*arrow*), hemangioma (*He*)

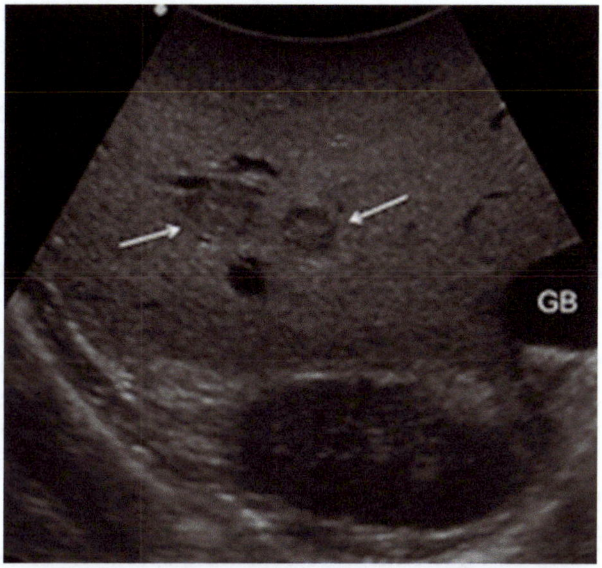

Fig. 22.10 Example of patient treated with oxaliplatin-based systemic chemotherapy with very small focal nodular hyperplasias (*arrows*) with an hypoechoic pattern and a central scar not detectable by IOUS which mimics a small liver metastasis; gallbladder (*GB*)

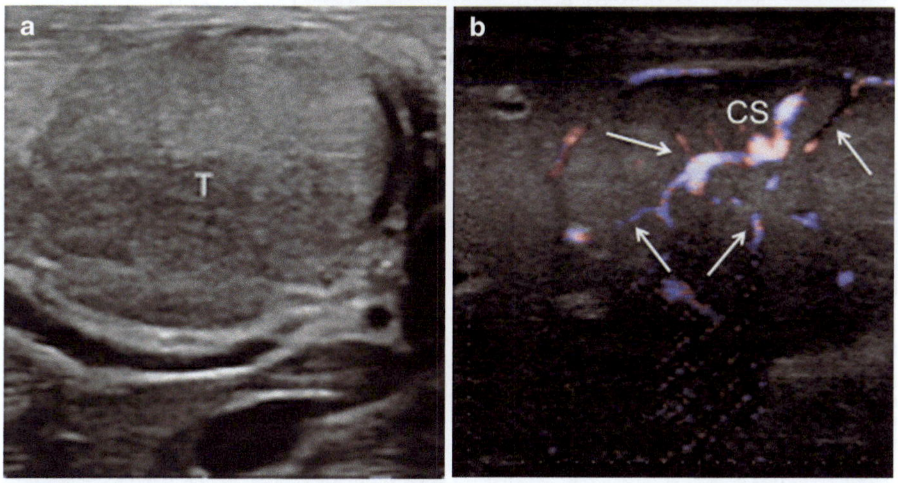

Fig. 22.11 (**a**) IOUS scan shows a inhomogeneous focal liver lesion, *tumor* (*T*); (**b**) color Doppler help to reveal the real nature of the FNH showing the typical spoke-wheel pattern (*arrows*) determined by vessels radiating from the vascularized central scar (*CS*)

22.5 Role of Contrast-Enhanced Intraoperative Ultrasound in Differential Diagnosis

IOUS's ability to recognize small new nodules is biased by the lesions' echogenicity compared to the echogenicity of the background liver (cirrhosis and steatosis).

However, this drawback has been limited by the introduction of contrast agents injected intravenously during ultrasound examination. We first introduced this new modality in the practice of the IOUS during liver surgery establishing its application for both HCC and CLM [15, 16].

The most adopted contrast agent in Europe is based on sulfur hexafluoride microbubbles stabilized by a phospholipid shell (SonoVue, Bracco Imaging, Milan, Italy). Recently, another contrast agent, but available only in Japan for clinical practice, has been introduced (Sonazoid, GE Healthcare, Norway). This new contrast agent provides a hepato-specific phase which may mimic the behavior of the hepato-specific contrast agents available for magnetic resonance imaging (MRI).

CEIOUS in general is used for characterizing new lesions initially detected by IOUS and helps in discriminating among regenerative or dysplastic nodules and HCC based on tumor vascularity and in detecting nodules not visible in IOUS in patients carriers of CLM.

For patients with HCC, we introduced a classification of the pattern of enhancement by CEIOUS [15]. Any lesion appearing as hypoechoic in the late phase and in arterial phase as fully enhanced prior to the surrounding liver parenchyma, or well-visualized inner vessels (Fig. 22.12): this nodule is considered with a pathologic behavior and therefore removed. In contrast, those lesions disappearing once the contrast enhances the liver parenchyma are considered nonneoplastic (i.e., regenerative and dysplastic nodule), and therefore they are not removed (Fig. 22.13). Based on these criteria we obtained a specificity of 69 % by CEIOUS for small lesions: this rate is encouraging as it means that we can provide proper information with this technique in seven out of ten lesions we detect at the time of laparotomy. For the remaining three, even histology may be lacking.

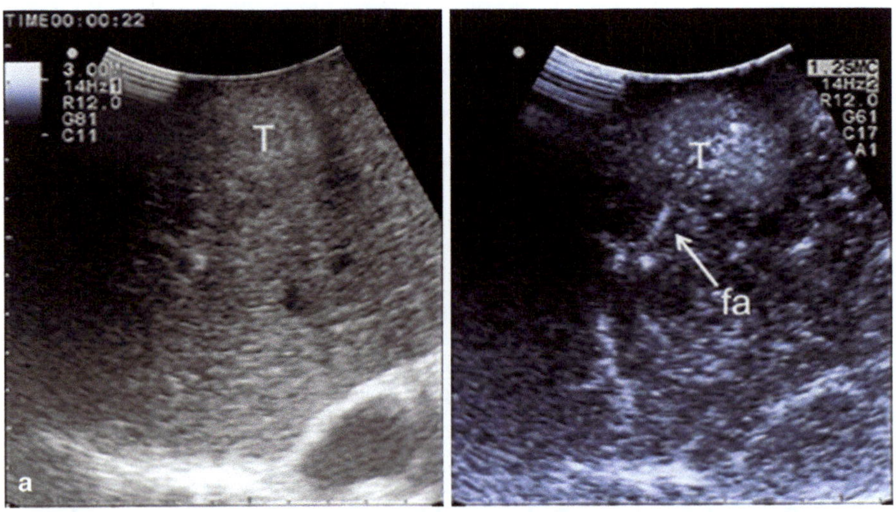

Fig. 22.12 (**a**) Typical pattern of HCC at CEIOUS in which the lesion uptakes the contrast before the surrounding liver parenchyma with nodular arterial enhancement; (**b**) the lesion is not completely enhanced in arterial phase but shows a pattern with a intranodular neoangiogenesis represented by inner vessels (arrows); (**c**) example of tiny lesion (*arrow*) which shows an atypical behavior at CEIOUS remaining hypoechoic in any phase (*circle*). Based on our criteria this lesion is considered malignant and removed; tumor (*T*), feeding artery (*FA*)

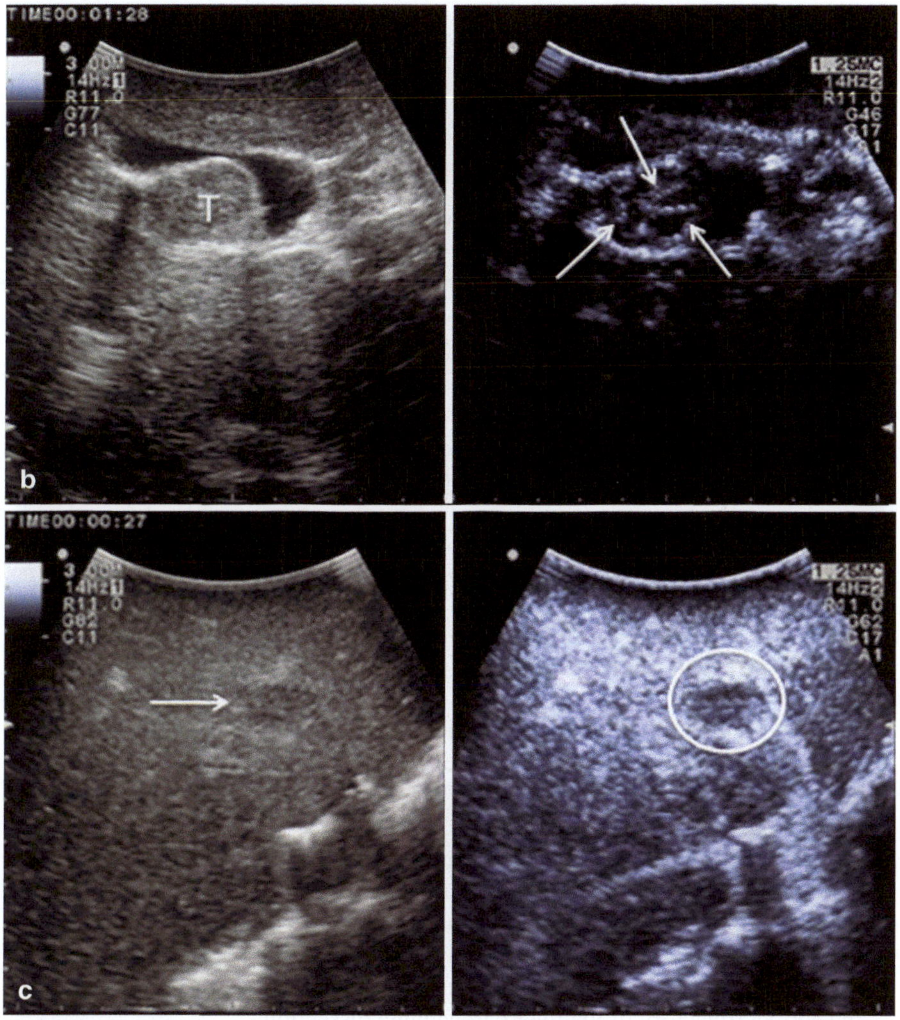

Fig. 22.12 (continued)

In patients who are carriers of CLM in a liver with cystic lesions, CEIOUS could be misleading if not preceded by a careful exploration with IOUS: indeed, cystic lesions may appear similar to metastatic ones during the delayed phases of contrast enhancement, then recognition and mapping has to be accomplished in the IOUS study. Therefore, any new lesions appearing as a "black hole" detected in a different positions from those previously mapped should be considered a potential new malignant lesion.

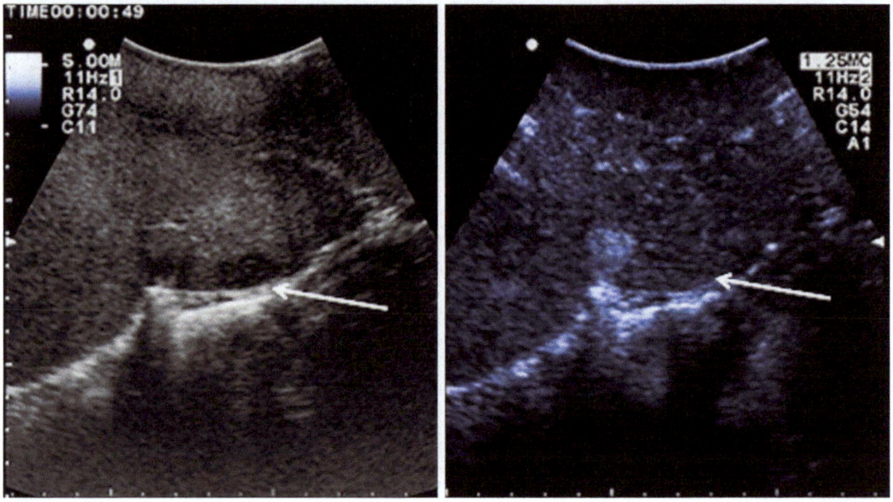

Fig. 22.13 In the delayed phase, the lesion (*arrow*) shows the same enhancement of the surrounding hepatic tissue becoming not clearly detectable. This lesion is not considered malignant and is not removed

22.6 Resection Guidance

As for IOUS-guided liver dissection done for liver malignancies, also for benign lesions undergoing surgery, two main steps can be recognized for an ultrasound-guided resection:

- Achievement of an adequate exposure of the surgical field implying adequate abdominal incision and liver mobilization for allowing proper maneuver both with the probe and the surgeon's left hand. The latter is used other than for sustaining or literally hanging the organ and limiting the blood loss, also as a landmark for keeping together with the information provided by the real-time IOUS, the correct trajectory of the liver parenchyma dissection.
- Proper IOUS-guided demarcation of the resection area.

Demarcation of the resective area for benign tumors can be accomplished in a non-anatomical fashion trying to maximize the parenchyma sparing. Anyway, also for limited resections, the IOUS guidance plays a fundamental role: indeed, although there is no need for identifying the area of the liver fed by the portal branch to be ligated, however, once the tumor is identified, the surgeon under IOUS control can relate the electrocautery positioned on the liver surface with the tumor edge and any eventual vascular structure close to the tumor itself drawing on the liver surface the optimal resection area to be confident of being able to remove the tumor and sparing the vessel he is planning to spare. To carry out this maneuver, the flat and thin tip of the electrocautery is positioned between the probe and the liver surface: this maneuver results in a shadow at the IOUS image which runs deeply just below the electrocautery (Fig. 22.14). Once marked on the liver surface, the adequacy of the marked

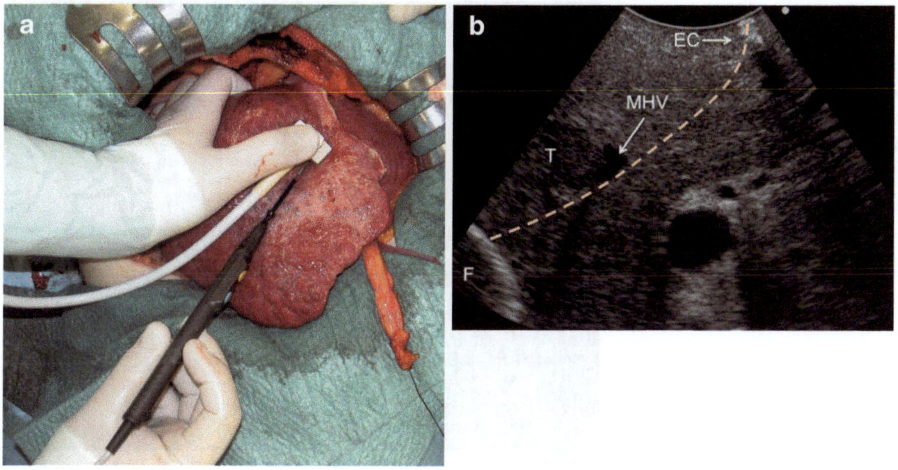

Fig. 22.14 (**a**) The surgeon's fingertip and the probe act simultaneously to draw the ideal dissection plane to be followed; (**b**) IOUS image showing the ideal plane connecting (*yellow dashed line*) the fingertip (*F*) and the shadow generated by the electrocautery (*EC*) interposed between the liver surface and the probe; middle hepatic vein (*MHV*), tumor (*T*)

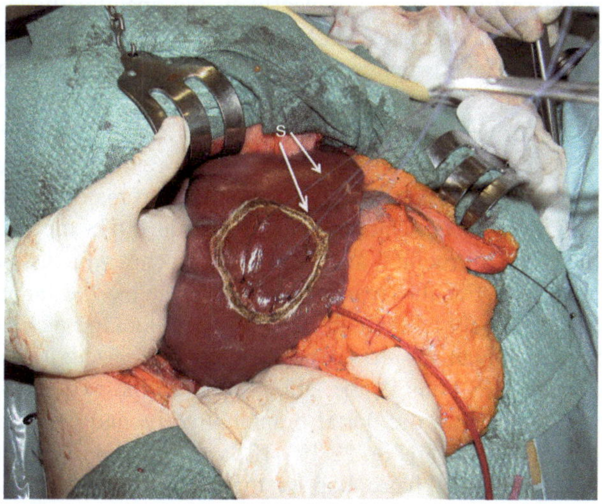

Fig. 22.15 Multiple stitches (*S*) are placed on the cardinal points of the resection area for pulling up the margins while the dissection is started

edge can be further checked with IOUS even without the aid of the electrocautery as the air trapped between the probe and the irregular surface of the demarcation line draw can be anyway visualized having at IOUS a similar aspect compared to the images obtained with the electrocautery itself [17].

At this point, in the event the selected area is on a flat portion of the liver surface, using stitches to pull up the dissected margin (parachute technique), the resection of the marked area is started (Fig. 22.15). IOUS allows to follow in real time the dissection plane, to put it constantly in relations with the tumor edge, with the

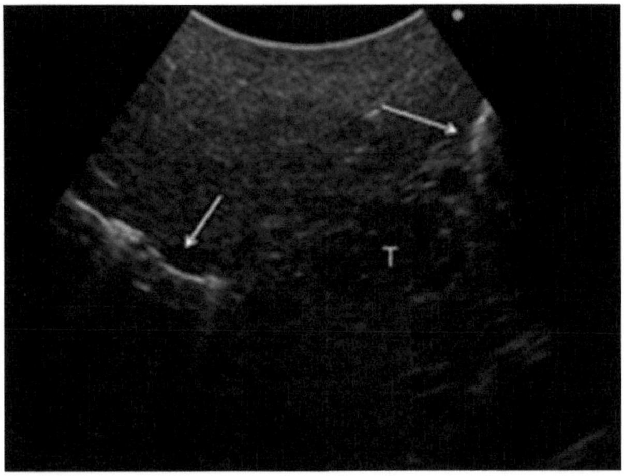

Fig. 22.16 At IOUS image the dissection plane (*arrows*) appears as an echogenic line obtained by the entrapment of air bubbles and clots between the faced cut surfaces; tumor (*T*)

fingertips of the left surgeon's hand positioned on the opposite side of the dissection plane "waiting" to its full accomplishment. The dissection plane is visible at the IOUS image appearing as a more or less intense echogenic line provoked by the entrapment of air bubbles and clots between the faced cut surfaces (Fig. 22.16). If the dissection plane is not clearly visible, specifically devised silicon gauze between the faced cut surfaces can be inserted or simply a common gauze can be used: the latter has the advantage of a better visualization but with the disadvantage of masking the structures laying posteriorly.

In this way it is possible to carry out a rounded trajectory of the dissection plane around the tumor allowing its complete removal: this results in more conservative but radical treatments and in a lower rate of major hepatectomies.

The artifacts, which allow showing at IOUS the dissection plane, could sometimes mask structures such as portal branches which should be ligated or conversely respected. For this reason to better visualize the targeted point where the portal branch should be divided, the so-called hooking technique is adopted [18]. When the Glissonian sheath is exposed and skeletonized, it is encircled with a stitch. Then under IOUS control, the stitch, hooking the exposed vessel, is gently pulled up, which stretches the portal branch slightly, and the traction point is demonstrated clearly by IOUS (Fig. 22.17). If the exposed portal branch is not clearly visible at IOUS because it has collapsed, the portal triad is unclamped. If the target site is correct, the portal branch is ligated and divided, and resection is completed under IOUS guidance; conversely, if the exposed vessel was not the targeted one, it is spared and useless sacrifice of further liver parenchyma is avoided.

During liver dissection, the backflow bleeding from the hepatic veins is an important source of blood loss: therefore, limiting its occurrence is a priority in liver resections. The surgeon's left hand hanging the liver other than driving the dissection contributes in controlling the backflow bleeding. However, IOUS can play a role in this sense too. Indeed, it has been recently described as an ultrasound-guided technique for backflow bleeding control from the RHV during right-sided liver

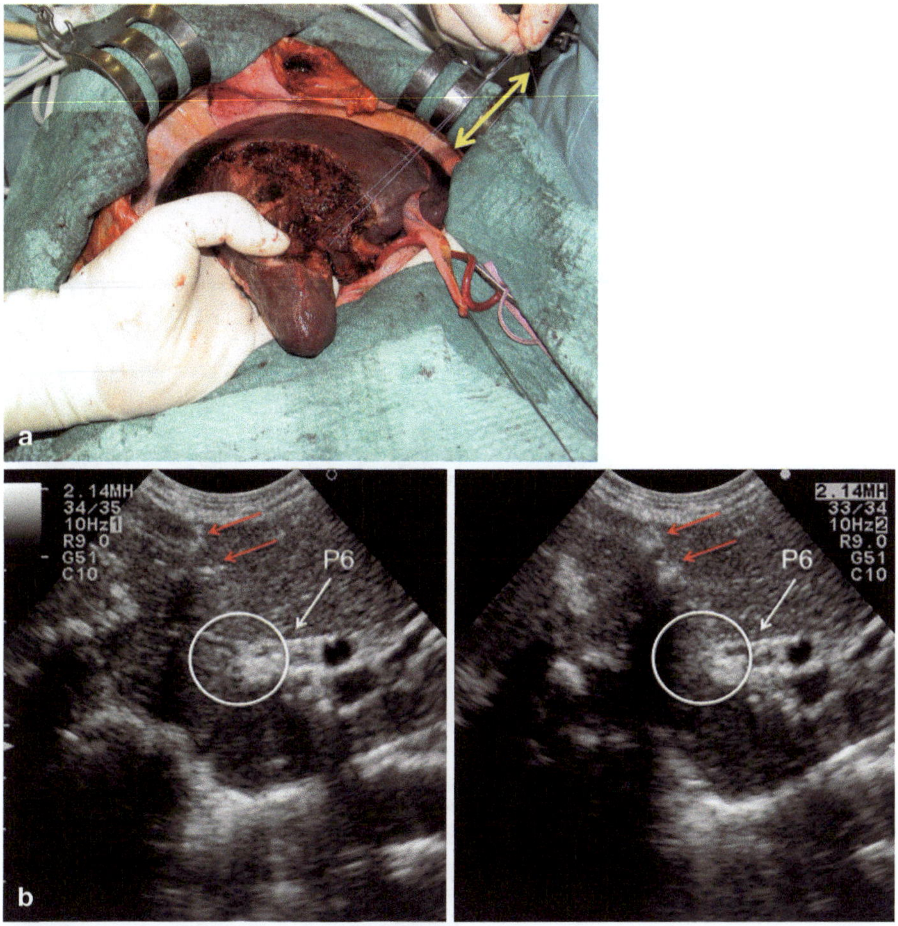

Fig. 22.17 (**a**) The Glissonian pedicle of segment 6 (P6) has appeared on the dissection plane and is encircled with a suture for ligation, but before ligating and dividing the pedicle, the suture is pulled up (*yellow arrow*) under IOUS control; (**b**) (*left*) in this IOUS image, the *red arrows* indicate the dissection plane through which the suture should have passed and the *circle points* out the site that should move in case the pedicle is the one the surgeon is thinking he has encircled (Glissonian pedicle to segment 6); (*right*) once the suture is pulled up, the site moves up (*circle*), stretching P6 and confirming that this is the encircled pedicle: then, its ligation and division can be carried out safely

resection [18]. The technique is very simple and is now applied to every hepatic vein. Once the hepatocaval confluence is exposed anteriorly, dissection is proceeded until the right surface of the extrahepatic RHV is exposed in case the RHV has to be controlled, the left surface of the extrahepatic LHV for the LHV itself, and the right anterior surface of the MHV for the MHV itself. The surgeon's fingertips compress the vessel at the exposed side, and the effectiveness of finger compression is checked by CF-IOUS (Fig. 22.18).

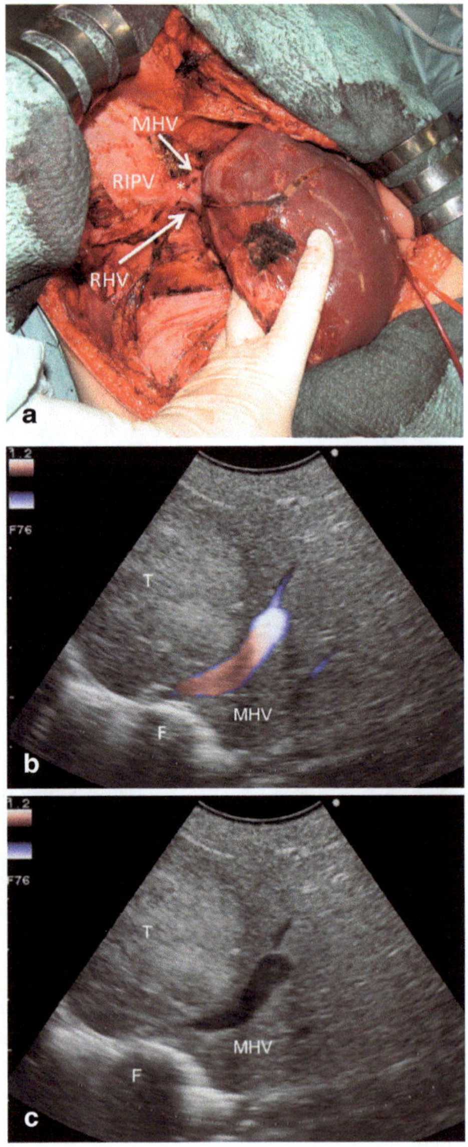

Fig. 22.18 (**a**) The *asterisk points* to the fossa between the right (*RHV*) and middle hepatic vein (*MHV*) in which the finger is allocated, enabling the surgeon to compress the MHV and reduce backflow bleeding if needed; (**b**) in this IOUS image, a hepatofugal flow into the MHV is well-documented; (**c**) once the MHV is compressed by the finger (*F*) at the hepatocaval confluence, the color flow disappears from its lumen; right inferior phrenic vein (*RIPV*), tumor (*T*)

22.7 Post-resectional Control

There are two possibilities given by IOUS after nodule removal: one is the "water bath" technique which consists of the real-time control of the proper resection of the targeted nodule, verifying its complete inclusion in the specimen just once removed from the liver (Fig. 22.19); the second is done checking the cut surface refilled with saline to avoid the artifacts generated by the residual air bubbles and clots (Fig. 22.20). The latter could be useful also for checking vessel patency in case of reconstruction.

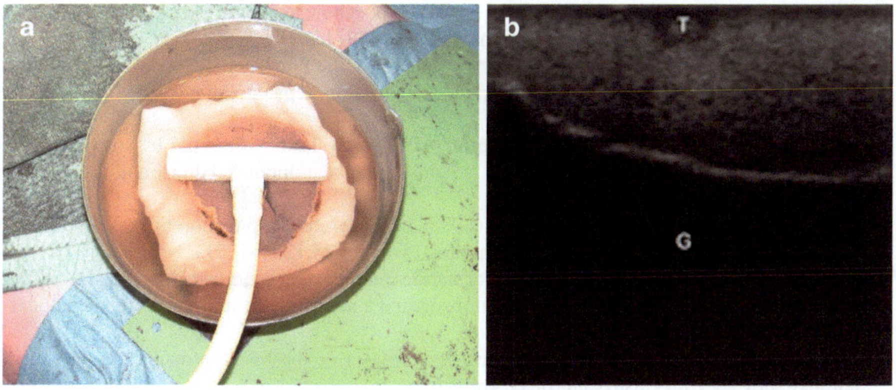

Fig. 22.19 The water bath technique used for checking the surgical specimen just removed (**a**) the whole inclusion of the targeted nodule, as confirmed by IOUS (**b**), gauzes (*G*), tumor (*T*)

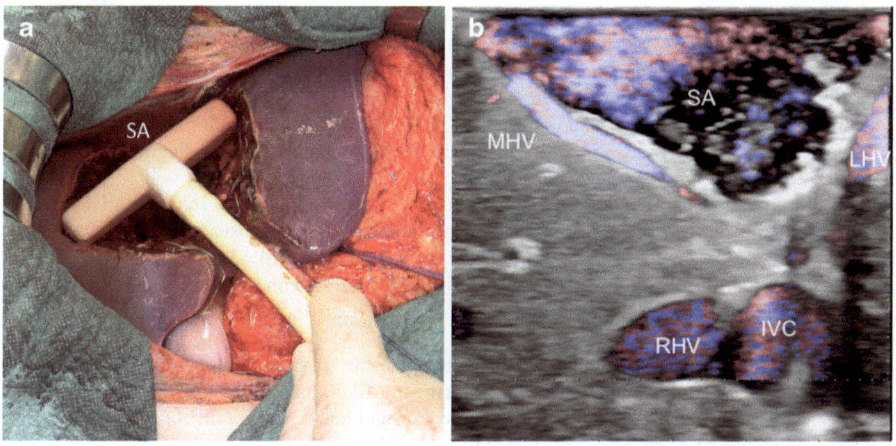

Fig. 22.20 In the in situ water bath technique, the cut surface filled with saline (*SA*) is explored by IOUS (**a**); exploration is here carried out in color-flow IOUS mode (**b**) confirming the absence of residual disease and the patency of the middle hepatic vein (*MHV*) and the left hepatic vein (*LHV*); inferior vena cava (*IVC*); right hepatic vein (*RHV*)

References

1. Kammula US, Buell JF, Labow DM et al (2001) Surgical management of benign tumors of the liver. Int J Gastrointest Cancer 30:141–146
2. Ibrahim S, Chen CL, Wang SH et al (2007) Liver resection for benign liver tumors: indications and outcome. Am J Surg 193:5–9
3. Choi BY, Nguyen MH (2005) The diagnosis and management of benign hepatic tumors. J Clin Gastroenterol 39:401–412
4. Hata S, Imamura H, Aoki T et al (2011) Value of visual inspection, bimanual palpation, and Intraoperative ultrasonography during hepatic resection for liver metastases of colorectal carcinoma. World J Surg 35:2779–2787

5. Caturelli E, Costarelli L, Giordano M et al (1991) Hypoechoic lesions in fatty liver. Quantitative study by histomorphometry. Gastroenterology 100:1678–1682
6. Kokudo N, Bandai Y, Imanishi H et al (1996) Management of new hepatic nodules detected by Intraoperative ultrasonography during hepatic resection for hepatocellular carcinoma. Surgery 119:634–640
7. Takigawa Y, Sugawara Y, Yamamoto J et al (2001) New lesions detected by Intraoperative ultrasound during liver resection for hepatocellular carcinoma. Ultrasound Med Biol 27:151–156
8. Kato K, Sugimoto H, Kanazumi N et al (2008) Intraoperative application of real-time tissue elastography for the diagnosis of liver tumours. Liver Int 28:1264–1271
9. Wanless IR (1990) Micronodular transformation (nodular regenerative hyperplasia) of the liver: a report of 64 cases among 2,500 autopsies and a new classification of benign hepatocellular nodules. Hepatology 11:787–797
10. Nakanuma Y (1990) Nodular regenerative hyperplasia of the liver: retrospective survey in autopsy series. J Clin Gastroenterol 12:460–465
11. Wicherts DA, de Haas RJ, Sebagh M et al (2011) Regenerative nodular hyperplasia of the liver related to chemotherapy: impact on outcome of liver surgery for colorectal metastases. Ann Surg Oncol 18:659–669
12. Donadon M, Di Tommaso L, Roncalli M et al (2013) Multiple focal nodular hyperplasias induced by oxaliplatin-based chemotherapy. World J Hepatol 5:340–344
13. Gupta RT, Iseman CM, Leyendecker JR et al (2012) Diagnosis of focal nodular hyperplasia with MRI: multicenter retrospective study comparing gadobenate dimeglumine to gadoxetate disodium. AJR Am J Roentgenol 199:35–43
14. Grazioli L, Bondioni MP, Haradome H et al (2012) Hepatocellular adenoma and focal nodular hyperplasia: value of gadoxetic acid-enhanced MR imaging in differential diagnosis. Radiology 262:520–529
15. Torzilli G, Palmisano A, Del Fabbro D et al (2007) Contrast-enhanced Intraoperative ultrasonography during surgery for hepatocellular carcinoma in liver cirrhosis: is it useful or useless? A prospective cohort study of our experience. Ann Surg Oncol 14:1347–1355
16. Torzilli G, Del Fabbro D, Palmisano A et al (2005) Contrast-enhanced Intraoperative ultrasonography during hepatectomies colorectal cancer liver metastases. J Gastrointest Surg 9:1148–1153
17. Torzilli G, Procopio F, Costa G (2014) Planning of the surgical strategy. In: Torzilli G (ed) Ultrasound-guided liver surgery: an atlas. Springer, Milan, pp 75–116
18. Torzilli G, Procopio F, Costa G (2014) Resection guidance. In: Torzilli G (ed) Ultrasound-guided liver surgery: an atlas. Springer, Milan, pp 117–168

Anesthesia and Intraoperative Management in Liver Surgery

23

Raffaella Reineke, Ambra Licia di Prima, and Luigi Beretta

Liver is one of the most complex organs in the body, and it is responsible for a huge range of important metabolic processes, such as coagulation factor synthesis, carbohydrate metabolism, bile acid synthesis, and drug metabolism. The presence of an underlying hepatic disease, such as cirrhosis, is an important determinant of intraoperative and postoperative outcome. Even in the case of benign tumors, the preoperative evaluation and the anesthetic management must consider the possible underlying liver dysfunction.

23.1 Planning

Hepatic resection is considered to be a high-risk surgery, with a perioperative mortality in high-volume centers estimated to 1–7 %, depending on the extent of the resection [1]. Risk factors associated with elevated mortality and morbidity include the extent and the complexity of the hepatic resection, the associated major biliary procedure, the amount of the intraoperative blood loss, the presence of thrombocytopenia and other comorbid conditions, as well as patient age.

Patients without chronic liver dysfunction or cirrhosis scheduled for hepatic resection should be evaluated as any patient scheduled for major noncardiac surgery.

R. Reineke (✉) • A.L. di Prima
Anesthesia and Intensive Care, S. Raffaele University Hospital, Via Olgettina, 60, Milan 20132, Italy
e-mail: reineke.raffaella@hsr.it; ambra.diprima@gmail.com

L. Beretta
Anesthesia and Neurointensive Care, S. Raffaele University Hospital, Via Olgettina, 60, Milan 20132, Italy
e-mail: beretta.luigi@hsr.it

L. Aldrighetti et al. (eds.), *Benign Tumors of the Liver*,
DOI 10.1007/978-3-319-12985-3_23

Planning should take into consideration monitoring, vascular access, type of anesthesia (drugs for induction and maintenance of general anesthesia), and postoperative pain control according to analgesic-scheduled programs, focusing the attention on the type of surgical incision and the potential hemorrhage, characteristic of this kind of surgery.

The anamnesis and physical examination of these patients include typical preanesthetic history, pointing up the cardiologic assessment. Surgical stress, in general, induces a proinflammatory condition; moreover, hepatic resection may be characterized by significant hemorrhage, leading to a hyperdynamic state (hypotension and tachycardia) conditioning an increase myocardial oxygen demand [2].

Thus, the patient should be carefully questioned about risk factors pertaining to coronary artery disease as well as the level of exercise tolerance. Symptoms of lipothymias or angina should be sought in details, and further examinations could be performed according to the American Heart Association (AHA) guidelines [2].

Laboratory examinations should assess the degree of the underlying hepatic disease, reminding that the liver is involved in the synthesis of proteins such as albumin and in the metabolism of many drugs.

The improvement in surgical technique and technology now allows shorter hepatic ischemic time and removal of less liver tissue, so that even patients with significant liver dysfunction may tolerate elective liver resections.

The anesthetic management must take into consideration the planned surgical technique and type of liver resection. In particular, the choice between laparoscopic or laparotomic resection can influence both the choice of type of monitoring and the intra- and postoperative anesthetic care.

In general, using a laparoscopic approach, the duration and the degree of postoperative pain is lower and mobilization and resumption of oral intake is earlier with a shorter and less expensive hospitalization.

The performance of a major liver resection using either a laparoscopic or a laparotomic approach presents several and different surgical difficulties; however, a clear understanding of the surgical technique and procedure is essential to predict and control the possible major risks of the operation.

The influence of anesthetic techniques and drugs on liver function following liver resection has never been investigated.

23.1.1 Antibiotics

Antibiotic prophylaxis suitable for clean surgery (Altemeier class 1) must be administered when a resection of a benign tumor, which has developed within a healthy or a diseased liver tissue, is scheduled. Intraoperative antibiotics prevent translocation of intestinal enterobacteria to the systemic circulation due to long operating time and large areas of postsurgery dead spaces and devitalized tissue [3, 4]. Usually, an intravenous first-generation cephalosporin before induction of general anesthesia and during prolonged surgical time is recommended [3]; if penicillin allergy is reported, the administration of macrolide or quinolone drugs is recommended. In case of biliary compression or obstruction, considered as a potential source of sepsis even without signs of clinical infection, piperacillin combined with an aminoglycoside or with a fluoroquinolone is suggested [4, 5].

23.1.2 Monitoring

Usual monitoring consists of standard noninvasive monitors and selected invasive monitors that are able to detect alterations of physiological parameters that may be explicable by the surgical procedure in order to prevent complications. Intraoperative monitoring should be adapted to the preoperative condition of the patient, the extent, and the technique of the liver resection.

Routine monitoring includes arterial pressure, electrocardiography (EKG), pulse oximetry, and capnometry.

An arterial catheter is usually inserted for invasive monitoring of blood pressure and for easy access to blood samples to check and eventually correct blood glucose values, plasma electrolytes, and potential metabolic acidosis.

The intraoperative placement of a nasogastric tube may prevent gastric distension during surgery, but it is usually removed after surgery according to ERAS guidelines.

In case of potential massive blood loss, a large-bore venous line may be used (14G). Central venous catheter (CVC) positioning is not always necessary; it provides an infusion line useful for vasopressor administration, and it allows to measure the value of the central venous pressure (CVP) to guide intravascular volume replacement and to assess hemodynamic changes when a large liver resection is planned.

During liver resection, there are some predictable variations of the CVP induced by surgical maneuver: the pressure of surgical refractors during laparotomic resection and the increased intra-abdominal pressure during laparoscopic procedure. Moreover, liver mobilization, twisting the vena cava, and clamping of the liver vessels through Pringle's maneuver reduce the venous return of blood to the right heart and therefore decrease the CVP [6, 7].

Hence, it could be better to monitor the trend of this value or simply use other devices.

Indication for pulmonary artery catheterization is reserved for patients with known preoperative left ventricular dysfunction, preoperative sepsis, or intricate circulatory impairment [8].

Nowadays, it is possible to monitor volemia and its hemodynamic changes, thus guiding infusion with a goal-directed therapy, through new minimally invasive devices which may be considered safe and reliable. This hemodynamic monitoring includes the esophageal ecodoppler monitor, the stroke volume variation, and the transesophageal echocardiography. They can provide information regarding volemia as well as cardiac performance, guiding both infusion of crystalloid or colloid and administration of vasopressors.

23.2 Anesthesia

Induction of general anesthesia may be done with standard methods. Generally, special attention is important with regard to the induction in patients with comorbidities (coronary artery disease, valvulopathies, esophageal reflux disease) and in patients with liver dysfunction. In these patients it is usually appropriate to avoid sedative premedication, benzodiazepines in particular, considering the pharmacodynamic and pharmacokinetic profile of these drugs.

23.2.1 Induction and Maintenance

Liver resections are usually performed under general anesthesia with tracheal intubation and controlled mechanical ventilation.

In case of patients with ascites or other causes of increased intra-abdominal pressure, a rapid sequence induction with cricoid pressure must be performed to avoid the risk of inhalation of gastric contents.

Paralysis may be obtained with a muscle relaxant.

Cisatracurium and atracurium are the nondepolarizing muscle relaxant of choice in patients with liver disease as they have no hepatic metabolic pathway but they are hydrolyzed by Hofman elimination. Moreover, cisatracurium is hemodynamically stable due to its scarce release of histamine [9].

Fentanyl and sufentanil pharmacokinetics are unlikely to be alternated even if liver impairment exists before surgery; liver function is not involved in remifentanil elimination [10] though the hyperanalgesia inducted by this opioid must be considered.

Anesthesia may be maintained with standard methods as well; it is usually granted with an halogenated volatile agent in air-oxygen mixture: isoflurane, sevoflurane, or desflurane at 0.2–1.0 age-adjusted minimum alveolar concentration (MAC) equivalents, titrated to hemodynamics.

Most commonly isoflurane and sevoflurane are used. Isoflurane has mild cardiodepressive effects but maintains hepatic oxygen supply, due to vasodilatation, and accordingly increases splanchnic blood flow [11]. Sevoflurane seems to decrease portal vein blood flow but increases hepatic artery blood flow [10]. In addition, Beck-Schimmer et al., in a randomized controlled trial on patients undergoing liver surgery [12], showed that ischemic preconditioning with sevoflurane before inflow occlusion limited postoperative liver injury.

However, there is no evidence that any one anesthetic agent should be preferred to another for the maintenance of anesthesia in elective liver resection [13].

During all the intraoperative period, patients must be warmed using more than one method. Warming is an important topic since it is involved in homeostasis of coagulation and clotting, thus reducing risk of hemorrhage; moreover, it is well known that hypothermia increases both the risk of surgical site infection and the time of recovery [14].

Usually it is applied on patient's upper chest and arms as a forced-air warming blanket; thermoreflectant units may be used on legs and head to prevent heating leakage. IV fluids should be warm or actively warmed through dedicated systems.

Temperature must be monitored both in the operative room and in the recovery room in order to maintain a value of Tcore >36 °C [14].

Postoperative nausea and vomit prophylaxis is usually performed, administering ondansetron at least 40 min before the end of surgery.

23.2.2 Ventilation and Oxygenation

Oxygen saturation measured using pulse oximetry may give early indication of impaired pulmonary gas exchange or inadequate function. Although it is unusual in patients to be submitted to hepatic surgery for benign lesions, approximately one-third of patients with cirrhosis or noncirrhotic portal hypertension has varied degrees of hepatopulmonary syndrome.

Hepatopulmonary syndrome is defined by the presence of hepatic dysfunction or portal hypertension and an elevated alveolar-arterial oxygen gradient. Hypoxemia in these patients is due to ventilation/perfusion mismatching, characterized by an increase in pulmonary perfusion secondary to capillary distension and accelerated transpulmonary blood flow [15]. Initially, hypoxemia can be treated by supplementation in inspired oxygen fraction and in ventilation.

Mechanical ventilation may be volumetric or pressumetric. A recent prospective randomized study on protective ventilation conducted by Pelosi and colleagues [16] showed that lower tidal volumes (7 ml/kg) with positive end-expiratory pressure (PEEP) and recruitment maneuvers improve pulmonary function and decrease post-operative pulmonary complications compared with high tidal volumes (9 ml/kg) and zero-positive end-expiratory pressure (ZEEP).

Regli and colleagues [17] reported an increase of end-expiratory lung volume and gas exchange with a reduction of pulmonary shunt and dead space fraction, when adequate level of PEEP was applied, especially in the presence of intra-abdominal hypertension. Although the application of high levels of PEEP carries the risk of barotrauma, PEEP itself may have a negative impact on hemodynamics.

During hepatic surgery, it would be better to avoid applying PEEP which might cause a congestion in the sovrahepatic venous district, thus increasing bleeding during hepatic transection. Furthermore, when PEEP is similar or higher than CVP, venous return is impaired and the decreased preload will result in a decrease of cardiac output [7].

On the basis of these studies, it is advisable to ventilate mechanically the patients to submit to hepatic surgery with relative low tidal volumes (7–8 ml/kg), avoiding PEEP and making recruitment maneuvers whenever it is possible in order to improve functional residual capacity (FRC) and pulmonary function in the first days after surgery, thus affecting also outcome.

Changes in fraction of inspired oxygenation and in ventilation result in changes in liver oxygenation and carbon dioxide elimination. This influences the pH that should be maintained normal.

In case of vascular exclusions (Pringle's maneuver commonly performed during hepatic transection to reduce bleeding), periods of hepatic ischemia occur affecting the pH, thus causing a metabolic acidosis state that must be corrected by administering bicarbonate. It seems reasonable to ventilate and oxygenate as better as possible to keep normal systemic conditions and normal pH values.

23.2.3 Hemodynamics

Hemodynamic changes due to clamping the portal vessels and the hypovolemic state induced with low CVP values are the major concerns.

The goals of a good hemodynamic management are to provide a satisfactory perfusion of vital organs and to maintain a vascular tone, a cardiac output, and a volemic status suitable during hepatic surgery. This is possible by integrating all available data monitored and registered intraoperatively.

Although general anesthesia is responsible for a transitory peripheral vasodilatation which may cause hypotension, the most important hemodynamic considerations must be done during the hepatic transection, when Pringle's maneuver is applied.

Clamping reduces venous return; in contrast, cardiac output and blood pressure do not decrease as one expected since there is a sudden increase in systemic vascular resistance by a neutrally mediated reflex [7].

On the other hand, total vascular liver exclusion through a vena cava cross-clamp causes a deep fall in venous return and a consequent reduction in cardiac output and blood pressure [18].

In case of cirrhotic patients, systemic vascular resistance is lower and their capability to increase it as response to clamping is not sufficient to maintain normal blood pressure values. Even hypovolemia induced to allow easier hepatic transection influences negatively. Hence, it could be necessary to administer vasopressor intraoperatively. Norepinephrine should be the vasopressor of choice, but each case should be discussed considering patient comorbidity.

As already mentioned, CVP during surgery should be maintained low in order to reduce blood loss [18] and transfusion rate, thus reducing hospitalization, morbidity, and mortality [19]. Hypovolemia may be considered safe, but a continuous monitoring of renal function to maintain a good renal perfusion throughout surgery must be done [8].

During hepatic resection, the anesthetist must be focused on both bleeding and air embolism which may occur. Air embolism is a common complication during hepatic resection, but it is rarely symptomatic [20].

23.3 Postoperative Issues

After hepatic resection for benign tumors, the anesthetist must consider these issues: airway management, eventual ICU transfer, and pain management.

Extubation at the end of surgery is guided by the same considerations done in case of any major abdominal surgery. The anesthetist must check and control patient temperature, muscle strength and residual sedation, and the presence of edema of the face and consequently of the upper airways. If these considerations are satisfactory, extubation is performed. Hence, the patient is monitored in a recovery room before going back to the ward [21].

In case of complicated operation or impossible early extubation, the intubated patient should be transferred and managed in ICU.

23.3.1 Postoperative Pain Management

Pain management for the postoperative period is a main topic, and it must be planned according to surgery that will be performed and to the preoperative assessment. The analgesic management must consider the extent of liver resection and the possible impairment of coagulation in the postoperative period.

It is well known that in case of large hepatic resection (more than three segments), the impairment of coagulation that results lasts more than 3 days [22, 23]; thus, it is not advisable to insert an epidural catheter before the induction of general anesthesia to grant postoperative analgesia.

In general, the anesthetist has got several approaches to assure postoperative analgesia. These approaches may be classified in two groups: central blocks and peripheral block. The easiest intravenous pathway in administering morphine through a patient-controlled system must be considered a further analgesic approach, useful in case of impossibility of performing any locoregional technique [24].

Among the central blocks, the anesthetist may choose between epidural and spinal blocks. The insertion of an epidural thoracic catheter (T7–T8) for the postoperative analgesia is recommended (Grade A evidence) [25, 26]. It is important to remind that it should be better not to use it intraoperatively, considering the hypotension that the sympathetic blockade may cause. In case of its intraoperative use (combined anesthesia), it should be better to administer low volume of diluted local anesthetic at low concentration or diluted mixture of local anesthetic combined with opioid [27]. Hypotension resulting from sympathetic blockade can be treated with administration of a vasopressor such as phenylephrine.

In the postoperative period, the epidural catheter is maintained until postoperative day 3 at least, administering a mixture of local anesthetic and opioid in continuous perfusion through a syringe pump, which is safer than an elastomer.

In case of large hepatic resections (more than three segments, such as in right hepatectomy), the insertion of the epidural catheter should be avoided considering the impairment of coagulation in the postoperative period which lasts more than 3 days, thus complicating its removal, since the risk of an epidural hematoma would be too high [25].

In this case, a peripheral block could be taken into consideration, such as a right paravertebral thoracic block with the insertion of a catheter in this space at T7 to have a continuous analgesic block for the first 2 or 3 days after surgery [28].

The paravertebral thoracic block is performed with a US guide, and it may be considered a block to be performed by a skilled anesthetist. Usually a T6 and T8 right paravertebral block is performed before inducing general anesthesia in order to reduce the administration of intraoperative opioids. In fact, this block allows a good analgesia in the dermatomes involved with the incision with better hemodynamic stability [29]. At the end of surgery, after restoring normovolemia, the continuous paravertebral block is started, previous administration of a bolus of local anesthetic at low concentration. Large volumes must be administered to ensure a satisfactory block.

Among the central blocks, a spinal block may be planned and chosen as an alternative to epidural or paravertebral block in case of laparoscopic hepatic resection [30]. In this case, pain could be considered moderate to severe only in the first 24–36 h after surgery. For this reason, it is possible to perform an analgesic subarachnoid block with morphine before induction of general anesthesia. Intrathecal morphine has a half-life of 24 h, thus resulting in a sparing effect of intravenous opioids and in a good postoperative analgesia. The dosage of intrathecal morphine is variable in literature. It is well known that the higher the dose of morphine (it is described even a dosage of 0.5 mg), the higher the risks of postoperative side effects like respiratory arrest, even at 24 h [31]. A spinal dose of 0.2 mg of morphine may guarantee a safe and satisfactory analgesia in the postoperative period, avoiding the necessity of an ICU postoperative management.

In case of any contraindications for regional techniques or of patient's refusal, the anesthetist could plan a postoperative pain management with intravenous administration of morphine, using a patient-controlled administration device (PCA), which will be set up by the anesthetist.

In order to reduce as much as possible the consumption of morphine, according to ERAS principles, a TAP (transversus abdominal plane) block could be performed in addition to general anesthesia.

TAP block is easy and it must be performed with a US guide by a skilled anesthetists. Among the different approaches (subcostal, lateral, and dual), the anesthetist will choose the best. It is a bilateral block where a large volume (20 ml) of local anesthetic is injected in the anterior fascia of the transversus abdominal muscle. The local anesthetic has a wide and long-time spreading which assures either a prolonged analgesia of the abdominal wall and of the incision or a very low risk of toxicity [32].

TAP block may be performed when an intravenous morphine PCA is planned, but it also may be taken into consideration in case of a laparoscopic approach to reduce pain related to the abdominal distention caused by inflated gas, even if a spinal block with morphine is performed [33].

Multimodal analgesic approach is ensured with the administration of paracetamol or an anti-inflammatory drug, reminding their risk of bleeding related to decreased platelet aggregation.

References

1. Jarnagin WR, Gonen M, Fong Y et al (2003) Improvement in perioperative outcome after hepatic resection: analysis of 1,803 consecutive cases over the past decade. Ann Surg 236:397–406

2. Eagle KA, Berger PB, Calkins H, Chaitman BR et al (2002) ACC/AHA Guideline Update for Perioperative Cardiovascular Evaluation for Noncardiac Surgery – Executive Summary. A report of the American College of Cardiology/American Heart Association Task Force on Practice Guidelines (Committee to Update the 1996 Guidelines on Perioperative Cardiovascular Evaluation for Noncardiac Surgery). Anesth Analg 94(5):1052–1064.
3. Kaiser AB (1986) Antimicrobial prophylaxis in surgery. N Engl J Med 315:1129–1138
4. Wu CC, Yeh DC, Lin MC, Liu TJ, P'eng FK (1998) Prospective randomized trial of systemic antibiotics in patients undergoing liver resection. Br J Surg 85:489–493
5. Lentschener C, Ozier Y (2002) Anaesthesia for elective liver resection: some points should be revisited. Eur J Anaesthesiol 19:780–788
6. Botero M, Lobato EB (2001) Advances in noninvasive cardiac monitoring: an update. J Cardiothorac Vasc Anaesth 15:631–640
7. Smyrniotis V, Kostopanagiotou G, Theodoraki K, Tsantoulas D, Contis JC (2004) The role of central venous pressure and type of vascular control in blood loss during major liver resections. Am J Surg 187(3):398–402
8. Redai I, Emond J, Brentjens T (2004) Anesthetic considerations during liver surgery. Surg Clin North Am 84:401–411
9. Servin FS, Lavaut E, Kleef U, Desmonts JM (1996) Repeated doses of rocuronium bromide administered to cirrhotic and control patients receiving isoflurane. A clinical and pharmacokinetic study. Anesthesiology 84:1092–2000
10. Dershwitz M, Hoke JF, Rosow CE et al (1996) Pharmacokinetics and pharmacodynamics of remifentanil in volunteers subjects with severe liver disease. Anesthesiology 84:812–820
11. Gatecel C, Losser MR, Payen D (2003) The postoperative effects of halothane versus isoflurane on hepatic artery and portal vein blood flow in humans. Anesth Analg 96(3):740–745
12. Beck-Schimmer B, Breitenstein S, Urech S et al (2008) A randomized controlled trial on pharmacological preconditioning in liver surgery using a volatile anesthetic. Ann Surg 248(6):909–916
13. Maze M, Bass NM (2000) Anesthesia and the hepatobiliary system. In: Miller RD (ed) Anesthesia, 5th edn. Churchill Livingstone, London, pp 1960–1972
14. Hart SR, Bordes B, Hart J, Corsino D, Harmon D (2011) Unintended perioperative hypothermia. Ochsner J 11(3):259–270
15. Hervé P, Lebrec D, Brenot F, Simonneau G, Humbert M, Sitbon O et al (1998) Pulmonary vascular disorders in portal hypertension. Eur Respir J 11(5):1153–1166
16. Severgnini P, Selmo G, Lanza C, Chiesa A, Frigerio A, Bacuzzi A, Dionigi G, Novario R, Gregoretti G, de Abreu MG, Schulz MJ, Jaber S, Futier E, Chiaranda M, Pelosi P (2013) Protective mechanical ventilation during general anesthesia for open abdominal surgery improves postoperative pulmonary function. Anesthesiology 118(6):1307–1321
17. Regli A, Mahendran R, Fish ET, Roberts B, Noffsinger B, De Keulenar BR, Singh B, Van Heerden PV (2012) Matching positive end-expiratory pressure to intra-abdominal pressure improves oxygenation in a porcine sick lung model of intra-abdominal pressure. Crit Care 16:R208
18. Jones RM, Moulton CE, Hardy KJ (1998) Central venous pressure and its effect on blood loss during liver resection. Br J Surg 85:1058–1060
19. Kooby DA, Stockman J, Ben-Porat L et al (2003) Influence of transfusions on perioperative and long-term outcome in patients following hepatic resection for colorectal metastases. Ann Surg 237:860–869
20. Koo BN, Kil HK, Choi JS, Kim JY, Chun DH, Hong YW (2005) Hepatic resection by the Cavitron Ultrasonic Surgical Aspirator increases the incidence and severity of venous air embolism. Anesth Analg 101(4):966–970, table of contents
21. Torossian A (2008) Thermal management during anaesthesia and thermoregulation standards for the prevention of inadvertent perioperative hypothermia. Best Pract Res Clin Anaesthesiol 22(4):659–668
22. Borromeo CJ, Stix MS, Lally A, Pomfret EA (2000) Epidural catheter and increased prothrombin time after right lobe hepatectomy for living donor transplantation. Anesth Analg 91(5):1139–1141

23. Siniscalchi A, Begliomini B, De Pietri L, Braglia V, Gazzi M, Masetti M, Di Benedetto F, Pinna AD, Miller CM, Pasetto A (2004) Increased prothrombin time and platelet counts in living donor right hepatectomy: implications for epidural anesthesia. Liver Transpl 10(9):1144–1149
24. Roy JD, Massicotte L, Sassine MP, Seal RF, Roy A (2006) A comparison of intrathecal morphine/fentanyl and patient-controlled analgesia with patient-controlled analgesia alone for analgesia after liver resection. Anesth Analg 103:990–994
25. Matot I, Scheinin O, Eid A, Jurim O (2002) Epidural anesthesia and analgesia in liver resection. Anesth Analg 95:1179–1181
26. Nishikawa K, Kimura S, Shimodate Y, Igarashi M, Namiki A (2007) A comparison of intravenous-based and epidural-based techniques for anesthesia and postoperative analgesia in elderly patients undergoing laparoscopic cholecystectomy. J Anesth 21(1):1–6
27. Ko JS, Choi SJ, Gwak MS, Kim GS, Ahn HJ, Kim JA, Hahm TS, Cho HS, Kim KM, Joh JW (2009) Intrathecal morphine combined with intravenous patient-controlled analgesia is an effective and safe method for immediate postoperative pain control in live liver donors. Liver Transpl 15(4):381–389. doi:10.1002/lt.21625
28. Ho AM-H, Karmakar MK, Cheung M, Lam GCS (2004) Right thoracic paravertebral analgesia for hepatectomy. Br J Anaesth 93(3):458–461
29. Luyet C, Siegenthaler A, Szucs-Farkas Z, Hummel G, Eichenberger U, Vogt A (2012) The location of paravertebral catheters placed using the landmark technique. Anaesthesia 67(12):1321–1326
30. De Pietri L, Siniscalchi A, Reggiani A, Masetti M, Begliomini B, Gazzi M, Gerunda GE, Pasetto A (2006) The use of intrathecal morphine for postoperative pain relief after liver resection: a comparison with epidural analgesia. Anesth Analg 102(4):1157–1163
31. Cole PJ, Craske DA, Wheatley RG (2000) Efficacy and respiratory effects of low-dose spinal morphine for postoperative analgesia following knee arthroplasty. Br J Anaesth 85(2):233–237
32. Børglum J, Maschmann C, Belhage B, Jensen K (2011) Ultrasound-guided bilateral dual transversus abdominis plane block: a new four-point approach. Acta Anaesthesiol Scand 55(6):658–663
33. Siddiqui MR, Sajid MS, Uncles DR, Cheek L, Baig MK (2011) A meta-analysis on the clinical effectiveness of transversus abdominis plane block. J Clin Anesth 23(1):7–14

Blood and Transfusion Management in Liver Surgery

24

Carlo Pulitanò

24.1 Introduction

Despite the significant progress made in the field of liver surgery, intraoperative blood transfusion is still required in 10–30 % of patients undergoing elective liver resection for benign tumors [1–3]. Transfusion of allogeneic (donated from another individual) blood is associated with an increased perioperative morbidity and possibly tumor recurrence, as well as carrying the inherent risk of transfusion-transmitted viral infections [1, 4]. In order to reduce the use of allogeneic blood, several pharmacological, anesthetic and surgical interventions have been tried with variable success. The decision to transfuse any patient for a given indication must balance the risks of not transfusing. While guidelines vary between centers and also between individual clinicians, generally accepted guidelines suggest that blood transfusion be considered at hemoglobin values <70 g/L, with a higher threshold (<90 g/L) reserved for patients with cardiovascular disease, or those suspected to have covert cardiovascular disease [5].

24.2 Predicting the Need for Blood Transfusion

Having an accurate method of predicting the need for blood transfusion preoperatively is useful when ordering allogeneic blood but particularly in the context of preoperative autologous blood donation (PABD).

The number of units of autologous blood obtained before surgery is most commonly based on the amount that would be cross matched before surgery if allogeneic blood were being used [6]. Algorithms have been proposed to stratify patients

C. Pulitanò
Department of HPB and Transplantation Surgery, Royal Prince Alfred Hospital, Missenden Road, Sydney, NSW 2050, Australia
e-mail: c.pulitano@centenary.org.au

L. Aldrighetti et al. (eds.), *Benign Tumors of the Liver*,
DOI 10.1007/978-3-319-12985-3_24

according to the likelihood of requiring transfusion, based on the preoperative hemoglobin level and type of operation planned [7]. However, an important limiting factor for this nonspecific approach is that similar surgical procedures can be accompanied by different amounts of blood loss. This concept is particularly important in liver surgery, where blood loss can range from a few milliliters to over 10 L [8].

Attempts have been made to predict the need for blood transfusion in liver surgery. We have previously identified 5 variables associated with blood transfusion which included preoperative hemoglobin concentration below 12.5 g/dl, largest tumor greater than 4 cm, need for exposure of the vena cava, need for an associated procedure, and cirrhosis. Using these variables we have developed a transfusion risk score highly predictive of the likelihood of needing blood transfusion [1]. A similar study from Cockbain et al. identified seven factors predictive of transfusion: coronary artery disease, hemoglobin <12.5 g/dL, preoperative biliary drainage, largest tumor greater than 3.5 cm, redo resection, cholangiocarcinoma, and extended resection. These studies have demonstrated that blood transfusion can be predicted with a high degree of accuracy [9]. These scores can be useful in order to estimate the amount of units likely to be required for preoperative cross matching or the need for PABD.

24.3 Preoperative Management

The patient's status should be optimized to reduce the risk of allogeneic transfusion. All patients undergoing liver resection should have a full blood count performed prior to surgery, and those patients presenting with anemia should be investigated and treated appropriately. Coagulation should be evaluated with a platelet count and clotting studies and corrected if necessary. Medication such as antiplatelet and anticoagulant drugs should be considered and stopped if the risk of bleeding outweighs the risk of discontinuing these drugs. Optimization of nutritional status with supplemental enteral feeding is usually not necessary in case of benign tumors, but can be considered in selected cases.

The use of PABD was once promoted to decrease allogeneic transfusion requirements but is only recommended when the risk of blood transfusion is more than 50 % [6]. The main advantage of PABD is avoiding exposure to allogeneic blood. However, PABD can only be considered when it is possible to guarantee admission and operative dates.

Preoperative hemoglobin levels can be improved in some patients with vitamin deficiencies by the use of pharmacological intervention such as iron, folate, and vitamin B12. Erythropoietin can also be considered and should be targeted at patients under 70 years of age who are scheduled for major liver resection and who have a presenting hemoglobin <130 g/l. Erythropoietin can also be used successfully in combination with PABD [10]. However, the efficacy and cost-effectiveness of preoperative erythropoietin and autologous blood donation to reduce allogeneic blood transfusion are still being debated, and their use remains limited [11].

24.4 Intraoperative Management

In the intraoperative period, measures should be aimed at decreasing blood loss and blood transfusion requirements. Low central venous pressure (<5 cm H_2O) is commonly used in liver surgery because it is thought to reduce hepatic venous pressure, resulting in a decrease in blood loss [8]. However, a recent meta-analysis concluded that low CVP reduces blood loss and fresh frozen plasma (FFP) requirements but not red cell transfusion requirements [12]. Hypoventilation through the reduction of tidal volume has been used as a method for decreasing blood loss because of its role in decreasing the CVP. However, the efficacy of this anesthetic technique remains controversial [13].

Acute normovolemic hemodilution (ANH) has been used to reduce the requirement of allogeneic blood [12]. The procedure consists in the removal of blood from the patient immediately before operation and replacement with a synthetic colloid. The removed blood is then reinfused as autologous whole blood later during the procedure. This method has several advantages: it is inexpensive, the chance of clerical error is reduced, and blood withdrawn during ANH does not undergo biochemical alterations unlike stored predonated autologous blood [14].

The use of cell salvage in liver surgery has been limited by the hypothetical risk of aspirating and reinfusing tumor cells to the patient and the supposed lower quality of cell-salvaged blood. However, considering that the unconfirmed risk of spreading tumor cell is not a problem in the case of benign liver tumors, the use of cell saver should always be considered [15]. Furthermore, Schmidt A. et al. have demonstrated that cell-salvaged blood in liver resection seems to be safe for retransfusion with respect to cytokine release and complement activation [16].

During a major liver resection, abnormalities of coagulation are common [17]. The use of thromboelastography and rotational thromboelastometry are more frequently used to detect coagulopathies even when the conventional coagulation profile is still normal. It can be expected that the use of these diagnostic methods will soon become standard of care in liver surgery [18].

Common blood products available for correction of intra- or postoperative coagulopathy include platelets, FFP, and cryoprecipitate. Aprotinin and tranexamic acid appear to be beneficial in decreasing the number of patients requiring allogeneic blood transfusion. Additionally, 4-factor prothrombin complex concentrate can significantly improve coagulation in a very short period of time and with lower volume than FFP [19]. Recombinant activated coagulation factor VII (rFVIIa) has been used to manage hemorrhage caused by severe traumatic injury or transplantation. However, there is no clear evidence to promote its use in liver resection [20]. Further randomized clinical trials are necessary to assess any pharmacological interventions aimed at decreasing blood transfusion and blood transfusion requirements in liver resections [19].

Surgical technique is also a determinant of blood loss and hence transfusion requirement. The choice of a special equipment to transect liver parenchyma, the use of portal clamping, and the way that the cut surface is managed depend on the preference of the operating surgeon. The use of fibrin glue sealants, local collagen, and cellulose pads have also been used to promote hemostasis and reduce the risk of postoperative bleeding [21]. However, the optimal treatment strategy for liver resection remains to be defined.

24.5 Postoperative Management

General postoperative care measures such as rapid rewarming, optimization of ventilation and oxygenation, rapid restoration of enteral feeding, and antibiotic therapy also apply to liver resection patients [22].

Derangements in conventional markers of coagulation and platelet count are common post liver resection and correlate with the extent of resection [17]. Prolongation of PT is usually self-limited and resolves without the need for transfusion of FFP. There is no consensus regarding the criteria for prophylactic FFP transfusion after liver surgery. However, in most centers prophylactic FFP is used for INR greater than 2.0, with a lower threshold for cirrhotic patients due to their higher risk of postoperative bleeding [22].

Transient postoperative anemia is partially a physiologic phenomenon. Torzilli et al. described the fluctuations in hemoglobin after liver resection. A steady and significant decrease is recorded until the third postoperative day, followed by a steady increase. Therefore, a decrease in the hemoglobin levels between first and fifth postoperative days without evidence of active bleeding does not justify blood transfusion [23]. The variations in blood transfusion rates after liver resection in different series could be in part explained by the different interpretations of postoperative anemia.

Conclusions

A multidisciplinary approach aimed at increasing preoperative red cell mass, decreasing surgical bleeding, and correcting coagulopathy may result in a substantial reduction in transfusion requirements in liver resection for benign disease. An evidence-based approach in defining optimal transfusion thresholds and employing these thresholds in the clinical setting will help to ensure that transfusions are only prescribed when clinically necessary. While transfusions form an integral part in many liver resections, transfusion is not a risk-free process and demands careful consideration.

References

1. Pulitanò C, Arru M, Bellio L, Rossini S, Ferla G, Aldrighetti L (2007) A risk score for predicting perioperative blood transfusion in liver surgery. Br J Surg 94(7):860–865
2. Ibrahim S, Chen CL, Wang SH, Lin CC, Yang CH, Yong CC, Jawan B, Cheng YF (2007) Liver resection for benign liver tumors: indications and outcome. Am J Surg 193(1):5–9
3. Kamphues C, Engel S, Denecke T, Bova R, Hippler-Benscheidt M, Puhl G et al (2011) Safety of liver resection and effect on quality of life in patients with benign hepatic disease: single center experience. BMC Surg 11(1):16. doi:10.1186/1471-2482-11-16
4. Kooby DA, Stockman J, Ben-Porat L, Gonen M, Jarnagin WR, DeMatteo RP et al (2003) Influence of transfusions on perioperative and long-term outcome in patients following hepatic

resection for colorectal metastases. Ann Surg 237(6):860–869. doi:10.1097/01.SLA.0000072371.95588.DA; discussion 869–870

5. Szczepiorkowski ZM, Dunbar NM (2013) Transfusion guidelines: when to transfuse. Hematology Am Soc Hematol Educ Program 2013:638–644. doi:10.1182/asheducation-2013.1.638
6. Thomas MJG, Gillon J, Desmond MJ (1996) Consensus conference on autologous transfusion. Preoperative autologous donation. Transfusion 36:633–639
7. van Klei WA, Rheineck Leyssius TA, Grobbee DE, Moons KGM (2002) Identifying patients for blood conservation strategies. Br J Surg 89:1176–1182
8. Melendez J, Arslan V, Fisher M, Wuest D, Jarnagin WR, Fong Y et al (1998) Perioperative outcome of major hepatic resections under low central venous pressure, anesthesia: blood loss, blood transfusion, and the risk of postoperative renal dysfunction. J Am Coll Surg 187:620–625
9. Cockbain AJ, Masudi T, Lodge JPA, Toogood GJ, Prasad KR (2010) Predictors of blood transfusion requirement in elective liver resection. HPB 12(1):50–55. doi:10.1111/j.1477-2574.2009.00126.x
10. Kato K, Nomoto S, Sugimoto H, Kanazumi N, Takeda S, Nakao A (2009) Autologous blood storage before hepatectomy for hepatocellular carcinoma. Hepatogastroenterology 56:802–807
11. Lentschener C, Gomola A, Grabar S, Soubrane O, Dousset B, Massault PP, Penhoud C, Ozier Y (2004) The effect of erythropoietin on allogeneic blood requirement in patients undergoing elective liver resection: a model simulation. Anesth Analg 98(4):921–926
12. Gurusamy KS, Li J, Vaughan J, Sharma D, Davidson BR (2013) Cardiopulmonary interventions to decrease blood loss and blood transfusion requirements for liver resection. Cochrane Database Syst Rev 5, CD007338
13. Hasegawa K, Takayama T, Orii R, Sano K, Sugawara Y, Imamura H et al (2002) Effect of hypoventilation on bleeding during hepatic resection: a randomized controlled trial. Arch Surg 137(3):311–315
14. Matot I, Scheinin O, Jurim O, Eid A (2002) Effectiveness of acute normovolemic hemodilution to minimize allogeneic blood transfusion in major liver resections. Anesthesiology 97(4):794–800
15. Waters JH, Yazer M, Chen YF, Kloke J (2012) Blood salvage and cancer surgery: a meta-analysis of available studies. Transfusion 52:2167–2173
16. Schmidt A, Sues HC, Siegel E, Peetz D, Bengtsson A, Gervais HW (2009) Is cell salvage safe in liver resection? A pilot study. J Clin Anesth 21(8):579–584
17. Pulitanò C, Aldrighetti L, Arru M, Finazzi R, Catena M, Guzzetti E et al (2007) Preoperative methylprednisolone administration maintains coagulation homeostasis in patients undergoing liver resection: importance of inflammatory cytokine modulation. Shock (Augusta, Ga) 28(4):401–405. doi:10.1097/shk.0b013e318063ed11
18. Durila M, Malošek M (2014) Rotational thromboelastometry along with thromboelastography plays a critical role in the management of traumatic bleeding. Am J Emerg Med 32(3):288.e1–3
19. Gurusamy KS, Li J, Sharma D, Davidson BR (2009) Pharmacological interventions to decrease blood loss and blood transfusion requirements for liver resection. Cochrane Database Syst Rev. 2009 Oct 7;(4):CD008085. doi: 10.1002/14651858.CD008085
20. Bezinover D, Kadry Z, Janicki P (2011) Contemporary anesthesia management for liver transplantation: a comparison of American and European methods. Middle East J Anesthesiol 21:251–258
21. Simillis C, Li T, Vaughan J, Becker LA, Davidson BR, Gurusamy KS (2014) Methods to decrease blood loss during liver resection: a network meta-analysis. Cochrane Database Syst Rev 4, CD010683
22. Wrighton LJ, O'Bosky KR, Namm JP, Senthil M (2012) Postoperative management after hepatic resection. J Gastrointest Oncol 3(1):41–47. doi:10.3978/j.issn. 2078-6891.2012.003
23. Torzilli G, Gambetti A, Del Fabbro D, Leoni P, Olivari N, Donadon M, Montorsi M, Makuuchi M (2004) Techniques for hepatectomies without blood transfusion, focusing on interpretation of postoperative anemia. Arch Surg 139(10):1061–1065

Fast-Track Programs

25

Francesca Ratti, Marco Catena, Michele Paganelli, and Luca Aldrighetti

25.1 Introduction

Over the last two decades, laparoscopic surgery has evolved to become the approach of choice for many abdominal procedures, involving even liver resections. The first wedge resection was carried out in 1992 by Gagner [1], and then this approach evolved to encompass more complex anatomical resections, including formal left and right hepatectomies, as well as extended ones [2, 3]. Multiple retrospective case series and reviews comparing open with laparoscopic liver resection indicate that laparoscopic liver resection can be applied safely for both malignant and benign liver lesions [4–6]. The widespread of minimally invasive liver surgery has not only contributed to the evolution of the surgical technique but also innovation of patient management. Indeed laparoscopic liver resection has been associated with shorter hospital length of stay, reduced intraoperative blood loss, less postoperative pain, earlier recovery, and better quality of life [2–6]. Nevertheless, the type of surgery/procedure itself is not the only variable that influences recovery and hospital length of stay.

Indeed, the application of multimodal perioperative care protocols, commonly referred as fast-track or enhanced recovery programs (enhanced recovery after surgery, ERAS), has achieved significant improvements in the outcome of a variety of surgical procedures. This multimodal program, derived from Kehlet's 1990s pioneer work in the multimodal surgical care field [7], involves optimization of several aspects of the perioperative management of patients undergoing major abdominal surgery. Targeting factors that delay postoperative recovery (pain, gut dysfunction,

F. Ratti (✉) • M. Catena • M. Paganelli
Hepatobiliary Surgery, San Raffaele Hospital, Via Olgettina 60, Milan 20132, Italy
e-mail: ratti.francesca@hsr.it; catena.marco@hsr.it; paganelli.michele@hsr.it

L. Aldrighetti
Hepatobiliary Surgery Unit, San Raffaele Hospital, Vita-Salute San Raffaele University, Via Olgettina 60, Milan 20132, Italy
e-mail: aldrighetti.luca@hsr.it

L. Aldrighetti et al. (eds.), *Benign Tumors of the Liver*,
DOI 10.1007/978-3-319-12985-3_25

and immobility) and combining a series of interventions to reduce perioperative stress and organ dysfunction, such programs have shown to accelerate postoperative recovery and reduce length of stay, without affecting rate of postoperative complications or even reducing them.

25.2 Principles of Fast-Track Surgery

In order to accelerate functional recovery and reduce length of hospital stay, a uniform and evidence-based perioperative management is fundamental: this is the reason why a structured and detailed program with well-defined recovery and discharge criteria has been developed and is currently introduced into clinical practice of centers involved in this program. This also allows improved comparability of clinical outcomes in clinical trials. It is also presumable that improvement of these programs will have a synergetic effect with minimally invasive surgery, as already experienced in colorectal surgery [8].

The ERAS multimodal evidence-based recovery program protocol was originally developed for elective colonic surgery and then modified to cover all aspects of elective liver resection. ERAS liver protocol is reported in details in Table 25.1.

As evident, one of the factors targeted by enhanced recovery is gastrointestinal function: the employment of thoracic epidural anesthesia, early mobilization, avoidance of excessive saline, and early feeding may shorten length of postoperative ileus and promote passage of stools [9].

Furthermore, carbohydrate loading and early oral nutritional supplements may interact with laxatives to enhance gastrointestinal recovery further allowing earlier

Table 25.1 Principles of fast-track perioperative management in liver surgery

Preoperative	Perioperative	Postoperative days 1–3
Counseling	Thoracic epidural analgesia	Daily review of discharge criteria
Minimal preoperative fasting (solid food up to 6 h? clear fluids up to 2 h)? carbohydrate loading	Prevention of hypothermia	Ileus prevention (MgO/Macrogol/lactulose)
No anxiolytic premedication	CVP monitoring (CVP\5 mmHg)	Free fluids/normal diet POD 1
	No routine drainage of the peritoneal cavity	Intravenous fluids discontinued POD 1
	No standard nasogastric drainage	Oral analgesia POD 1
	Start intake of water and free fluids	Normal diet POD 2
	Early mobilization	Removal of urinary catheter POD 2
	Postoperative nausea and vomiting (PONV) prophylaxis	Stop epidural/intravenous analgesia POD 3
	Antithrombotic prophylaxis	Full mobilization POD 3
	Antibiotic prophylaxis	

oral intake and therefore intravenous fluid discontinuation. Thanks to these principles, postoperative catabolism may be attenuated, and insulin resistance abated. Even the incidence of minor postoperative complications proved to be reduced by improved nutritional status [10].

As stated previously, the main goal of fast-track programs is to enhance functional recovery: definition of this item is based on several criteria that are defined as follows (when all of these five criteria are met, the patient is considered functionally recovered):

- Adequate pain control with oral analgesics: patients rate the intensity of their current pain on a scale of 0 ("no pain") to 10 ("worst possible pain"). A score of 1–3 is considered to be mild, 4–6 to be moderate, and 7–10 to be severe. An adequate pain control is considered when the patient rates pain 1–3 with oral analgesics only.
- Independently mobile (mobile at preoperative level): in order to report the difference between pre- and postoperative level of mobility, the "ERAS Mobility Scale," which is inferred from the "Groningen activity restriction scale" [11], was developed. The EMS utilizes ten items of basic actions to compare the level of mobility before and after surgical intervention. When the patient is able to perform 8 out of 10 items, they are independently mobile.
- Tolerance of solid food: fluid and solid food intake is monitored and must be returned to normal tolerance level. Tolerance is considered to be normal when oral intake of water or normal food is resumed and continued for at least 24 h. Furthermore prophylaxis of postoperative nausea and vomiting (PONV), which obviously influences the intake, is always performed.
- Normal or decreasing serum bilirubin
- No intravenous fluids

25.3 Results of Fast-Track Programs in Liver Surgery

In patients undergoing colonic surgery within ERAS® program, an earlier recovery and consequently shorter hospital length of stay was registered [12, 13]. Furthermore, a reduction of postoperative morbidity in patients undergoing intestinal resection was reported too [14]. These results stimulated liver surgeons of the ERAS® group (Maastricht, Edinburgh, and Tromsö) to adapt the ERAS program to patients undergoing open liver resection. Van Dam et al. [15] prospectively collected data from 61 ERAS patients and compared them with a historical series of 100 patients: patients belonging to the first group were able to drink fluids after 4 h from surgery and eat normally on the day after the operation; furthermore, patients were independently mobile after 3 days and were therefore discharged after a median of 5 days, reducing length of stay from 8 to 6 days (25 %), without any negative effect on surgical safety. Authors even postulated that a further reduction of stay could be achievable, given the delay between functional recovery and discharge. The explanation of this delay is often linked to social problems, problems in home care support, or logistic problems.

Stoot et al. [16] investigated the additional value of laparoscopy in the context of enhanced recovery programs and reported retrospectively a further reduction in length of stay from 7 to 5 days when patients were operated laparoscopically and managed within an ERAS program, even confirming the delay between recovery and actual discharge of the patients. Furthermore the same authors reported a reduced blood loss in ERAS group that could be explained both to fast-track principles of low central venous pressure and avoidance of excessive fluid administration and to learning curve acquisition by operating surgeons.

A reduced postoperative morbidity in liver surgery within the ERAS context never managed to be demonstrated in the literature until now, indeed in van Dam [15] and Stoot [16], series morbidity was comparable between groups, but it is also true that no specific study regarding this issue has been developed so far.

Thanks to these encouraging results, together with recent development in surgical field, many elements of the ERAS program have been more widely introduced into many tertiary centers performing hepatobiliary surgery worldwide. In order to deepen this issue, a recent report by Wong et al. [17] was developed to assess adhesion to ERAS principles in 11 hepatobiliary centers in Europe: "Compliance" of centers was defined according to fulfillment of 22 ERAS protocol core items. The author observed that the median number of implemented items per center was 9 and compliance was partial in preoperative and perioperative phases, while it was still poor during postoperative course, so they concluded that implementation of fast-track protocols is desirable in order to standardize care and improve recovery after surgery even further, but it requires multidisciplinary efforts.

25.4 Fast-Track Surgery in Management of Patients with Benign Disease

Patients affected by benign disease requiring hepatic surgery seem to be particularly suitable for fast-track management since they are frequently young people needing fast postoperative recovery to come back to work and normal life as soon as possible, even reducing social costs of hospitalization. Furthermore they are frequently more careful to cosmetic result and body image that was always considered a secondary end point in oncologic surgery but needs to be revisited as a primary goal in this subset of patients. Finally, patient consciousness regarding benefits of laparoscopy frequently stresses the desire to perform surgery for benign lesions through minimally invasive approach. No report exists in the literature specifically addressing the topic of fast-track surgery in patients with benign disease nor outcome in terms of quality of life and cosmetic results after laparoscopic surgery.

Despite this, interesting results will be provided by ORANGE II trial [18] that was developed to provide evidence on the merits of laparoscopic surgery in patients undergoing a left lateral hepatic sectionectomy and participating in an enhanced recovery program in terms of time to functional recovery, hospital length of stay, readmission percentage, morbidity (liver-specific), quality of life, body image, hospital costs, and the incidence of incisional hernias.

References

1. Gagner M, Dubuc J, Rheault M (1992) Laparoscopic partial hepatectomy for liver tumor. Surg Endosc 6:97–98
2. Pulitanò C, Aldrighetti L (2008) The current role of laparoscopic liver resection for the treatment of liver tumors. Nat Clin Pract Gastroenterol Hepatol 5:648–654
3. Nguyen KT, Gambin TC, Geller DA (2009) World review of laparoscopic liver resection – 2,804 patients. Ann Surg 250:831–841
4. Aldrighetti L, Guzzetti E, Pulitanò C et al (2010) Case-matched analysis of totally laparoscopic versus open liver resection for HCC: short and middle term results. J Surg Oncol 102:82–86
5. Lee KF, Cheung YS, Chong CN et al (2007) Laparoscopic versus open hepatectomy for liver tumours: a case control study. Hong Kong Med J 13(6):442–448
6. Troisi R, Montalti R, Smeets P et al (2008) The value of laparoscopic liver surgery for solid benign hepatic tumors. Surg Endosc 22(1):38–44
7. Kehlet H, Wilmore DW (2002) Multimodal strategies to improve surgical outcome. Am J Surg 183(6):630–641
8. Vlug MS, Wind J, Hollmann MW et al (2011) Laparoscopy in combination with fast track multimodal management is the best perioperative strategy in patients undergoing colonic surgery: a randomized clinical trial (LAFA-study). Ann Surg 254(6):868–875
9. Hendry PO, van Dam RM, Bukkems SF et al (2010) Randomized clinical trial of laxatives and oral nutritional supplements within an enhanced recovery after surgery protocol following liver resections. Br J Surg 97:1198–1206
10. Smedley F, Bowling T, James M et al (2004) Randomized clinical trial of the effects of preoperative and postoperative oral nutritional supplements on clinical course and cost of care. Br J Surg 91:983–990
11. Suurmeijer TP, Doeglas DM, Moum T et al (1994) The Groningen Activity Restriction Scale for measuring disability: its utility in international comparisons. Am J Public Health 84(8):1270–1273
12. Fearon KC, Ljungqvist O, Von Meyenfeldt M et al (2005) Enhanced recovery after surgery: a consensus review of clinical care for patients undergoing colonic resection. Clin Nutr 24(3):466–477
13. Lassen K, Soop M, Nygren J et al (2009) Consensus review of optimal perioperative care in colorectal surgery: Enhanced Recovery After Surgery (ERAS) Group recommendations. Arch Surg 144(10):961–969
14. Delaney CP, Zutshi M, Senagore AJ et al (2003) Prospective, randomized, controlled trial between a pathway of controlled rehabilitation with early ambulation and diet and traditional postoperative care after laparotomy and intestinal resection. Dis Colon Rectum 46(7):851–859
15. van Dam RM, Hendry PO, Coolsen MM et al (2008) Initial experience with a multimodal enhanced recovery programme in patients undergoing liver resection. Br J Surg 95(8):969–975
16. Stoot JH, van Dam RM, Busch OR et al (2009) The effect of a multimodal fast-track programme on outcomes in laparoscopic liver surgery: a multicentre pilot study. HPB (Oxford) 11(2):140–144
17. Wong-Lun-Hing EM, van Dam RM, Heijnen LA et al (2014) Is current perioperative practice in hepatic surgery based on enhanced recovery after surgery (ERAS) principles? World J Surg 38(5):1127–1140
18. Van Dam RM, Wong-Lun-Hing EM, van Breukelen GJ et al (2012) Open versus laparoscopic left lateral hepatic sectionectomy within an enhanced recovery ERAS programme (Orange II-trial): study protocol for a randomised controlled trial. Trials 13:54